The Schwarzbein Principle II

THE SCHWARZBEIN PRINCIPLE II
The Transition

A REGENERATION PROCESS TO PREVENT AND REVERSE ACCELERATED AGING

Diana Schwarzbein, M.D.

with Marilyn Brown

Health Communications, Inc.
Deerfield Beach, Florida

www.hci-online.com

**Library of Congress Cataloging-in-Publication Data
is available from the Library of Congress.**

©2002 Diana Schwarzbein

ISBN 1-55874-964-0

Publisher: Health Communications, Inc.
3201 S.W. 15th Street
Deerfield Beach, FL 33442-8190

Cover design by Lisa Camp
Inside book formatting by Dawn Von Strolley Grove

For Larry,
Mami y Papi,
Viviana, Sergio, Gabriella,
Audrey, Dick, Danielle, Jacob,
Alexis, Keith, Rachel and Jaclyn

WITH LOVE
—DIANA SCHWARZBEIN, M.D.

Contents

PART II: THE TRANSITION

PART III: HOW TO

Acknowledgments

T his book would never have gotten started without the help of my sister Alexis Sersland and would never have been finished without the help of the following people.

An unbelievable amount of gratitude goes to those who opened up their lives and shared their stories. You know who you are!

A special thank-you to my parents, Edison and Martha Schwarzbein, who gave up their plans to come and give me emotional, scientific and literary support!

Thank you to my sister Viviana Ortolani, whose incessant questions helped to add clarity.

Steven Brown, thank you for reading and editing this book a countless number of times, but more importantly, thank you for letting me have Marilyn on your time! I know it was not always easy.

Dan Taylor, thank you for commenting, organizing and truly caring.

Cameron Bonney, thank you for the literature research and your right-on constructive criticisms.

Karin de la Peña, thank you for your amazing command of the English language. You truly are a dear friend.

Kathleen Unger, thank you for your enthusiasm and expertise. As usual, your input was invaluable.

Many a heartfelt thanks to Angel L. Iscovich, M.D. and Lisa A.

Iscovich, M.S., Janet Miller, David Dennis, Eric Smith, Diana Estes, Ron Mousouris, Barbara Mousouris and Theresa Grumet, R.D.—your thorough comments and analysis of each chapter have definitely improved this book.

For always being there whenever I needed technical support, thank you, my dear cousin, Horacio Hojman, M.D.

For help with meal plans, food lists and supplement suggestions, thank you to my present and past dietician staff—Theresa Grumet, R.D., Betsy Reynolds, M.S., R.D., and Geri French, M.S., R.D.

Many thanks to my staff at the Endocrinology Institute, both past and present, who put up with me during this latest project—Olga Barraza, Miranda Braid, Chin, Mark Duhamell, Geri French, R.D., Tana Grenz, PA-C, Theresa Grumet, R.D., Betsy Reynolds, R.D., Gina Syslo, LVN. Jane Westerman, R.N. and Doris Vargas.

Peter Vegso, thank you for saying "yes!" That was one of the easiest negotiations I have been through and I appreciated it. And thank you again to your wonderful staff. It was great working with all of you again; Christine Belleris, editorial director; Allison Janse, senior editor; Kim Weiss, public relations director; Kelly Maragni, marketing director; Dawn Von Strolley Grove, typesetter; Larissa Hise Henoch, art department director; Terry Burke, vice president of sales and marketing; and Lori Golden, general sales manager.

An amazing amount of gratitude and thanks to Nancy Burke, whose superb editing surpassed all my expectations. You really do not miss a thing!

Thank you, thank you, thank you. I cannot thank you enough, Marilyn Brown. Your expertise was invaluable, and you made me grammatically correct. What else could I have asked for? I could not have done this without you.

And last but not least, thank you to Larry Mousouris, my loving husband, who was there to comfort, feed me and put up with my long hours (most of the time). You are the best and I love you very much!

Preface

A ging is inevitable. We all know it is happening to us every time we look in the mirror.

You probably think that there is nothing you can do about aging, but that is not true. This book has been written to show you that there is a great deal that you can do about it—and it will teach you how to age successfully.

It may seem strange to think of success in terms of aging, but you can be as successful at aging as you can in any other area of your life. Successful aging is not only possible; it is crucial if you are going to live a long, healthy, active life. You can control your aging process by adopting the nutrition and lifestyle habits that bring your body's systems back into balance, thus promoting health and longevity.

Part of successful aging is the ability to heal your metabolism or keep it running efficiently if you already have a healthy metabolism. As you adopt good habits and your metabolism begins to heal, you will go through a transition time where your body repairs the damage caused by your previous years of poor nutrition and lifestyle habits. This transition will take some of you longer than others, but the good news is that everyone can heal. You will have optimum health, ideal body composition, and increased longevity when you complete your transition.

To help you through your transition, I have put together a "How

To" section in Part III of the book that contains a five-step regeneration program based on what I recommend in my clinical practice depending on your current metabolism type. There are four individual programs based on the four different current metabolism types: insulin-sensitive with healthy adrenal glands; insulin-sensitive with burned-out adrenal glands; insulin-resistant with healthy adrenal glands; and insulin-resistant with burned-out adrenal glands. These metabolism types are acquired and not genetic. If you implement the five areas outlined in the How To section into your daily lifestyle, as described in your individual program, you will heal your metabolism or keep it healthy and achieve successful aging. It does not get much better than that.

If you are going to skip to the back of the book and read the How To section to learn the Schwarzbein Principle II (SPII) program first, come back and read the first half of the book that deals with the Why To and the Transition process. By reading the case studies, you will learn why you need to change certain habits and what you may experience along the way. This will help you make the necessary changes and then stick to them. This book is not intended to be a quick fix but a life-changing tool that will help you enjoy your remaining years to their fullest.

Hormonal Disclaimer

For the purpose of simplicity, the actions of adrenaline, norepinephrine and glucagon are consolidated into one hormone, adrenaline. Though this is not 100 percent correct, it is sufficient for the purpose of this book, which is to inspire you to improve your nutrition and lifestyle habits. If you would like more specifics, refer to *Williams Textbook of Endocrinology 9th Edition,* Saunders.

Terminology

The term "biochemical" is used herein to describe chemicals that your body needs for regeneration, and the term "toxic chemical" is used in reference to chemicals that are not needed for regeneration and have the potential to cause cellular damage.

PART I

Why To

One

Successful Aging

D id you know that the maximum life span for the human race is 120 years, yet most of us do not even live to be 100 years old? Why is that? What is keeping you from reaching *your* potential life span? Is it your genetic makeup, or your poor nutrition and lifestyle habits? From my knowledge of physiology and from my clinical experience, I have no doubt that daily habits, not genetics, play the most important role in determining how well people age.

Most of us are concerned about growing older because we do not want to be dependent on others or have to live with a debilitating disease for many years until we die. We want to age successfully and remain as healthy as we can for as long as we can, but we are getting conflicting information about how to do this. We wonder if it is even possible.

I have good news for you. Though it is normal for some of your bodily functions to decline with age, your quality of life does not have to diminish as well. You *can* remain healthy, vital and happy for a longer time by aging successfully, and this book will be your guide.

The Schwarzbein Principle II (SPII) program contains five steps that will teach you how to improve your nutritional and lifestyle habits so you can age successfully. These steps include:

1. Healthy nutrition, including supplementation with vitamins, antioxidants, minerals, and amino and fatty acids, if needed

2. Stress management, including getting enough sleep

3. Tapering off toxic chemicals or avoiding them completely

4. Cross-training exercises

5. Hormone replacement therapy (HRT), if needed

If you feel it is too late for you to age successfully, do not despair. This book will also guide you through a process of healing called the *transition* that will help restore your health. **You will learn how to begin this healing process in part II of the book.**

What Is Aging?

There are two types of aging: genetic aging and metabolic aging. You have a predetermined maximum total life span because the cells of your body are genetically programmed to die. Though the life span for the human species is 120 years, length of life varies for the individual. This is what is known as genetic aging. You cannot live longer than your preset genetic age, but you can certainly die earlier from accidents, infections or metabolic aging.

Metabolic Aging

Metabolic aging is the type of aging that occurs in relation to daily nutrition and lifestyle habits. You are in control of your metabolic aging process because stress, food, toxic chemicals and exercise can either speed up or slow down this process. If you speed up your metabolic aging through poor nutrition and lifestyle choices, you are going to die prematurely before reaching your genetic age. This is what is known as *accelerated metabolic* or *premature* aging.

You can reach your preset genetic age by preventing or reversing accelerated metabolic aging, and living a healthier life will help you do just that.

Living Longer, Not Better

Not too long ago the average life expectancy was between thirty and forty years. Today most Americans can count on living to at least seventy years of age or longer because research and education about sanitation and health along with advances in medical technology have helped to prolong our lives.

However, the simple act of being alive does not ensure being healthy, nor does it guarantee that we will be performing at our highest physical, mental and social capacity. While most people are living longer, many are also developing the degenerative diseases of aging (see chart, "Degenerative Diseases of Aging").

Those who do not have degenerative diseases may still have physical and mental ailments such as achy muscles and joints, allergies, anxiety, constipation, decreased memory and concentration, depression (short-term), emotional lability (abrupt mood changes), headaches, heartburn, low energy levels and sleep disturbances. With ten thousand baby boomers a day reaching age fifty, the number of people with these ailments and degenerative diseases is guaranteed to rise.

Although the decline of organ and immune system function together with a loss of flexibility occurs with normal aging, you can completely avoid developing a degenerative disease at a younger age. You just need to learn a few simple principles about how the body works and then make the necessary changes to slow down your aging process.

> ## Degenerative Diseases of Aging
>
> Abnormal cholesterol levels
> Cancer (almost all types of cancer can be caused by aging, but breast, prostate and colon are the most common types)
> Dementia
> Depression (long-term)
> Early menopause
> Heart disease
> High blood pressure
> Morbid obesity (weighing 30 percent or more above your ideal body weight)
> Osteoarthritis
> Osteoporosis
> Stroke
> Type II diabetes

Dr. Schwarzbein's Healing Story

While I was in the process of writing this book, I ran into an acquaintance of mine, Andrew Klavan, a bestselling author of fiction books. Coincidentally, he had just started reading my first book, *The Schwarzbein Principle*, and he had been talking to a physician friend of his about the fact that since I looked so healthy, maybe I was on to something. The physician replied, "No, I do not think so. It is all in her genes; she is genetically fortunate." After hearing this comment again, I have decided to include my own success story to illustrate how habits play a more important role in health than genetics. Genetically, the women in my family are healthy until their eighties. I became ill long before then because of my poor eating habits. My story illustrates how changing your nutrition and lifestyle habits can improve health and reverse accelerated metabolic aging.

When I was growing up I was a very poor eater. I would have a bowl full of sugar mixed in hot milk with a few oats (my version of oatmeal) for breakfast every morning. I would have a tuna sandwich on white Wonder Bread for lunch. And then at around 3:00 P.M. every day I would eat cotton candy, Pixi-Stix, Sweet Tarts, a box of sugar cookies and several Popsicles. I also drank half a quart of milk every day. Needless to say, by dinner I was pretty filled up with junk and ate very little, much to my mother's dismay. A green vegetable never passed my lips, and I did not eat birthday cake or ice cream because they were not sweet enough for me.

You would think that I would have been overweight from eating so much junk food, but that did not happen until later in my life. At first I was painfully underweight—so underweight that I would wear a T-shirt over my bathing suit at the beach to hide my ribs. I would then push my stomach out when I was lying down just to try to get it to be flat and not caved in. I was so thin that the doctors recommended that my parents try to fatten me up by increasing the number of vanilla milk shakes I drank every day. "What a problem!" you might think.

Actually, being underweight was a problem—it was a health problem. I was constantly sick with bronchitis and asthma. I had terrible menstrual periods with lots of cramps. This menstrual problem later was diagnosed as Stein-Leventhal syndrome (SLS).* I also had severe cystic acne that required cortisone injections in the acne lesions as well as radiation therapy to my face. I developed an intestinal problem that the doctors could never diagnose, so they called it "irritable bowel syndrome." I was in abdominal pain all day long, and I had to constantly be near a bathroom because I had multiple loose bowel movements each day. My doctor said I was probably going to end up with Crohn's disease (an autoimmune, inflammatory intestinal disease). He kept asking me if there was blood in my stool! Thankfully, that never happened.

I was a metabolic mess, but at least I was thin. If I was going to be unhealthy, I certainly thought that it was better to be thin and unhealthy than fat and unhealthy. Little did I know how wrong I was.

I was seeing several different doctors for all my problems, and none of them ever asked me about my diet. In fact, the dermatologist specifically said that sugar and chocolate did not cause my acne or make it worse. I

---

*Stein-Leventhal syndrome (SLS) is a female clinical condition of insulin resistance, fat-weight gain around the midsection, infertility, menstrual cycles without ovulation, acne and/or facial hair.

was so relieved to hear this news because at that time the rest of my doctors were telling me that all my other health problems were genetic, and I did not want anyone to take away my comfort foods. I was a sugar addict and if I had to be sick, I wanted to be sick but still be able to eat all the sugar I wanted.

I was lucky that I was born after the discovery of antibiotics because I had to take a lot of them to treat my chronic lung infections. If it were not for antibiotics, I believe I would have succumbed to an infectious disease at an early age because of my poor nutrition and lifestyle habits.

Now you, too, have a chance to reach your potential life span thanks to medical and cultural advances.

No Longer the Survival of the Fittest

Before modern medicine and plentiful food supplies, only the "fittest" people survived. Infections and malnutrition were the number-one killers of people in the past. The "fittest" people were those with the strongest immune systems, who were able to fight off infections, and those who had a "thrifty" gene that enabled them to utilize less stored food as energy in times of famine.

The good news is that with modern advances, it is no longer the survival of the "fittest" but the survival of everyone. We no longer have to fight off infections or survive famines on our own because we have antibiotics and year-round access to food. In our time people are succumbing to the degenerative diseases of aging rather than infectious diseases or starvation.

Today, how long and how well you live is more dependent on your daily nutrition and lifestyle habits and their influence on the aging process than on your genetic makeup. When these degenerative diseases occur, quality and quantity of life are shortened.

This does not mean that your genetic makeup does not matter—it does. If you are born with "bad" genes, you may die young. But once you become an adult, your daily nutrition and lifestyle habits play the biggest role in determining when and how you will die.

By learning how the body works and how your nutrition and lifestyle habits determine your health, you can take control of your quality and quantity of life. This will give you the opportunity to feel great and to live to your genetic potential.

My Healing Story Continues

When I was seventeen, I felt like I would not live past the age of twenty-five. This is when I finally decided I needed to do something about my health. You might think that I am exaggerating, but I did not know a person could feel as sick as I did and live a long time. I only found this out years later from hearing my patients' stories. By the time I was seventeen years old I had already badly damaged my metabolism and was on my way to a degenerative disease of aging. I felt terrible, and I knew that I did not want to spend the rest of my life feeling this way. So I started to read books about nutrition. This is when I began to take control of my health and my aging process.

I changed my destiny, and now it is time for you to change yours.

Change Your Destiny

In my first book, *The Schwarzbein Principle*, I introduced my principle: *Degenerative diseases are not genetic but acquired. Because the systems of the human body are interconnected and because one imbalance creates another imbalance, poor eating and lifestyle habits, not genetics, are the main cause of degenerative diseases of aging.*

Remember, bad habits, not genetic defects, catch up with us over time and cause accelerated or acquired metabolic aging, and many studies* are backing this up. These longevity studies are showing that lifestyle has a greater influence on our health than genetics and that living longer does not have to equate to the development of degenerative diseases of aging.

The Nun study, the Okinawa study and the MacArthur study.

This is very exciting news since these recently published studies are proving what I have been advocating since the early 1990s—it is never too late to improve your nutrition and lifestyle habits. You *can* change your own destiny by improving your daily habits.

In other words, someone who is genetically destined to die at age one hundred may not live past age sixty because of poor nutrition and lifestyle choices that cause accelerated aging and premature death. Conversely, a person can live to one hundred and be functionally intact. This is successful aging.

My Healing Story Continues

At age seventeen, I clearly remember reading Adele Davis, a dietitian who is famous for coining the phrase, "You are what you eat," and thinking, *Oh boy, I am in trouble. If that is true, I am nothing but a bag of cotton candy.* No wonder I was so sick. I did not eat well.

Now I am not going to lie and tell you that I knew that my "genetic diseases" were all acquired. I had no idea. I never thought I would cure myself. I just hoped I could help myself to feel better if I ate better.

The first thing I did was switch from drinking two Cokes a day to drinking two 7-Ups a day. My thinking was that since I could see through 7-Up, it must be better for me than Coke, a murky dark liquid. I also substituted a half a jar of honey a day for all the candy and other sugary junk I was eating—I thought honey was good for me since it was natural. I had to stop drinking milk at the same time because I had become lactose intolerant.

Big steps, right? Well, not really. Though it turned out to be fortunate that I could no longer drink milk because I could no longer digest lactose (milk sugar), and I unintentionally stopped my entire caffeine intake by switching from Coke to 7-Up, I was still drinking sugar by drinking 7-Up. Also, eating honey was better for me because honey has some nutrients and refined sugar does not, but honey is still sugar! So I did make some initial improvements to my habits, but not many. I was still ingesting too much sugar.

Because I was so ill, I became interested in learning more about how food could affect my health, so I started taking nutrition classes in college. I had my first green vegetable and started eating pastas and cereals instead of cookies and candy because I was learning how important it was to eat more vegetables and complex carbohydrates. I started eating Grape Nuts cereal with a milk substitute for breakfast; falafel sandwiches filled with lettuce, tomatoes and hummus, and a frozen yogurt shake for lunch and pasta with butter and tomato sauce for dinner, along with a salad full of all types of green vegetables.

I began to feel better, and by eating this way I was able to stop my daily high consumption of honey. Of course, I still binged on chocolate and candy right before my period because I had such intense cravings at that time of the month, but overall I thought this was a much better meal plan than before. However, I was still eating too much sugar in the form of complex carbohydrates. Complex carbohydrates were definitely an improvement from simple sugars, but in order to balance out my meals I needed to lower my carbohydrate intake and increase my protein and healthy fat intake. I would learn this in the years to come.

Despite being far from perfect, my new eating habits were a step in the right direction in helping me slow down and reverse my metabolic aging process. By making positive changes in my habits, I was starting to take control of my own aging process.

By improving your nutrition and lifestyle habits, you, too, can take control of your own aging process.

Taking Control of Aging

Now that you know that you have more control over your own aging process than you were ever led to believe was possible, the next step is to take that control. You can slow down the aging process and remain healthy by keeping your metabolism working efficiently.

Understanding Your Metabolism

To keep your body alive and functioning well, you need to have chemicals that are used for structure, function and energy. These chemicals are known as biochemicals. Cells, cell membranes, organs, glands, teeth, hair, skin, nails, muscles, bones and connective tissue are examples of structural biochemicals. Hormones, neurotransmitters, enzymes, cell mediators and antibodies are examples of functional biochemicals. Some of the energy biochemicals are sugar, ketones, triglycerides and glycogen. They are burned for fuel to keep biochemical reactions occurring.

Your body is made up of all these biochemicals that are continuously undergoing chemical reactions in order to carry on all the functions of the body. For example, for your heart to beat you need to have a heart (made up of structural biochemicals), signals to your heart that it should beat (functional biochemicals) and energy to contract the muscles of the heart to cause the heartbeat (energy biochemicals). All your bodily functions require the use and building back up of all the different biochemicals needed to keep you functioning and to sustain life.

This combination of using up and rebuilding biochemicals is called *regeneration*. Think of it this way—every time you breathe, think, go for a walk, read a book, eat a meal, watch a movie or do any other activity during your day, you are using up biochemicals. Your body must then rebuild the same biochemicals so that you can engage in all your life activities again. What you use up you must replenish, and you get the materials you need to rebuild your biochemicals from the food you eat.

The sum of these regeneration reactions, all the using-up reactions plus all the building-up reactions that are occurring, is what you know as your *metabolism*. You have an efficient metabolism if all of these chemical reactions are occurring on a continuous basis and you rebuild just as many biochemicals as you use up.

Every system and function in the body is connected, so when these chemical reactions occur efficiently your metabolism runs efficiently, helping you reach your preset genetic age. When regeneration is not efficient (use is greater than rebuilding, or rebuilding occurs more than using up), premature disease and death occur because of accelerated metabolic aging.

My Healing Story Continues

I had never counted calories before. After all, I was the one who was told I had to have more calories on a daily basis to try to gain weight. So when my weight shot up thirty pounds in three months after I improved my eating habits, I was stunned.

I had to keep a daily calorie count for the nutrition class I was taking and discovered that I was eating one thousand to fifteen hundred fewer calories on my new eating plan than I had when I ate sugary foods all the time. So I was eating fewer calories and healthier foods, but I still got fat! My thighs rubbed together and I went from wearing a size 6 to barely fitting into a size 14 in as little as three months. I remember thinking, *Thanks a lot, Adele Davis!*

Up until that point I thought that I had been born with the best metabolism in the whole world—I could and did eat anything I wanted for seventeen years, and I could not put a pound on to save my life. Then my world was turned upside down. For the first time in my life I was making an effort to improve my eating habits, and I gained fat weight. I became very distressed and confused. And to make matters worse, my family—who had always told me to eat more calories to gain weight—started telling me to eat fewer calories because I was fat!

I am sure that you can guess how close I came to going back to eating all that sugar, junk and cotton candy. In fact, I came very close to doing just that except for one tiny little fact: I felt that my health was getting appreciably better. I had been a far cry from being healthy, and now I was unhealthy and fat, but I had an instinctive feeling that my body was trying to heal.

Also, I knew intellectually that eating better types of food had to be better for me than eating tons of refined, sugary ones. I really had no choice. I needed to continue to eat this way if I had any chance at all of regaining my health. I believed I was destined to be overweight because I thought it was a trade-off—I could either be thin and unhealthy or fat and healthy.

The mistake I made was that I believed it did not matter what I ate as long as I stayed thin. If you think the same way I used to, you may be destroying your metabolism and not even know it.

Metabolism Myth

Because our culture has come to equate thinness with health, you may think that someone has a healthy metabolism when that person can eat what he or she wants and does not gain weight. However, this is not always true because the physiological definition of a healthy metabolism refers to *all* the processes of efficient regeneration— building up and using functional and structural proteins and fats— not *just* to the ability to burn off sugar and stored fat as energy. The chart below lists some functional, structural and storage biochemicals and what they are made of.

The Composition of Functional, Structural and Storage Biochemicals

Functional	Structural	Storage
Antibodies (P)	Bones/Muscles/Teeth (P)	Glycogen (S)
Cellular products (P & F)	Cells/Cell membranes (P & F)	Triglycerides (F)
Enzymes (P)	Connective tissue (P & S)	
Hormones (P & F)	Glands/Organs (P)	
Neurotransmitters (P)	Hair/Skin/Nails (P)	

(P = Protein, F = Fat, S = Sugar)

Many people equate using energy only with exercise and weight loss. However, you also require energy during all regeneration processes—when you use up and rebuild your functional and structural biochemicals.

An inferior metabolism—the kind that leads to accelerated metabolic aging—is a mismatch between rebuilding and use. In other words, you rebuild your functional, structural and storage biochemicals at a faster rate than you can use them, or you use up more than you can rebuild. So you can be overweight *or* thin and have an inferior metabolism.

In summary, a healthy metabolism occurs when efficient regeneration of body parts is occurring—when what you use up is being replaced or rebuilt. An inferior metabolism—the kind that leads to accelerated metabolic aging—is a mismatch between using up and rebuilding.

My Healing Story Continues

I could not figure out what was going on if eating fewer calories made me gain weight, and it was at this point that I became very fearful. You can bet that I made sure that I did not drop any more calories as recommended by my well-intentioned sisters. I was too afraid to eat less. I never started dieting after I gained weight because I was so afraid that I would end up gaining another thirty pounds of fat in three months' time.

I was afraid to lower my caloric intake, but I still thought that energy in was supposed to equal energy out, so I began exercising more to try to lose weight and boost my energy levels. Most days I ran a few miles, I swam about a half a mile and took at least one other gym class such as volleyball, tennis or track. Although I was exercising more than ever before, I did not lose any weight. By overexercising, I accomplished exactly the opposite of what I was trying to do. I did not know that too much exercise, just like eating the wrong foods, also creates a mismatch between using up and rebuilding. This imbalance delayed my healing process.

The slight increased feeling of well-being that I experienced kept me from going back to all my bad habits, and I cannot tell you how thankful I am that I listened to my body. Once I stopped overexercising I was able to heal without dieting. I never eliminated food groups; I just improved the types of food I ate from each food group. Because I had experienced it firsthand, I learned early on that eating too many calories is not the reason people become fat, and counting calories will never make a person thin. Never dieting turned out to be one of the most important components to my own healing.

Today I have the body composition I want because I listened to my body, continued to improve upon my food choices and put in the time I needed to heal. I no longer have asthma, chronic bronchitis, Stein-Leventhal syndrome, acne or irritable bowel syndrome. I am completely cured of my "genetic" diseases because I healed my metabolism by improving my nutrition and lifestyle habits. You can read about my *transition* later in chapter 8.

Because of my willingness to learn about and take control of my own health, I now have a healthy metabolism. Do you?

Take the Metabolism Quiz

Since a healthy metabolism cannot be measured by how much you weigh, you can determine if you have a healthy metabolism by evaluating the following signs and symptoms. Check off any that describe you.

1. ☐ Poor energy and stamina
2. ☐ Poor memory and concentration
3. ☐ Poor mood
4. ☐ Poor sleep habits
5. ☐ Poor digestion and bowel movements
6. ☐ Poor strength
7. ☐ Weak bones, teeth, hair and nails
8. ☐ Addiction(s) to refined sugars, artificial sugars, caffeine, nicotine, alcohol and/or illicit drugs
9. ☐ Allergies, asthma, chronic pain (not due to trauma), frequent severe headaches, daily heartburn and/or frequent infections
10. ☐ Degenerative disease(s) of aging

If you checked off none of the items, you have a healthy metabolism. If you checked off any of the first seven items, you have a fair metabolism. If you checked off three or more of the first seven items or items 8 or 9, you have a damaged metabolism. If you checked off item 10 because you already have a degenerative disease of aging, you have a *badly* damaged metabolism.

No matter how awful this sounds, you now know that there is hope. You can heal your metabolism just like I did and thousands of others have.

My Healing Story Continues

So what did happen to me? Because I am an endocrinologist, I have a hormonal explanation for you, of course.

Because of my poor eating habits, I was unable to rebuild the functional and structural biochemicals I was using on a day-to-day basis. When I started to eat better, my body responded by catching up on rebuilding my biochemicals and not letting me use up as much. My hormones directed my body to rebuild functional and structural proteins and fats and also determined whether I would store or use them. My rebuilding hormones came out in full force to help heal me from all the past damage I had done to myself. Unfortunately, once the damage is done, you cannot rebuild functional and structural proteins and fats without also rebuilding storage fats. This is why I put on so much fat weight—my body was trying to heal itself. Once my body healed, I burned off the fat weight for energy.

Controlling Your Hormones

Slowing down or reversing the aging process is related to improving your metabolism, and your metabolism is related to your body's ability to regenerate efficiently. Your ability to regenerate efficiently requires that all the biochemical reactions in your body are occurring simultaneously and in conjunction with one another—and *it is the hormones of the body that regulate these biochemical reactions.*

You have control over your hormones when you change your nutrition and lifestyle habits. Therefore, you have control over whether or not you have an efficient metabolism, and thus control over the quality of your health and your aging process.

In summary, the key to preventing accelerated aging is to achieve and/or maintain an efficient metabolism by balancing your hormones. You do this by following the five steps of the SPII program.

The Transition to Healing

You, too, can have a healthy metabolism and achieve your ideal body composition, but if you begin as unhealthy as I did, you have to go through a *transition* process. This process is explained in more detail in chapter 8, but it is the key to healing your metabolism so I will introduce it briefly here.

The *transition* is a journey of healing, and you enter your *transition* when you begin improving your nutrition and lifestyle habits. During your *transition* your hormones will be changing in response to your new habits, which enables you to heal, but you will not attain balanced hormones immediately. There are sequential steps of healing that everyone must go through.

1. You must first improve your nutrition and lifestyle habits to initiate your *transition.*

2. When you improve your habits, your body will begin to rebalance its hormones. This is when your body rebuilds all the functional and structural biochemicals that have not been made as efficiently because of your *past* poor nutrition and lifestyle habits. The more damaged your current metabolism is, the longer it will take for this process to be completed.

3. You will heal your metabolism by taking the necessary steps

outlined in the SPII program and by allowing enough time to balance your hormones.

4. When you have healed your metabolism, you will be primed to lose fat weight—if necessary.
5. Once you have lost all your stored fat, you have completed your *transition*.

Most importantly, there are no shortcuts in this process if you need to heal your metabolism. However, if you have poor nutrition and lifestyle habits, but you have not yet destroyed your metabolism, you will go through a fairly quick *transition*. You are already primed to lose stored fat and achieve your ideal body composition because you do not have to put in the time to heal your metabolism first.

Summary

- To age successfully, you must stay as healthy as you can for as long as possible.
- Daily habits—not genetics—play the most important role in aging.
- There are two types of aging: genetic aging and metabolic aging.
- By improving your diet and lifestyle habits, you can prevent accelerated metabolic aging.
- A healthy metabolism is the result of efficient regeneration (using up and rebuilding) of your body's biochemicals. An inferior metabolism—the kind that leads to premature aging—is a mismatch between use and rebuilding.
- Hormones regulate your body's biochemical reactions—and therefore your metabolism.
- Controlling and balancing your hormones will lead to an efficient metabolism.
- Since a healthy metabolism cannot be measured by how much you weigh, you can determine if you have a healthy metabolism by taking the metabolism quiz.

- Healing a badly damaged metabolism takes time.
- Once your metabolism is damaged, you cannot rebuild functional and structural proteins and fats without also rebuilding storage fats.
- The *transition* is a journey of healing from a damaged metabolism to a healed one. During your *transition* your hormones will be changing in response to your improved nutrition and lifestyle habits, but you will not attain balanced hormones immediately.
- The SPII program will guide you in improving your nutrition and lifestyle habits, so that you can balance your hormones, move into your transition, age successfully and avoid premature degenerative diseases of aging.

* * *

Because your hormones regulate regeneration, it is important that you familiarize yourself with them so that you will understand what will happen to you as you go through your *transition*. Learning to balance your hormones so that your body can regenerate efficiently is the key to successful aging.

Chapter 2 explains hormones—what they are, what they do and how they work to help your body regenerate.

Two

Hormones and How They Work

Your body maintains a highly sophisticated communication system with hormones acting as messengers between the different cells and systems of your body. As discussed in chapter 1, your hormones regulate all the biochemical processes in your body, including life-sustaining functions. If your hormones are not delivering the right messages, you will initially feel lousy. As time progresses, this imbalance will not only make you feel bad and cause accelerated metabolic aging, but it will also increase your risk for developing a degenerative disease of aging.

Hormones: The Great Communicators

Hormones relay messages to your cells, which in turn respond by changing the biochemical reactions that are occurring within those cells. These cells then secrete new hormones that relay messages to other parts of the body. It is through these constant and simultaneous hormone signals that all your cells are able to stay in contact with each other and keep the systems of your body aware of what is going on in other systems of your body. All of these signals keep your body communicating effectively.

When Communication Breaks Down

If hormonal communication breaks down between cells because of hormonal imbalances, your body will not be able to regenerate efficiently. For you to remain healthy, you need to keep your hormones balanced so they can communicate effectively with each other and with your cells. Unfortunately, life itself is antibalance—your hormones are constantly changing to meet your daily demands. This means you have to work at keeping your hormones balanced in order to age successfully.

Where Hormones Come From

Hormones are functional biochemicals that are made by the cells of your body. Contrary to popular belief, you do not get hormones *in* your food! In order to produce new hormones, you have to eat the right food that has the necessary material for your body to make them. Since hormones are mainly made from proteins, cholesterol and essential fats, eating a balanced diet is essential for keeping up the production of your hormones. (Nutrition is discussed in detail in chapter 11.)

The Balancing Act

In order for you to slow down the aging process and remain healthy, your body's hormones need to be kept in balance so that controlled regeneration can occur.

How do you keep your hormones balanced? You improve your nutrition and lifestyle habits to bring hormone levels that are too low or too high back to normal levels. If a hormone is missing, you take hormone replacement therapy (HRT) to replace it to normal levels.

It sounds simple, but there is one small catch. Since all the hormone systems of the body are interconnected, if one hormone system is out

of balance, they are all out of balance. On the other hand, the opposite applies. I cannot emphasize this enough. Nutrition and lifestyle
habits that balance one hormone will help balance out all hormones.
By following the five steps of the SPII program, you can ultimately
balance all your hormone systems and be in control of your health.

Hormone Classifications—
Major and Minor Hormones

There are two classifications of hormones: major and minor. As
stated previously, *all* hormones regulate all the biochemical reactions
that are occurring in your body. Think of the major hormones as having the greater role in determining what happens within your cells and
the minor hormones as having the lesser role, and you now understand their primary difference. For example, though both major and
minor hormones play a role in keeping you alive, the major hormones
have a greater influence than the minor ones.

The major hormones are also the first hormones to be secreted in
response to your constantly changing nutrition, lifestyle and environmental signals. How the major hormones respond in turn determines
how the minor hormones will respond to the same situations. And the
response of the minor hormones will cycle back to regulate the
response of the major ones and so forth. It is a continuous cycle of
communication with the major hormones having the greatest
influence.

Major Hormones

Three of the major hormones are adrenaline, cortisol and insulin.
Among their many other purposes, these hormones are crucial for
maintaining immediate life-sustaining functions, such as regulating
your heartbeat and blood pressure and also maintaining the pH (the
balance between acidity and alkalinity) of your blood. So if you are

missing any one of the major hormones, you will get sick quickly and not live for very long. Since these hormones keep you alive and also determine how you feel daily, their importance to your health and well-being are obvious; therefore, there is no controversy about whether or not these hormones need to be replaced if they are low or missing.

Minor Hormones

There is, however, a controversy surrounding some of the minor hormones, such as estradiol, dehydroepiandrosterone (DHEA) and human growth hormone (HGH). Should you replace them or not? If any of the minor hormone levels fall too low, you may have many complaints, such as fatigue, mood changes and weight gain, but your heart keeps beating, your blood pH remains reasonably balanced and your blood pressure is still present. Therefore, you are alive, but you may not feel as well as you could if you balanced your minor hormones by taking hormone replacement therapy. More importantly, the loss of a minor hormone will shorten your life span. However, because the loss of any one of the minor hormones does not cause immediate death, it is harder to understand their roles in sustaining health and promoting longevity.

In short, with the loss of a major hormone you absolutely know that something is medically wrong with you, and if the major hormone is not replaced you will die rather quickly. With the loss of a minor hormone, you will not feel well, but you are likely to attribute your poor health to normal aging and not seek medical attention. You will eventually die from the loss of a minor hormone, but when you die ten to fifty years later, who is to know that the minor hormone loss contributed to your death?

Make no mistake—every hormone, major or minor, plays a role in health and longevity. You need to keep all of your hormones balanced so that you can be healthy and live a long time. And sometimes the only way to achieve balance is through hormone replacement therapy—taking the hormone that is missing.

Hormones and Regeneration

Hormones control regeneration in the body; when your hormones are not balanced, your body's ability to regenerate is compromised. Remember, regeneration involves using up and then rebuilding the same structural, functional and energy biochemicals—such as cells, neurotransmitters, hormones, enzymes and glycogen—that are used again and again. (See chapter 1 for more information on biochemicals.)

How Hormones Control Regeneration

Some hormones regulate destruction, while others regulate construction. The "using up" hormones regulate destruction by activating the body to get rid of old cells or functional, other structural and energy biochemicals. The "rebuilding" hormones regulate construction by activating the chemical pathways that make new cells or functional, other structural and energy biochemicals. All of this is occurring in your body simultaneously. When "destruction" hormones are secreted to use up your chemicals and cells, these hormones in turn trigger the secretion of the rebuilding hormones and vice versa.

This is a good thing. You want your body parts to communicate with each other. If they did not communicate, your body would use up its biochemicals and not be aware that it needed to rebuild them. Or your body would rebuild your biochemicals but then not use them.

As you can imagine, this coupling process is an area of potential chaos. What if using up exceeds rebuilding? What if rebuilding exceeds using up? Both cases could lead to health problems or a degenerative disease of aging.

For example, if the brain uses more serotonin than your body can produce, the imbalance created can lead to memory loss or depression. Or if more energy is consumed in the form of carbohydrates than is needed at a given moment, the excess energy will be stored as fat, and morbid obesity or Type II diabetes can occur over time.

Pathways of Regeneration

Your body regenerates functional, structural and energy biochemicals in two ways. Either you use up your functional and/or energy biochemicals during a chemical reaction and then they are replenished by new production from fresh material, or your body gets rid of old structural biochemicals to make room for new structural biochemicals. The first pathway has a faster turnaround time than the second. There is usually a greater need for more functional and energy biochemicals than there is for more structural biochemicals on a daily basis.

For example, in the process of thinking, functional biochemicals called neurotransmitters are secreted into special areas of the brain; after they are used, some of these functional biochemicals are broken down and disposed of by the body. You then must rebuild new neurotransmitters in order for you to be able to think again. Or in order for you to be able to be active, energy biochemicals are used up and need to be replaced so that you can move again. This type of regeneration can occur over a period of hours.

An example of the second pathway of regeneration is when cells called *osteoclasts* literally chew up and get rid of old bone tissue (structural biochemicals), and then cells called *osteoblasts* come in and build new bone. This type of regeneration occurs over a period of weeks to months.

Food and Regeneration

Food is the material that your body uses to regenerate itself; all your structural, functional and energy biochemicals are made from food nutrients. Your hormones regulate all the chemical reactions that your body undergoes to regenerate. Because the systems of the body are all interconnected and hormones direct all chemical reactions, every function of your body is tied into the changing of food into hormones, which then regulates the changing of other food into the different biochemicals. That is why eating well is essential to efficient regeneration and successful aging.

You probably understand that if you were to stop eating altogether you would die because your body would not be able to rebuild. But are you aware that poor nutrition habits such as skipping meals, eating junk food and eliminating food groups may not cause immediate death, but your body is not getting what it needs to rebuild efficiently? These bad habits can lead to illness and accelerated metabolic aging.

My patients are often embarrassed to show me their three-day food journals because they have such bad eating habits. Then they ask me why they do not feel well and wonder if they have a terrible disease! These patients do not have a disease. They are ill from the hormone imbalances that have occurred because of their poor eating habits and their inability to regenerate efficiently.

Regeneration

In industrialized nations like ours, people's regeneration needs have increased. Our day-to-day busy lifestyles mean people use up more biochemicals every day, and they also need to rebuild them.

The more physically and mentally active you are, the more you need to regenerate. A high-powered executive who works long hours or a parent who is constantly on the go needs to regenerate more than a Tibetan monk who sits on a mountaintop and meditates all day long.

If you led a monklike existence, your regeneration needs would be much less because you would not be using up your biochemicals as much. This means you would not need to eat as much to rebuild. But most people do not want to live a monklike existence; therefore, they need to change their habits to meet their bodies' needs.

Taking Regeneration for Granted

Though you are not aware of it, your body is constantly regenerating. We take it for granted that regeneration occurs as it needs to, but this is not always true. A high-powered executive who works long hours, and is also a parent constantly on the go, needs to pay more attention to healthy eating and lifestyle habits so that her body's regeneration matches her fast-paced lifestyle.

If your life is too hectic, your body will not be able to keep up. You can live hard and fast and burn out sooner, or you can work to achieve moderation in all aspects of your life and age successfully. As simplistic as it sounds, it is true.

However, if you want to live a fast and busy lifestyle, you can still improve your quality of life by working on other aspects of your health such as eating well and taking hormone replacement therapy (HRT) if you need to. You do not have to follow all five steps of the SPII program to obtain some benefits and improve your health.

To put it briefly, if you are going to slow down your aging process and remain healthy, you need to keep your hormones in balance. Only then can controlled regeneration occur, and controlled regeneration leads to an efficient metabolism.

Summary

- Hormones are your body's messengers. If they are not delivering the right messages, you will feel lousy, and with time you will develop a degenerative disease of aging.

- Since hormones are mainly made from proteins, cholesterol and essential fats, eating a balanced diet is essential for keeping up the production of your hormones.
- Sometimes the only way to achieve hormonal balance is by taking the hormone that is missing (called hormone replacement therapy or HRT).
- Since all the hormone systems of the body are interconnected, if one hormone system is out of balance, they are all out of balance.
- Every hormone, major or minor, plays a role in health and longevity.
- Hormones control regeneration in the body and if your hormones are not balanced, your body's ability to regenerate will be compromised.
- Regeneration needs have increased; our day-to-day busy lifestyles mean we are using up more biochemicals on a daily basis that then need to be rebuilt.
- In order for you to slow down the aging process and remain healthy, you need to improve your nutrition and lifestyle habits to balance your hormones. This will keep you regenerating efficiently, for it is your body's ability to effectively regenerate that determines the rate of aging.

* * *

In chapter 3, I introduce the concept of "lifestyle-based" endocrinology and explain how hormone imbalances caused by poor nutrition and lifestyle habits can affect your health.

Kelley's story in chapter 3 illustrates how someone with a lifestyle-based endocrine disorder can get immediate results on the SPII program. She was fortunate; she had not yet damaged her metabolism.

Three

Lifestyle-Based Endocrinology—How Hormone Responses Lead to Illness

---

Glandular-Based Endocrinology

Your hormone systems are made up of glands that produce and secrete hormones into the bloodstream. The study of these hormone systems and their role in the functions and vital processes of the body is the science of endocrinology. If any of these glands malfunction, you will end up with a "glandular-based" endocrine disorder.

Glandular-based endocrine disorders or diseases can result in either a hormone deficiency or excess. A deficiency state occurs when a gland produces too little of a hormone, and an excess state occurs when a gland produces too much of a hormone.

But glandular-based disorders are not the only causes of hormonal imbalances. This chapter introduces "lifestyle-based" endocrine disorders and explains how, just like glandular-based endocrine disorders, lifestyle-based disorders can cause many symptoms and problems that make it impossible for you to lead a healthy and happy life.

Lifestyle-Based Endocrinology

Most glandular-based endocrine diseases of the body are not that common. In fact, some are pretty rare.* But the hormonal imbalances that I see in my office every day are very common. These imbalances are not caused by diseases of the glands but by long-term daily poor nutrition and lifestyle habits. I have named these types of endocrine abnormalities "lifestyle-based" endocrine disorders.

For the purposes of this book, we will define *lifestyle-based endocrinology* as the study and treatment of the cumulative hormone changes related to chronic over- or underproduction and/or secretion of hormones in response to any or all of the following:

- Poor nutrition, including lack of vitamins, minerals, and essential amino and fatty acids

- Stresses such as lack of sleep and being overly busy

- Exposure to toxic chemicals, such as food additives, alcohol, artificial sugars, prescription and over-the-counter medications, refined sugars, stimulants and street drugs

- Excessive exercise, or not enough exercise

- Aging (your body's ability to make different hormone changes at different stages in your life)

- Genetics (Although everyone shares the same physiology, the amount of any hormone secreted in response to various factors is different for everyone.)

---

*For example, the diagnosis of Hashimoto's thyroid disease in the population is approximately 4.3 people per 1000/year or 0.43 percent/year. The diagnosis of Cushing's disease is 5 to 25 people per 1 million/year or 0.0025 percent/year.

All these factors determine which hormones will be secreted and in what amounts throughout the day. If one or more of these factors is present every day, you will end up with hormonal imbalances that lead to regeneration problems.

Here's an example. It is not harmful for you to be stressed for a few hours, but if you are stressed for a few hours every day for many years, the effects add up. The hormone changes that occur in times of repetitive stress cause you to use up your biochemicals faster than you are able to rebuild them. As you already know, this imbalance in using up and rebuilding leads to accelerated metabolic aging, degenerative diseases and premature death.

Glandular Versus Lifestyle-Based Hormone Disorders

I have compiled a comparison list to illustrate the differences between glandular-based and lifestyle-based endocrine disorders. In each case, the first example listed is a glandular-based endocrine disease. The second example is the normal response of the endocrine system to your daily habits. Though these responses are normal, you will end up with a lifestyle-based endocrine disease if they occur day in and day out.

Disorders Caused by High Insulin Levels

Glandular-Based:	Lifestyle-Based:
Insulinoma, a tumor in the pancreas that overproduces and secretes insulin.	The pancreas secretes a high level of insulin in response to a high-carbohydrate meal. Years of high insulin levels increase your risk for Type II diabetes, plaque buildup in your heart arteries, high blood pressure and strokes.

Disorders Caused by Low Thyroid Levels

Glandular-Based:	Lifestyle-Based:
Hashimoto's thyroid disease, an autoimmune process that causes destruction of the thyroid gland and therefore low or no thyroid hormone production.	Eating a low-calorie diet signals the cells of the body to deactivate thyroid hormone, which can cause metabolic hypothyroidism— i.e., low-thyroid function. (See Metabolic Hypo- thyroidism sidebar, page 45)

Disorders Caused by High Adrenaline Levels

Glandular-Based:	Lifestyle-Based:
Pheochromocytoma, a tumor in the adrenal glands that overproduces and secretes adrenaline.	The adrenal gland secretes higher levels of adrenaline in response to skipping meals, low-calorie diets or other stressors. Chronic high levels of adrenaline increase your risk for many problems such as asthma, allergies, migraine headaches, severe bone loss and depression.

Disorders Caused by High Cortisol Levels

Glandular-Based:	Lifestyle-Based:
Cushing's disease, a pituitary tumor that overproduces and secretes adrenocorticotropic hormone (ACTH), which then stimulates the adrenal glands to overproduce and secrete cortisol.	Chronic life stressors stimulate the pituitary gland to over-produce ACTH, which in turn tells the adrenal glands to overproduce and secrete cortisol. Sustained high cortisol levels can lead to many problems, including Type II diabetes, severe bone loss, fat-weight gain, high blood pressure and depression.

Disorders of High Blood-Sugar Levels

Glandular-Based:	Lifestyle-Based:
Type I diabetes, an autoimmune disease that causes destruction of the cells of the pancreas that make and secrete insulin, leading to hypo- or low insulin levels and high blood-sugar levels.	Chronic poor nutrition (e.g., high-carbohydrate, low-fat diets or chronic low-calorie dieting) and poor lifestyle habits (too much stress, not enough sleep, ingesting too much alcohol or caffeine, smoking and overexercising) are signals to the body to release high amounts of insulin (hyperinsulinemia). Over a long period of time these high insulin levels cause your cells to be overfilled with sugar and fats (triglycerides).

Disorders Caused by High Blood-Sugar Levels

Glandular-Based:	Lifestyle-Based:
	When this happens, your cells do not let as much sugar or triglycerides inside when insulin is present. This is known as early insulin resistance and is a prediabetic condition.
	If nothing is done to correct this early insulin resistance, your pancreas over time will not be able to secrete enough insulin to overcome your cells' resistance to insulin. You will be unable to normalize your blood-sugar levels and they will rise, resulting in high blood-sugar levels. This is Type II diabetes. (See chapter 5 for more details on insulin resistance.)

The similarities between glandular-based and lifestyle-based endocrine disorders are that an over- or underproduction and secretion of hormones exist in both cases. The difference is that glandular-based endocrine disorders are caused by diseased or damaged glands, while lifestyle-based endocrine disorders initially are normal responses that arise from healthy glands.

When a gland is diseased, the treatment is surgical, pharmaceutical or hormonal replacement therapy. When a hormone imbalance is caused by daily bad nutrition and lifestyle habits, the prescription is a change in habits, which is exactly what the SPII program is designed to help you do.

Kelley's Hormonal Imbalances

Kelley is a perfect example of someone with a lifestyle-based endocrine disorder. It was years before the real cause of her illnesses was found.

Kelley: Around the age of ten I lost three grandparents, and I comforted myself with food. I ate mostly sweets and carbohydrates. By the time I was twelve years old I was the largest kid in my sixth-grade class, and it really bothered me a lot. I was bigger than everyone, including the boys. I was about five feet tall and weighed 130 pounds—which made me feel pretty fat.

I was very unhappy and wanted to do anything I could to change my appearance. I spoke to my mother about taking me to our doctor, and he put me on the "grapefruit diet." I lost thirty pounds in a month and a half. I also lost half of the hair on my head. But I was thin, and I felt really good about myself.

After going off my first diet, I ate one meal a day because I was so weight conscious. Since I wasn't eating sweets, I thought I was being healthy.

Within two years of starting my period, I started having excruciating menstrual pain. I was fourteen years old. Every month I would faint from the pain and have to miss school. So my mom took me to the doctor again, and he put me on birth control pills to regulate the severe cramps. They worked. I was able to function normally because I wasn't cramping anymore. It was like a miracle.

At age twenty-one I moved from Florida to California and started developing allergies and sinus problems, so my doctor put me on some allergy medication. I also started having yeast infections, and I became quite run-down. I was weak and didn't have much energy. I felt like I was dragging myself to work. My doctor ran blood tests, including thyroid tests that came up negative, and he diagnosed me with chronic fatigue syndrome. He said that there was nothing medical that could be done for chronic fatigue syndrome except to take better care of myself and have a positive attitude. His advice at that time was to exercise, to eat right and to get plenty of sleep. Since I thought that I was already exercising enough,

I tried to get more sleep. Although I felt that I was eating pretty well, I was concerned about heart disease, so I lowered my fat intake, thinking I was making a healthy change.

Dr. Schwarzbein: Kelley's problems all began when she ate to comfort herself from the stress of her grandparents' deaths and then went on her first diet to "solve" her fat-weight gain. Since she lost weight when she cut her calories and she felt good about herself, she thought if she focused on staying thin she would be healthy. However, she was very mistaken because eating a low-fat, low-calorie diet over a period of years is one of the quickest ways to develop a lifestyle-based endocrine disorder.

Some of the first signs of Kelley's lifestyle-based endocrine disorder were her hair loss and painful menstrual cycles. Instead of treating the cause of her problems, which would have entailed changing her poor nutrition habits, she was given birth control pills to treat her symptoms. The birth control pill, however, led to additional symptoms of allergies, sinus problems and yeast infections—it was not the answer to her problems.

Because her blood tests all came back negative, she was diagnosed with chronic fatigue syndrome*, a "catchall diagnosis" given to many patients when the root problem cannot be found. When Kelley tried to further "improve" her eating habits by eliminating almost all the fat from her diet, she inadvertently worsened her problems because healthy fats are important for good health and healing.

Over the years, her hormone levels continued to fluctuate dramatically because of her continuing poor nutrition and lifestyle habits, and she continued to feel worse, until she believed she had a serious disease. In reality, Kelley had a lifestyle-based endocrine disorder that easily could have been treated by changing a few habits.

Kelley: I really didn't think my nutrition habits caused my feelings of weakness and other symptoms because I ate at least one decent meal a day. I was still trying to keep my figure, so when I was up a few pounds I

*Though I believe in the concept of chronic fatigue syndrome, I do not believe that we should label patients with syndromes. I think it is better to get to the root cause of what is occurring and treat the problem, not the symptoms.

would have a glass of wine and popcorn for dinner instead of a meal. I began to notice that I would have a hard time sleeping when I ate this way, though. Sometimes my heart would pound and my skin would crawl and itch. I felt like I was having a reaction to food, and I gave this feeling a name. I called it a "food hangover." I felt toxic. I had my doctor give me a test for hypoglycemia, but the test results were negative. So I just kept eating the same way.

My symptoms were intensified in my early thirties when I began to notice that my hair was falling out like it had when I went on my first diet. I was losing my hair through the temple area, and my doctor diagnosed it as male pattern baldness. I was told there was nothing I could do about it.

With time I got to the point where I was coming home from work and plopping down on the couch exhausted, but I still didn't think that my eating habits were my problem. I was getting weaker and weaker even though I could still work and exercise.

I could always come up with a reason for what was happening to me. I thought I felt weak from all the stress of running a business, or that my hair was falling out because I colored it. But deep down inside I think I knew that I was always fooling myself. I just wanted to stay thin.

Dr. Schwarzbein: Kelley kept hanging on to the notion that being thin meant that she was healthy. However, it was her poor nutrition habits such as skipping meals, eating junk food and eliminating fats from her diet to stay thin that caused her to become weaker. Kelley, like many of my patients, became ill from the hormone fluctuations caused by her poor eating habits.

Glandular- and Lifestyle-Based Endocrine Disorders Cause Disease

Both glandular- and lifestyle-based endocrine disorders cause serious problems, but the timing and severity of the initial symptoms are very different.

Type I Diabetes—Glandular-Based Disorder

For example, when a person acquires Type I diabetes because of destruction of the cells of the pancreas that produce insulin, the loss of insulin immediately causes extremely high blood-sugar levels and rapid weight loss. These high sugar levels in turn cause excessive thirst, fatigue and urination. It is obvious that something is wrong, and the laboratory blood work will reflect the problem with high blood-sugar levels and low insulin levels. A glandular-based endocrine diagnosis is made.

Type II Diabetes—Lifestyle-Based Disorder

Type II diabetes, however, is diagnosed many years after the initial hormone imbalance begins. High insulin levels, not low insulin levels, are the problem originally associated with Type II diabetes, and high insulin levels are harder to detect because it is normal for insulin levels to rise under many circumstances. The slightly higher insulin level causes slow weight gain, small increases in blood pressure, slow changes in cholesterol numbers and the beginning of artery plaque formation. One by one, diagnoses of obesity, hypertension, cholesterol abnormalities and heart disease are made without taking into account that these are all related to higher insulin levels and to each other.* If the underlying physiology is not corrected, Type II diabetes will likely be the next diagnosis.

The physical changes that occur when you have higher insulin levels are so subtle and cause damage over so many years that it takes approximately ten to thirty years for your blood-sugar levels to rise after the initial changes in insulin levels begin. By the time Type II diabetes is diagnosed, chronic high insulin levels have done a lot of metabolic damage—though it will seem to happen overnight.

---

*The good news is that the association between fat-weight gain, blood pressure, cholesterol, heart disease and Type II diabetes is finally being widely recognized as a "metabolic" syndrome. More advances in prevention and treatment of this syndrome are being researched because there is no longer any dispute that higher insulin levels play a central role in the cause of this epidemic problem.

Why Lifestyle-Based Hormone Problems Are Difficult to Diagnose

It is much harder to diagnose a lifestyle-based hormone problem than it is to diagnose a glandular-based hormone disease because you will experience the symptoms of a lifestyle-based hormonal imbalance long before your blood tests register the imbalance. This discrepancy between symptoms and lab work is seen in all lifestyle-based disorders.

Here are some more reasons that it is hard to diagnose a lifestyle-based hormone problem.

Normal Hormone Levels Cover a Wide Range

The normal ranges of hormone levels in the population are very wide. So if one of your glands is over- or underproducing a hormone in response to poor nutrition and lifestyle habits, it may be very difficult to detect in the blood work because the normal ranges for a population are not the same as for an individual.

For example, if the normal range of a hormone blood level in a population runs between 60 and 500 units, and your blood level measures 250 units, it registers as within normal limits but could actually mean high, low or normal levels for you.

Hormone Levels Vary in Different Parts of the Body

Some of the hormone levels measured are meaningless because the blood levels do not accurately reflect the levels in other parts of the body.

For example, the blood levels of serotonin are not the same as the brain levels of serotonin. Measuring the blood level of serotonin does not give you an accurate level of serotonin in the brain where most of the action of serotonin exists. Unfortunately, there is no easy way to measure brain levels of serotonin.

Certain Hormone Levels Fluctuate Regularly

Other hormones, such as cortisol and human growth hormone (HGH), have normal, daily fluctuations. Unless a *series* of levels is measured, the individual level is meaningless, even if it is very high or very low.

Free Hormone Levels Are Difficult to Measure

Some hormones are bound to proteins in your bloodstream. The bound plus the free hormone levels equal the total hormone count. It is the *free* hormone that is active and needs to be measured, not the total hormone level, to get an accurate assessment of the hormone's activity in the body.

Hormone Quantities Are Difficult to Measure

Hormones are found in such small quantities in the body to begin with that accurate testing in general is difficult to accomplish.

Hormone Levels Do Not Always Reflect Hormone Action

Hormone levels do not necessarily correlate with hormone actions because hormones must first bind to specific receptor sites on individual cells to communicate. Hormone measurements do not reflect this binding. Therefore, a hormone level will tell you how much of a hormone is in your bloodstream at a given moment, but not what it is doing within your body.

Kelley: I badly injured my back when I was thirty-five. Now I was not only feeling bad, but I also had an injury. I could not exercise because of the pain, and I was even more determined to keep my fat intake low so that I could keep my weight down. I was sleeping only three or four hours a night, my skin felt like it was crawling, my heart felt like it was pounding out of my chest and my hair was still falling out. Because my lab tests were normal, I was told, "Oh, it's allergies, oh it's stress—allergies and stress." I live in the San Joaquin Valley where a lot of people have allergy problems, so it kind of made sense to me, but not a whole lot. I began to think that there was something really wrong with me that nobody could figure out.

I was depressed, and I knew that I needed to find some answers. All I knew was that I didn't feel right for somebody my age. I was feeling horrible all the time, so I went to see another doctor who did blood tests on me that showed a positive ANA [a screening test for lupus], and he had me do further testing for lupus. The additional tests were all negative, but I was still having a lot of lupuslike symptoms such as fatigue, hair loss, muscle weakness and skin rashes. The doctor told me that I might have lupus and that it could show up at any time [subclinical lupus].

Dr. Schwarzbein: After Kelley's blood tests came back showing that there was nothing seriously wrong with her, she became more distraught and confused. She was told, "It's stress; it's allergies; it's just that you are getting older." No wonder she did not know what to do to make herself better.

Just like Kelley, many women are being misdiagnosed with lupus or subclinical lupus because one of the tests that frequently comes up positive is the ANA test—*if* they have a lifestyle-based endocrine disorder from using birth control pills (BCPs) and are starving themselves to stay thin. Here's an important point, though—a positive ANA screening test is *not* the definitive test for lupus. There are many criteria that have to be met in order to diagnose someone with lupus. Even though women like Kelley who have lifestyle-based endocrine disorders do not meet the strict criteria for a lupus diagnosis, a lot of them are still being diagnosed as having subclinical lupus. They are told that they will probably meet all the criteria for lupus someday. What someone should be telling all these women is that the same symptoms that are associated with lupus can be caused by poor eating and lifestyle habits. They should be told to stop taking BCPs and start eating healthy balanced meals—then these symptoms will all go away.

Throughout her life, Kelley was diagnosed with chronic fatigue syndrome; screened for hypoglycemia, thyroid problems and lupus; told she had male pattern baldness; suffered from painful periods, allergies, hair loss and insomnia; and suffered a severe back injury. What she really had was a lifestyle-based endocrine disorder because she was on BCPs and had starved herself trying to stay thin.

Her symptoms were all due to fluctuating hormone levels that resulted from her body trying to keep her alive from starvation and chemical stresses.

Your body's job is to keep you alive despite your poor habits. It will do this at the expense of your well-being by slowing or shutting down nonvital systems such as good mood and good energy. Being alive has nothing to do with feeling good and being healthy. It is *your* job to keep yourself feeling good while you are alive. So, if you want to stay alive, remain healthy *and* feel good, you need to take better care of yourself by improving your nutrition and lifestyle habits in order to balance your hormones.

Your Thyroid: It Is *Not* Always the Problem

Even more common than misdiagnoses of lupus or subclinical lupus are misdiagnoses of thyroid disease or subclinical thyroid disease. In fact, the thyroid system is usually the most common hormone system to be tested when someone is overweight, cold, tired, achy, constipated, experiencing hair loss and/or feels depressed. Most of the time these symptoms are not caused by a thyroid glandular-based disease but to an acquired, reversible, lifestyle-based metabolic disorder.

Once a glandular-based thyroid gland disease is excluded through normal blood tests, the most common diagnoses are subclinical thyroid disease, depression or old age. People are told something like, "You have a borderline thyroid condition that the lab tests cannot detect. Here is a prescription for thyroid medicine," or, "Maybe you should see a counselor or psychiatrist to determine if you are depressed," or, "You are just getting older; learn to accept how poorly you feel."

Chances are, however, that you are not suffering from a borderline thyroid condition, depression or genetic aging, but that you have poor nutrition and lifestyle habits. Therefore, you do not have to learn to adjust to low energy levels, body aches and pains, and changes in mood. Nor should you take thyroid hormone replacement* or any other medication. These are just Band-Aids to cover up symptoms. They do nothing to restore balance to your body.

Thyroid hormone replacement therapy should be used by those with real thyroid hormone disease. Do not stop taking your thyroid medication because you are reading this book. You may actually have a real thyroid condition that requires therapy.

Metabolic Hypothyroidism:
A Lifestyle-Based Thyroid Disease

The pituitary gland secretes a hormone known as thyroid stimulating hormone or TSH, which travels through the bloodstream to the thyroid gland and stimulates the thyroid gland to produce and secrete mainly T4, one of the thyroid hormones. The T4 that is secreted into the bloodstream travels back up to the brain and signals the pituitary to stop making and secreting as much TSH. If your thyroid gland cannot make enough T4, you have primary hypothyroidism. This is a glandular-based endocrine disorder.

There is a lifestyle-based counterpart to thyroid disease. When T4 is secreted into the bloodstream, it also travels to specific cells of the body where T4 is chemically converted into T3, the more biologically active thyroid hormone. It is T3 that conveys to the cells what to do. Some of the functions of T3 are to tell your cells to increase their adrenaline receptors and to burn energy for warmth. However, instead of converting to T3, T4 can also convert to a biologically inactive form of the hormone called reverse T3 (rT3).

If T4 is efficiently converted to T3, you burn off more sugar and fat as energy; if most of the T4 is converted into the inactive rT3, you may experience all of the signs and symptoms of glandular-based hypothyroidism. However, you do not have a glandular disease but a metabolic or lifestyle-based one.

T4 is converted mainly to rT3 when the body perceives that it is under stress and responds as if it were in the middle of a famine to conserve energy. Poor nutrition and lifestyle habits are the most common reasons that T4 is converted to rT3.

(continued)

The appropriate treatment of glandular-based hypothy-roidism is thyroid hormone replacement. If you need to take a hormone because your body can no longer make it, it is important to take it to balance your hormone systems.

The correct treatment of the inability to convert T4 effi-ciently into T3 is to change your nutrition and lifestyle habits. Lifestyle-based hypothyroidism should not be treated with thy-roid hormone therapy because there is no thyroid hormone deficiency. If you take thyroid hormone replacement therapy for a lifestyle-based endocrine disorder instead of improving your nutrition and lifestyle habits, you will actually create more hormonal imbalances and further destroy your metabo-lism. You will be pushing your body to burn off more energy when it should be conserving energy because of your poor habits.

Educate yourself about the differences between glandular- and lifestyle-based hypothyroidism. Take thyroid hormone replacement if you need to, but do not take thyroid hormone replacement therapy if what you really need to do is change your poor nutrition and lifestyle habits.

Your Wake-Up Call

It is time for you to take a different approach to your health and consider all the various hormone systems of the body and what you can do to restore their balance. You need to realize that years of poor eating and lifestyle habits have caught up with you—this is your wake-up call. Like Kelley, you can change your nutrition and lifestyle habits and still heal. And now is the time to begin.

If you have any of the following symptoms and your lab tests are normal, and/or if you have been tested for organ failure and cancer and found to be "healthy," and/or if you have been diagnosed with a borderline thyroid condition or told to seek psychiatric help when you know you were not emotionally depressed, then you, like Kelley, probably have an early lifestyle-based endocrine disorder.

Achy and swollen joints

Body aches and pains

Bowel troubles

Decreased strength and energy

Fatigue (both physical and emotional)

Hair loss and/or changes in your skin and/or nails

Headaches

Inability to sleep well

Loss of lean body mass

Menstrual abnormalities, including irregular periods and PMS

Mood changes

Poor memory and concentration

Your daily "bad" habits are causing some hormones to be oversecreted and others to be undersecreted. *Your daily hormonal imbalances are causing all your symptoms.* However, because you do not have a tumor that is overproducing a hormone, nor do you have failure of a gland causing an underproduction of a hormone, your hormone levels will never get dramatically too high or too low at any given moment.

Although you feel lousy, your lab tests will show that your blood and urine chemistry is normal. (Remember, it is hard to diagnose these types of fluctuations with blood or urine tests.) You will either be escorted to the nearest psychiatrist, or worse yet, you will be diagnosed with a syndrome that is a collection of symptoms, such as chronic fatigue syndrome, for which there is no "cure." You will be told that you will have to adjust your lifestyle in order to live with your condition, instead of being taught how to improve your lifestyle habits to cure your condition.

Kelley: I was thirty-eight years old when I connected with a personal trainer and started working with her to try to strengthen my back. I was in pain almost constantly and losing all my muscle tone. My back pain was keeping me awake at night.

I tried doing resistance exercises, and they helped. I became stronger and my back wasn't bothering me so much. However, I felt that for all the exercise I was doing that I should be toning up better and quicker. I could see some improvement, but for the amount of working out I was doing, my body did not seem to be responding as well as it should have been. My overall health did not improve, either.

When I was about forty years old, I went off my birth control pills (BCPs) because I wanted to get pregnant. Since I did not marry until I was thirty-six, and I wanted to have a child, I was absolutely hysterical when my periods did not resume after I stopped the pill. I went to an internist in Santa Barbara to see if he could help me get my periods started again; I figured at this point that my problems probably had something to do with hormones. He checked my pituitary gland, and that was okay. He thought I might have lupus. I already knew that wasn't the problem, but I let him do another test anyway—it was negative. He sent me away telling me I was in perimenopause.

I became desperate and had my primary physician check my hormones. He put me back on BCPs to try to get all of my hormone levels up so that I could get pregnant, but that did not work.

Then my father was in a bad accident; he sustained a head injury. Getting pregnant was no longer my main concern. My mother and I slept in the hospital for the first three months that my father was there. I was even more sleep-deprived then, so to keep going all day I drank lattes and tried to calm down at night with wine. I was in shock and extremely stressed. I gained around twenty pounds and felt like I was going to have a nervous breakdown. I was feeling hopeless, and I ended up on three different antidepressants.

I got off two of my three antidepressants when I went to a two-week health institute that a friend recommended. It focused on the connection between the body, mind and soul, and only vegetarian meals were served. I stopped drinking coffee and alcohol, and I came back from there feeling so good that I thought I had cured my health problems. When I got home I ate mostly vegetarian meals, but I did resume drinking wine in moderation. However, after a few months of eating this way, I began to feel worse again. I had to quit working because I felt so sick and I was not sleeping well. At this point I really could not figure out what was wrong because I thought I was being so healthy. I thought I must be going crazy.

Dr. Schwarzbein: Poor nutrition, overexercising, BCP use and personal trauma all caught up with Kelley. Her major hormones were fluctuating wildly, causing her to have a myriad of symptoms. When she took a two-week break from her life at the health institute, she was able to stop the toxic chemicals that she had been using to make herself feel better. But, when she went back to reality all the stresses were still there, and all her symptoms resumed once more.

You Are Not Going Crazy

While it is true that these lifestyle-based endocrine disorders are not full-blown glandular diseases, what you are experiencing is very real and leads to multiple symptoms that make it impossible for you to live a healthy, happy life. To make matters worse, an inaccurate diagnosis will probably mean you are prescribed medication that may make you feel better for the moment, such as an antidepressant, but the medication will not cure you—it only masks your symptoms. (It is appropriate to take an antidepressant if you need one as long as you also work on your poor nutrition and lifestyle habits.)

If no one recognizes that poor nutrition and lifestyle habits have led to your hormonal imbalances and symptoms, and you keep up the same "bad" habits, your symptoms will only get worse over time. You will end up with an inefficient metabolism and an increased risk of the degenerative diseases of aging.

Worse yet, you could have prevented all of this from the onset with a few changes in your nutrition and lifestyle habits.

Kelley: I finally went to see Dr. Schwarzbein because I felt I was too young to be in perimenopause. I had read her first book, and I thought that my problems were hormonal.

When I was there for the exam, my heart was pounding out of my body, and it was not from fear but from my problem. I was so weak that I almost fainted in her office. She talked with me about what she thought was wrong with me, and I was surprised that my hormones were being affected by my lifestyle. She sent me home with a list of supplements to take and a nutrition plan to follow. She told me to eat butter, olive oil, meat and fish. She taught me about the omega-3 and omega-6 oils that are in fish and vegetables and told me to take flaxseed oil. I followed her advice.

She mentioned that I might gain weight initially, but at this point I didn't care, even though staying thin had been my focus my whole life. I mean, even my infertility was not a concern at this point. I knew I was sick, very sick. I felt so bad that all I wanted to do was feel good again.

I decided I was going to focus on the sleeping and nutrition parts of the program first. So I came home and I started the supplements, and I took her advice to rest. I slept a lot. I had been taking lorazepam [an antianxiety drug] before I saw Dr. Schwarzbein, and she changed that and put me on desyrel [a nonaddicting drug used to reset the sleep cycle] to help me sleep. I was actually sleeping all night for the first time in years. I took my supplements and my B vitamins every day and within a week I could feel a difference.

Dr. Schwarzbein: All of Kelley's problems were caused by years of her poor nutrition and lifestyle habits. I told her to concentrate on improving her eating habits, getting enough sleep, stopping her BCPs and taking a few supplements. Because she had not damaged her metabolism, she experienced immediate results.

Determining Your Treatment Plan

If, like Kelley, you are feeling lousy all the time, you first have to identify whether you have a glandular-based endocrine disorder or a lifestyle-based one. This determines your treatment plan.

If you have a glandular-based endocrine disorder in which there is an *overproduction* of a hormone caused by a diseased gland, you should be treated with medicine or surgery and improve your nutrition and lifestyle habits. For glandular-based hormone problems where a hormone is *low* or *missing* because of a diseased gland, you will need hormone replacement therapy—as well as changes in your nutrition and lifestyle habits that will keep the replaced hormone in balance.

How do you fix or balance hormone problems in lifestyle-based endocrine disorders? The description of the solution itself is very simple. If a hormone is being oversecreted, it needs to be brought down into balance; if a hormone is being undersecreted, it needs to be brought up into balance. These changes will allow your body to reestablish efficient regeneration and therefore you will be able to heal.

Implementing the solution is more involved as it necessitates making the necessary changes in your nutrition and lifestyle habits to reregulate your hormones. It takes longer to bring a hormone back up into balance than down into balance because you have to reestablish hormone production for the former to occur. The SPII program is specifically designed to help simplify the process. Healthy nutrition, including supplementation with vitamins, antioxidants, minerals, and amino or fatty acids; stress management, including getting enough sleep; tapering of toxic chemicals or avoiding them completely; and cross-training exercises balance out the hormones your body can still make.

Kelley: Within two months of seeing Dr. Schwarzbein, I felt so much better! I started sleeping through the night, and now I wake up full of energy. My depression is a lot better. I haven't started my period yet again, but I can see such a difference in how I feel. I'm so much more level-headed and I can handle stress so much better. The difference is like night and day.

I am eating three balanced meals and one to two snacks a day, but I am not gaining weight. I'm feeling stronger, and I've started working out again. I noticed a big difference in my muscle tone right away.

I can't even begin to explain how much better I feel. I was so down before. I was depressed, I was moody—I was so many ugly things. I didn't like myself very much, but now that I feel good again, I do. This program saved my life, and I would recommend it to anyone.

I feel that I've finally gotten to the root of all the symptoms that no one could diagnose, and it was so simple. I just needed to eat right and stop taking BCPs. It's so hard to believe, but it really was that simple. And the sad thing is that all those years I thought I was eating well and taking care of myself.

Dr. Schwarzbein thinks that within a year I'll be well, and I'll probably be able to conceive if I so desire, though there is no guarantee of that because of my years of using BCPs. Having a baby would be wonderful, but right now I'm just so happy to feel better.

Dr. Schwarzbein: Birth control pills (BCPs) are not hormones; they are drugs that disrupt a woman's sex hormone balance. Since all of the hormones of the body are connected, BCPs affect all your hormone systems. The longer you take BCPs, the greater your hormonal imbalances.

Most women do not recognize their problems as being related to the use of BCPs because BCPs cause hormone imbalances that are insidious. It is not until several years after they begin taking the pill that their symptoms become more pronounced. I have treated many women in my clinical practice who, just like Kelley, have multiple system complaints related to their BCP use. [See Common Risks of Birth Control Pill (BCP) Use, page 53.] One of the easiest "cures" is having them stop the pill. Read the package insert of the BCP that you are currently taking or are thinking of taking for a complete list of associated risks.

Common Risks of Birth Control Pill (BCP) Use

Acne

Ankle swelling

Deep vein blood clots

Depression

Dry skin

Emotional lability (severe
  mood swings)

Facial and abnormal body
  hair growth

Fatigue

Gallbladder disease

Hair loss

Headaches

Heart attacks

High blood pressure

High blood sugars

High triglycerides, low high-
  density lipoprotein (HDL)
  levels

Infertility

Irritable bowel syndrome

Loss of sex drive

Lupuslike symptoms

Pulmonary embolism (blood clot
  to the lungs)

Rosacea

Stroke

Vaginal yeast infections

Weight gain

Do Not Wait to Change Your Habits!

You can have the beginning of a lifestyle-based endocrine disorder and never feel as bad as Kelley did. Her story illustrates a worst-case scenario. Kelley's wildly fluctuating hormone levels—which resulted from her poor eating habits and use of BCPs—caused her to have many dramatic symptoms. Now is the time to improve your nutrition and lifestyle habits so that you never experience severe symptoms like Kelley's.

Balancing Your Hormones

It is beyond the scope of this book to discuss all of your body's hormones since there are so many of them. However, because the hormones of the body are interconnected, you can balance all your hormones by concentrating on the nutrition and lifestyle changes that will keep adrenaline, insulin, cortisol, HGH, DHEA and the thyroid hormones balanced. By focusing on balancing these few essential hormones, you will balance all your hormones.

Patterns of Hormonal Imbalance

In general, the major hormones—adrenaline, insulin and cortisol—are oversecreted because they are the first hormones that are secreted in response to your nutrition and lifestyle habits. Therefore, the changes you make in your habits will bring the major hormones back *down* into balance.

The minor hormones—HGH, DHEA and the thyroid hormones—tend to be undersecreted because of your normal aging process and the disruption of their production caused by the oversecretion of the major hormones. The changes you make in your nutrition and lifestyle habits will cause the minor hormones to be produced more efficiently, and this will bring the secretion of these hormones back *up* into balance.

Healing a Damaged Metabolism: It Takes Time

It is easier to balance your hormones through nutrition and lifestyle changes when you have not badly damaged your metabolism yet.

Unfortunately, this is not the case for many people. Long-term bad habits that lead to the oversecretion of major hormones can eventually lead to a *decrease* in the production of both major and minor hormones. When this occurs, you have badly damaged your metabolism, and you have to work on habits that increase the production of *all* the lowered hormones, as well as correct the habits that caused the oversecretion of the major hormone to begin with. This is where time comes in.

With a badly damaged metabolism, reestablishing normal hormone production becomes the step that determines the rate of your healing process. It does not happen overnight, and this is where many people fail to heal. No one wants the healing process to take time. Everybody is looking for a quick fix. But believe me—that quick fix does not exist. And the longer you put off healing your metabolism, the worse things will get.

This is exactly what happened to Mary in chapter 4. By the time she first saw me, she was no longer able to avoid coming to terms with her lifestyle-based endocrine disorder that caused severe imbalances of adrenaline.

Summary

- Endocrinology is the study of the hormone systems and their role in the functions and vital processes of the body.
- For purposes of this book, the diagnosis and treatment of glandular diseases is called glandular-based endocrinology.
- For purposes of this book, lifestyle-based endocrinology is defined as the study and treatment of the cumulative hormone changes related to chronic over- or underproduction and/or secretion of hormones in response to poor nutrition, stress, exposure to toxic chemicals, excessive or insufficient exercise, aging and genetics.
- The similarities between glandular- and lifestyle-based disorders are that an over- or underproduction and/or secretion of hormones exists in both cases. The difference is that glandular-based endocrine disorders are caused by diseased or damaged glands, and lifestyle-based endocrine disorders are normal responses that arise from healthy glands.
- Both glandular- and lifestyle-based endocrine disorders cause serious problems, but the timing and severity of the initial symptoms are very different.
- If you experience unexplained symptoms, have been tested for organ failure and cancer and are found to be "healthy," you may have a lifestyle-based endocrine disorder.

- To balance hormone problems in lifestyle-based endocrine disorders, if a hormone is being oversecreted, it needs to be brought down into balance; if a hormone is being undersecreted, it needs to be brought up into balance.
- Metabolic thyroid disease is a lifestyle-based endocrine disorder that should not be treated with thyroid hormone replacement therapy.
- Birth control pills (BCPs) are not hormones; they are drugs that disrupt a woman's sex hormone balance and cause a lifestyle-based endocrine disorder.
- An unrecognized and untreated lifestyle-based endocrine disorder leads to an inefficient metabolism and increased risk for the degenerative diseases of aging.

* * *

In the next three chapters, we will take a look at each of the major hormones (adrenaline, insulin and cortisol) individually, beginning with adrenaline in chapter 4. You will learn what adrenaline is, how your nutrition and lifestyle habits affect its secretion, and the problems you can develop if your adrenaline levels remain too high for many years.

Four

Adrenaline and Adrenaline Addiction

Adrenaline: Not Just a Stress Hormone

You may know adrenaline as the "fight/flight" hormone and think that it is only secreted when you are under stress. So you might be surprised to learn that adrenaline is being secreted constantly to help your body perform various functions. For instance, it sustains life by keeping your heart beating.

Additionally, adrenaline helps your body access its biochemicals so that you can use them to think, move and do all of the activities of daily living such as breathing, eating and having bowel movements. It also allows you to break down and use your food for energy so that your body can perform all these functions.

Furthermore, adrenaline signals the breakdown of old cells to make room for new ones, and this turnover process keeps your cells younger and functioning better.

While adrenaline is important to help your body access and use up your functional, structural and energy biochemicals, you do not want too *much* adrenaline in your body over a long period of time because your body will use itself up faster than it can rebuild. This causes accelerated metabolic aging.

On the other hand, you do not want too *little* adrenaline, either. Adrenaline is such an important hormone that you cannot survive for very long if your adrenaline levels drop to zero. Fortunately, this is not going to happen. Although your adrenaline levels can become low because of poor nutrition and lifestyle habits, your body is not going to stop making adrenaline altogether. This is a good thing because adrenaline cannot be replaced if you stop making it.

If your adrenaline levels are too low, your body will not be able to access your biochemicals, which leads to an inefficient metabolism and accelerated metabolic aging.

Balancing your hormones, including adrenaline, is essential for good health. Too much or too little of any hormone can lead to accelerated metabolic aging.

Glandular-Based Adrenaline Disorders

The glandular-based endocrine disorder that causes your adrenal glands to produce too much adrenaline is a *rare* disease called pheochromocytoma. There is no glandular-based endocrine disorder that causes you to secrete too little adrenaline. (You would die without enough adrenaline.)

The Effects of High Adrenaline Levels

For the purpose of simplicity, we are going to consider the actions of adrenaline as though it were the only hormone in your body telling your cells what to do. But remember—adrenaline like all hormones does not act alone; all the hormones of the body are connected, and they are helping each other regulate all the same biochemical reactions simultaneously.

Early on, if your adrenaline levels are higher than they should be all day because of poor nutrition and lifestyle habits, you will continuously secrete and use up your functional and energy biochemicals—which gives you a sense of well-being. This feeling can be as addicting as any drug. You will also increase the turnover of your structural biochemicals, and this will keep you looking younger in the short-term. For example, you will have shinier hair, softer skin and stronger nails. Because you look and feel good, you will think that your poor habits are working for you. But do not be fooled—they are not. You can be destroying your health while you feel good. The following explains why.

If you were to continue secreting, using up and turning over your biochemicals because of the actions of adrenaline, you would completely deplete your body of biochemicals, break down your structure and die. Luckily, your body has built-in stopgaps. There are many hormones and other cell changes that counteract adrenaline, and these protective mechanisms *slow down* the utilization of energy and functional biochemicals and the destruction of structural biochemicals.

Unfortunately, these protective mechanisms cannot completely counter the damage done by *chronic* high adrenaline levels. By continuously secreting, using up and breaking down your biochemicals through the action of *chronic* high adrenaline levels, you will end up "broken." This means you will look older and develop health problems, including the degenerative diseases of aging that will compromise the quality and decrease the quantity of your life. It is only a matter of time before your habits catch up to you.

Warning Signs

There are no early warning signs of high adrenaline levels. In fact, the opposite occurs. Because it feels good to use up your biochemicals, this feeling of well-being is what you strive for on a daily basis. You end up addicted to using yourself up before you start to experience some of the ill symptoms of intermittent high adrenaline levels (see list below).

The same holds true for recognizing the short-term low adrenaline levels that can occur at any given moment from increased demand. You may not recognize the symptoms as intermittent low adrenaline secretion because they are not occurring with any frequency, and you can come up with many reasons that you may have an ache here, a pain there or a headache (see list, next page).

Also, when you feel poorly from low adrenaline levels, you usually self-medicate with caffeine (aspirin or coffee or soda), which is one of the chemicals that helps whatever adrenaline you have at the moment become more potent; or you may use sugar to get your adrenal glands to put out more adrenaline. Again, you are seeking that feeling of well-being. It feels good to use up your biochemicals. The problem is that these daily, short-term bursts of higher adrenaline levels can become long-term spikes of higher adrenaline levels.

Symptoms of Intermittent High Adrenaline Levels

All these symptoms occur for short periods of time.

Agitation	Interrupted sleep (the inability
Anxiety	to fall asleep or stay asleep)
Bladder urgency	Light-headedness/dizziness
Blurry vision	Loose bowel movements
Burning feet	Nausea
Emotional intensity	Nervousness
Excessive sweating	Short emotional fuse/
Heartburn	uncontrollable anger
Heart palpitations	

Symptoms of Intermittent Low Adrenaline Levels

All these symptoms occur for short periods of time.

Allergies	Insomnia
Asthma attack	Mental exhaustion
Flulike symptoms	Shingles attack
General aches and pains	Short emotional fuse/
Headaches	uncontrollable anger
Increased susceptibility to	Short-term fatigue
infections	Weepiness

The signs and symptoms of intermittent high or low adrenaline levels are not mutually exclusive. You can have any combination of the symptoms listed above because your adrenaline levels can fluctuate widely from high to low throughout the day. Sometimes, both high and low adrenaline levels cause the same symptoms, such as a short emotional fuse.

Chronic High or Low Adrenaline Levels Cause Lifestyle-Based Endocrine Disorders

If high adrenaline levels continue unchecked, these temporary symptoms can become constant. Your occasional heartburn symptoms begin to occur daily, and you develop acid reflux disease or ulcers. The occasional nights of interrupted sleep become constant and you end up with insomnia. Intermittent heart palpitations become heart arrhythmias, and feelings of agitation and anxiety become panic attacks leading to panic disorder. If your high adrenaline levels continue to occur over many years, you will end up with the degenerative diseases of aging. These are all lifestyle-based endocrine disorders of too much adrenaline resulting from years of high adrenaline levels.

Adrenaline Burnout

Or you may end up with burned-out adrenal glands. This means that your adrenal glands can no longer produce enough adrenaline on a daily basis to keep up with your body's demands for the hormone. This is a lifestyle-based endocrine disorder of too little adrenaline resulting from years of excessive demand for adrenaline. It is manifested by one or a combination of the following chronic symptoms:

Allergies, including skin allergies	Depression
Arthritis	Fibromyalgia
Asthma	Headaches
Candida infections	Insomnia
Chronic fatigue syndrome	Interstitial cystitis
Degenerative diseases of aging	Irritable bowel syndrome
	Suppressed immune system

The disorders of chronically high or low adrenaline levels are not mutually exclusive. Both adrenaline states lead to an increased risk for insomnia and the degenerative diseases of aging.

Chronic High Versus Chronic Low Adrenaline Levels

Your ability to rebuild adrenaline from food is one of the factors that determines whether you will eventually end up with high or low adrenaline levels.

If you are intermittently stressed, using stimulants and eating well, you are more likely to end up with high adrenaline levels over time and to develop high blood pressure, strokes and heart attacks.

If you are constantly stressed, using stimulants and not eating well, you are more likely to end up with burned-out adrenal glands and/or osteopenia/osteoporosis (bone loss).

Mary, a Story of Adrenaline Addiction

By the time Mary came to see me, she was suffering from the effects of years of living a high adrenaline lifestyle. Her story is a perfect example of someone whose adrenaline addiction caused a lifestyle-based adrenaline disorder of burnout and bone loss.

Mary: I was a vegetarian on a high-carbohydrate/low-fat diet on and off for twenty-four years because I initially felt good when I ate that way and believed that it was good for me. I also thought that the amount of exercise I was doing was healthy for me.

I used to get up every single weekday morning at about 4:30 to exercise. I would swim five times a week, work out at the gym three times a week, do the cycling class at the gym once a week and run at other times. I thought I was doing quite well because I could keep up my exercise program.

I first heard about Dr. Schwarzbein when I began working out with Liz, a trainer at my local gym. I'm sure Liz saw a frazzled, worn-out me, but I thought I was doing very well. I was very thin, and I think Liz was concerned about me. She kept encouraging me to go see Dr. Schwarzbein because she felt I did not eat well and that I exercised too much.

Dr. Schwarzbein was the one who told me that I suffer from this adrenaline addiction thing. I'd see other people who were workout-aholics, and I'd think, *Oh, those poor people.* I had never put myself in the same category as them.

Dr. Schwarzbein: When you are an adrenaline junkie like Mary was, you do not realize what you are doing to yourself. Years of a high adrenaline lifestyle can lead to biochemical changes in your personality. Being intense and extreme are both manifestations and causes of high adrenaline levels, and it becomes a vicious cycle.

In Mary's case, her high-adrenaline levels from undereating and overexercising caused her body to "eat" itself for energy, resulting in, among other problems, her depression.

Mary: I suffer from intermittent depression, and I take antidepressants for it. Until I started talking to Liz, I didn't know my habits might be making my depression worse. Intuitively I knew that something needed to change, and I was willing to try. This is one of the main reasons I finally listened to Liz and went to see Dr. Schwarzbein. Dr. Schwarzbein told me that I might be able to stop the antidepressant medication in the future if I could get my hormones balanced by eating more protein and healthy fats, *decreasing* my exercise and taking hormone replacement therapy for menopause.

Dr. Schwarzbein: The most likely cause of Mary's depression is malnutrition. Because Mary did not eat enough protein and calories for the amount of exercise she was doing, she was unable to rebuild enough functional biochemicals. Instead of being used for rebuilding neurotransmitters, the small amount of protein she did eat was diverted into energy for exercise. The good news is that this type of depression is 100 percent curable if she continues to follow her improved nutrition and lifestyle habits—but it will take time.

When Mary's metabolism is healed, she will be able to quit taking her antidepressants. Unfortunately, until that time, she cannot stop her medication because she would unmask her underlying damaged metabolism and feel depressed. There is no need for her to feel poorly as she goes through her healing process, and as long as she is working on improving her nutrition and lifestyle habits, being on an antidepressant will not harm her. It is when people take antidepressants to feel better, but do not change their habits to heal themselves, that these drugs are harmful.

Malnutrition and Depression

There are many causes for depression, but what I have been seeing clinically since 1993 is a dramatic rise in the amount of depression caused by malnutrition, especially in women. This is in part caused by the low-fat movement and also by women trying to stay thin by counting calories. I know that these women are not intentionally trying to harm themselves; they just do not understand the connection between low-calorie and/or low-fat dieting and mood disorders. Since the brain is mostly made from structural fats, and you need functional fats to help your brain produce neurotransmitters, eating healthy fats is essential for a healthy brain.

Mary: Some years ago I was having back trouble and went to see an orthopedic surgeon who took X rays and said, "Oh, hmm. It could be osteoporosis." It went in one ear and out the other for me. I believed that I was such a healthy and athletic person that I thought he had to be kidding. He said, "Well, it could just be the way you were born, too." He didn't make a big deal about it or say I should have it checked out further, so I didn't take him seriously.

Many years later, I was diagnosed with severe osteopenia [bone loss]. My bone scan came back with 35 percent bone loss in my hips, and it just about blew me away. I researched about bone loss and did everything I learned to try and improve my bones. I increased my exercise, ate a vegetarian diet and made sure I was getting enough calcium. When I had another scan a year later, it was 7 percent worse!

Dr. Schwarzbein also wanted me to go on hormone replacement therapy [HRT] for menopause because of my continuing bone loss. I was upset because I thought I had been doing all the right things for my bones and that I could avoid HRT in menopause. Dr. Schwarzbein said that HRT could prevent further bone loss and would help balance my other hormones. I finally decided to give it a try because she said it might help my bones and my depression.

Dr. Schwarzbein: Mary, like many people, believed that bones are made from calcium and if you take or eat enough calcium and also exercise you will build bones. She also had read that too much protein causes bone loss and that is why she became a vegetarian. So she was very surprised to find out that her bone loss was caused in part by not eating *enough* protein and by overexercising.

Adrenaline and Strong Bones

Bones are made mainly from proteins. All structural proteins need to turn over—that is, they need to be broken down and then rebuilt to maintain their structural integrity. The faster the bone turnover rate, the more likely you are to develop some bone loss because your body will not have enough time to rebuild completely before you start breaking down again. One of the most often ignored causes of faster bone turnover is high adrenaline levels over many years.

Anything you do to chronically increase adrenaline levels will decrease your bone mass since adrenaline causes structural proteins to break down. And *if you do not eat enough protein*, you will not have enough material to rebuild your bones.

However, *if you eat too much protein*, you can also end up with bone loss because one of the triggers of adrenaline secretion is high protein intake. That is why one of the things that you can do to keep your bones healthy and strong is to eat balanced meals that include enough protein and carbohydrates to keep your adrenaline levels balanced.

Overexercising is another cause of higher adrenaline levels, and women marathon runners are noted for having a high incidence of bone loss.

To be healthy and have strong bones, you need to keep your adrenaline levels balanced. To do this, you need to know the nutrition and lifestyle habits that cause adrenaline to be oversecreted.

Causes of High Adrenaline Levels

In general, almost anything and everything raises adrenaline levels in your body because adrenaline is one of the hormones that is needed to access your biochemicals for use in the activities of daily living. If you do not eat well, do not get enough sleep, do not manage stress well, overexercise, ingest too many stimulants and/or have other hormone imbalances, you still need to function. So your adrenaline levels go higher as your body secretes, uses and breaks down its biochemicals to keep you functioning as best as it can, given the stressful circumstances.

The secretion and effects of adrenaline throughout a person's life are caused by any or all of the following:

Anemia

Being awake

Fight/flight syndrome

Genetics

High DHEA levels

High progestogen levels

High protein intake

High testosterone levels

High thyroid-hormone levels
(High T4 or high T3 levels for any reason, including taking Armour thyroid)

Hypoglycemia (low blood-sugar levels)

Infections

Learned responses to stress

Low caloric intake (dieting)

Low carbohydrate intake

Low estrogen levels

Low-estrogen or high-progestogen birth control pills

Overexercising

Pain

Skipping meals

Stimulants, such as caffeine, nicotine, ginseng, ma huang or ephedra, Dexedrine, cocaine, ephedrine and pure white sugar

Stress (both good and bad)

Let me explain how each of these factors affects your adrenaline production, secretion and/or action.

Anemia

When the amount of red blood cells in your bloodstream is low, you are anemic. This means you carry less oxygen to your cells because your red blood cells are oxygen carriers. It also means that your heart rate has to increase so that your cells receive enough oxygen—and your body must release adrenaline to increase your heart rate. If you are anemic, discuss the type you have with your medical provider because there are different causes of anemia that I will not discuss here. Whatever type you have, it is important to get it treated. Otherwise you will have chronic high levels of adrenaline from your anemia, and this causes you to age faster.

Being Awake

Your body secretes more adrenaline when you are awake because you are more active and using up more biochemicals than when you are asleep. Since your adrenaline needs are higher when you are awake, it is important to get enough hours of sleep every night or you will age faster. You can read more about sleep in chapter 12.

Fight/Flight Syndrome

During times of extreme stress—that is, during the fight/flight syndrome when your body senses that you are being "threatened"—your body is geared to run faster to get away from your threat, to clot your blood faster in case you sustain an injury, and to concentrate and think more clearly to tackle the life-threatening situation. All of this requires that your heart beat faster and that you are able to access and use your biochemicals. Your adrenal glands pour out more adrenaline to help you accomplish all of these functions.

In the short-term, if the stress is life-threatening, the adrenal gland response is crucial for your survival. If the stress is chronic and not life-threatening, the adrenal gland response becomes detrimental. Stress management is important for your health in these chronic non-life-threatening types of stressful situations.

Genetics

We all share the ability to make the same types of biochemicals, but we differ genetically in how much of a particular biochemical we can make. For example, the amount of adrenaline you are able to produce and secrete in given situations is under genetic control. Some people put out more adrenaline than others in the same situations because they are more genetically adrenaline-sensitive. If you are adrenaline-sensitive, you will need to incorporate stress management techniques into your daily lifestyle habits. Overresponding with increased levels of adrenaline leads to accelerated metabolic aging.

High DHEA Levels

DHEA is a rebuilding hormone made from cholesterol. Recently it has been getting more popular press as an antiaging hormone, and people are taking it even if they do not need to. Ironically, too much DHEA can do just the opposite of helping you rebuild; it can cause you to use yourself up more because it increases adrenaline's effect.

If you think that you may be DHEA-deficient, have your DHEA sulfate (DHEA-S) levels measured to determine if you need to take it or not. If you have been on a low-cholesterol diet, correct your diet before you take DHEA replacement. If you still need DHEA therapy, take a pharmaceutical-grade DHEA, not an over-the-counter form. Then have your DHEA-S levels retested to be certain you are not taking too much. As explained more fully in chapter 15, taking too much of a hormone can be just as damaging as having too little of a hormone.

High Progestogen Levels

Progestogens are a class of hormones, and progesterone is the naturally occurring progestogen in the body. Medroxyprogesterone acetate (Provera) is the most common synthetic progestogen drug used for progesterone hormone replacement therapy. Both natural and synthetic progestogens increase the release of adrenaline by decreasing the action of both natural and synthetic estrogens. When estrogen action is low, adrenaline levels are higher.

Recently, lay books have stated that you can use all the natural progesterone that you want because it cannot harm you. *This is not true.* Too much progesterone over the long-term causes too much adrenaline over the long-term. If you take too much of any hormone, you will end up with a hormone imbalance. Too much progesterone is no exception and can lead to accelerated metabolic aging.

High Protein Intake

If you eat too much protein, your body will secrete higher amounts of adrenaline to convert proteins into sugar for brain fuel and also to detoxify the amino acids so that your blood does not get too acidic. Amino acids are the building blocks of proteins: Proteins are made up of different amino acids linked together chemically. When you eat proteins, you digest them into amino acids in your intestinal tract, and these amino acids are absorbed and travel to the liver where they are broken down and converted into sugar or into waste chemicals that are eliminated from your body in your urine. The last part of this process (converting to sugar or eliminating the waste) happens if you eat too many proteins so that your blood does not get too acidic. Your body does not function at its best when you are too acidic, and this results in an inefficient metabolism. Eat balanced meals to prevent your body from becoming too acidic.

High Testosterone Levels

Testosterone is a hormone found in much higher quantities in men than in women. Higher testosterone levels equate to higher overall adrenaline levels. Because men naturally have higher testosterone levels, they usually are able to burn off fat better than women, but they also have more heart attacks at a younger age because chronic high-adrenaline levels cause heart attacks. (Low levels of testosterone in men have also been associated with increased heart attacks.)

There are now both natural and synthetic preparations for testosterone hormone replacement. If you need to take testosterone, make sure you do not get too much of it, and make sure you use natural testosterone, not methyl-testosterone, a synthetic version. As stated throughout this book, balancing your hormones is essential for good health.

High Thyroid-Hormone Levels (high T4 or high T3 levels for any reason including taking Armour thyroid)

Thyroid hormones regulate the action of adrenaline by changing the number of adrenaline receptors on cells. Higher levels of thyroid hormone increase the number of adrenaline receptors, making the same amount of adrenaline more active. It is the binding of hormones to their specific receptors that determines the activity of that hormone.

The more binding, the more activity. Too much thyroid hormone, in any form, is bad for you because it causes you to use up your biochemicals faster than you usually can rebuild them. This mismatch in regeneration leads to accelerated metabolic aging.

Hypoglycemia (low blood-sugar levels)

The brain uses sugar for energy. If the brain cells are deprived of enough sugar fuel, they die off very easily. Because sustained low blood-sugars are not compatible with life, your body responds to low blood-sugar levels in multiple ways because this is an emergency. Hypoglycemia signals the release of adrenaline, which then signals the liver to break down glycogen (a storage form of sugar in the liver) into sugar to feed the brain. At the same time, adrenaline also signals the body to break down proteins into amino acids, which the liver then converts into sugar. Both of these immediate actions keep your blood sugar from getting too low when you do not eat enough or you skip meals, thereby preventing brain damage. If you are repeatedly hypoglycemic, you are using up your functional and/or structural proteins so they can be used as brain food. Over the long-term, this damages your metabolism.

Infections

Your immune system helps you fight off infections. When you have an infection, you release more adrenaline to signal the cells of your immune system to come and fight. Also, adrenaline increases body temperature, and when you develop a fever you have another way to kill off viruses and bacteria in your body. Multiple infections will age you faster. Therefore, it is important to rest and take antibiotics, if indicated, when you have a severe infection. The sooner your body gets rid of the infection, the sooner your adrenaline levels can return to normal.

Learned Responses to Stress

Your body can learn to put out more adrenaline for a given stress if you have responded poorly to that same situation in the past. For instance, if you have become angry or stressed by a particular person, your body may produce more adrenaline when you encounter that person again. You can learn to control your adrenaline response by practicing stress management techniques such as deep breathing, meditation or visualization. These techniques are discussed further in chapter 12. Constantly oversecreting adrenaline is harmful to your health.

Low Caloric Intake (Dieting)

If you do not get enough food into your body because you are restricting calories, your brain will run out of fuel. This causes your body to secrete adrenaline to "eat itself up" in order to keep your brain alive. This means that you are using up your functional and structural biochemicals and causing more damage to your metabolism. To keep this from happening, it is important that you never diet another day in your life.

Low Carbohydrate Intake

If you do not eat enough carbohydrates, you will secrete more adrenaline to convert the proteins you eat and your body's own proteins into sugar for brain fuel. This is why it is important to match the amount of carbohydrates you eat to your current metabolism and activity level. Eating too few carbohydrates is just as damaging as eating too many. Balance is essential to good health. Many people count nonstarchy vegetables as their carbohydrate selection. However, nonstarchy vegetables do not have enough carbohydrates to count as the carbohydrate in your meal. It is important to eat enough *real*, not refined or man-made, carbohydrates so that your adrenaline levels do not get too high. You can read about real carbohydrates in chapter 11.

Low Estrogen Levels

Estradiol is the human estrogen made by the ovaries. Estradiol levels are inversely proportional to adrenaline levels; when estradiol-levels are lower, adrenaline levels are higher; when estradiol levels are higher, adrenaline levels are lower.

Low estradiol levels are seen in females before puberty and during menopause. Before puberty, most girls are thinner because they have low estradiol levels and therefore naturally higher adrenaline levels.

When puberty begins, the body produces a lot more estradiol, which lowers adrenaline levels. If a girl does not start ovulating soon, she will not produce higher levels of progesterone.

Progesterone levels are proportional to adrenaline levels; the higher the progesterone levels, the higher the adrenaline levels. Therefore, if a girl is not ovulating she will have higher estradiol levels and lower progesterone and adrenaline levels. This imbalance promotes weight gain. When this happens, many girls start their first diet and dieting causes higher adrenaline levels. The higher adrenaline levels seem to "be working" since the girl loses weight, but all she is doing is setting herself up to destroy her metabolism. A girl who eats better before and throughout puberty will have a better chance to begin ovulating and, therefore, less chance of weight gain.

Low-Estrogen or High-Progestogen Birth Control Pills

Birth control pills (BCPs) contain chemical estrogens and progestogens. The BCPs that are low in estrogens and high in progestogens increase the secretion of adrenaline. Initially, using a BCP that raises adrenaline will not cause weight gain and in fact usually causes weight loss.

However, chronic high levels of adrenaline can cause weight gain because adrenaline results in the loss of functional and structural proteins and fats as well as storage fats—and destroys your metabolism over time. Unfortunately, by the time this weight gain occurs, a woman will have been on BCPs for years and will not recognize the connection. BCPs are harmful. Read more about why you should not take them in chapter 13.

Overexercising

You *can* overexercise. Overdoing exercise, especially cardiovascular activity, makes your body secrete too much adrenaline. A workout routine that maintains your heart rate at more than ninety beats per minute puts you in a higher adrenaline-secretion mode. While you are exercising you are using up your biochemicals and breaking them down. It usually feels good at the time, but all that excess adrenaline leads to the using up of your functional and structural biochemicals, which destroys your metabolism. To compound the problem, most people who overexercise have a difficult time eating enough food to match their activity level because adrenaline is a natural appetite suppressant. If they are already "eating themselves up," they will not be hungry for food later on. The combination of overexercising and undereating destroys their metabolism faster. Find out more about overexercising in chapter 14.

Pain

Pain triggers the release of adrenaline because pain is a stress to your body, and all stresses raise adrenaline levels. Adrenaline helps control the severity of the pain. For example, an athlete can continue to play with a broken bone during a high-intensity game because he is full of adrenaline. However, chronic pain will lead to adrenaline "burnout," and this can cause more pain. It is important and easier to treat pain before it becomes chronic. If you already have chronic pain, you should work with a pain management specialist. You will not be able to heal your metabolism if you have pain on a daily basis.

Skipping Meals

Skipping meals signals the release of adrenaline just as if you were becoming hypoglycemic or dieting. See Low Caloric Intake and Low Carbohydrate Intake on page 72.

Stimulants

Stimulants such as caffeine, nicotine, ginseng, ma huang or ephedra, ephedrine, Dexedrine, Ritalin, cocaine and refined sugars mimic adrenaline, raise adrenaline levels or make adrenaline more active. This causes your body to use up more biochemicals, which can destroy your metabolism.

Caffeine is a drug that keeps whatever amount of adrenaline you have in your bloodstream around longer. Remember that hormones act through binding with their own receptors. After adrenaline binds to its receptors it is usually broken down and disposed of by your body. However, caffeine blocks the breakdown of adrenaline, so adrenaline continues to bind, causing your body to respond to adrenaline. This makes adrenaline more potent.

Some of you may have to stay on stimulants until you have worked on other areas of your life such as eating better, stress management and HRT, if needed. Find out more about why you may need to continue stimulants in the How To section. Taper off stimulants if you are addicted to them, so that you can avoid feeling worse as you try to stop using them.

Stress (both good and bad)

Stress of any kind, good or bad, increases adrenaline in your body. The more intense the stress, the higher the secretion of adrenaline. Good stress still increases adrenaline levels, but levels will not be as high as during bad stress.

Being busy and multitasking in the course of a normal day are also stresses—but it is okay to use up your biochemicals from the normal stresses of living as long as you understand your need to eat well on a daily basis to rebuild your biochemicals.

Unfortunately, both good and bad chronic stresses lead to an increase in the amount of biochemicals you need on a daily basis, and as you age your body's ability to rebuild biochemicals efficiently declines. Therefore, you need to learn how to manage stress better as you age so that you do not use up your biochemicals faster than your body can rebuild them again. Refer to chapter 12 for stress management.

Mary: After I had been on the SPII program for a couple of weeks, I started to slow down. I was so tired that I could barely make it across the pool. I was out of breath and had absolutely no energy. I felt so lousy that

I became discouraged and told Liz that I was not sure why I was doing this to myself. She told me to hang in there, that these awful feelings would pass very soon.

Even with Liz's encouragement, I went through a lot of soul-searching about why I was doing this. I knew exactly why I'd started when I started. After a few months on the program, however, I began to forget why I was on it because I felt worse than I ever had before. I began to wonder what was so bad about the way I was originally? Yes, I was kind of depressed and maybe I was running on high revs, but was that really so bad?

Dr. Schwarzbein: What Mary was experiencing is the adrenaline withdrawal that occurs whenever adrenaline levels are too high over many years. This is analogous to a drug addict coming off any stimulant drug. Emotionally and physically, it is very difficult to go through this withdrawal process.

Mary's problem was that she had had a high-adrenaline lifestyle that led to low adrenaline levels. Because she had been running on adrenaline for years, she had caused her own adrenal glands to burn out.

When you burn out your adrenal glands, you may experience fatigue and/or depression because you cannot produce enough adrenaline. You will usually look for ways to raise your adrenaline levels again so that you can feel better.

In Mary's case she was undereating and overexercising to feel better, and when she improved her eating habits and decreased her exercise, she experienced a major letdown because she exposed her underlying physiology of a low-adrenaline state. Mary's adrenal glands were finally able to rest and shut down to repair, and she felt worse than ever. This is when she began to question and wonder why she was continuing with the program.

Intellectually, Mary understood how harmful her habits had been to her. After all, they had led her to develop depression and severe bone loss. She realized that she needed to heal, but emotionally she did not want to go through the trauma of the healing process.

If you start to go on a healthy nutrition and lifestyle program and begin to feel worse, your adrenal glands are probably burned out like Mary's were. As you improve your habits to lower your high adrenaline levels back to normal, they will first dip below normal—this is really your starting physiology. Before you can normalize your adrenaline levels, you have to heal your adrenal glands, and this takes time.

Mary: Before I started seeing Dr. Schwarzbein, I thought I'd given up everything I had to give up. I had given up all my vices except for sugar. I gave up meat, cigarettes, coffee and alcohol. I didn't know that the biggest challenge was still to come. Carbohydrates and junk food had been a problem for me my whole life.

When I was first married to my husband, I'd go to the store and buy five candy bars and eat them all at once. Luckily he never said anything to me like, "Gee, why are you killing yourself?" Because he gave me permission to do anything I wanted, I was able to realize how stupid it was and started regulating myself. However, I was never able to stop bingeing completely.

Dr. Schwarzbein: As Mary kept trading one poor nutrition and lifestyle habit for another, she thought that she was completely improving her habits. But what she mostly was doing was exchanging one stimulant for another. Yes, giving up cigarettes, caffeine and alcohol were big improvements, but her low caloric intake, her lack of protein, her overingestion of sugars and her excessive exercise kept her adrenaline levels too high.

Mary thought she had gotten rid of all her vices because caffeine, alcohol and tobacco have been identified as poor lifestyle choices. What Mary did not realize was that substituting processed and refined carbohydrates for red meat pushed her further and faster into adrenal gland "burnout." Like many vegetarians, Mary did not eat enough plant proteins. This is why she was unable to repair her low-neurotransmitter state. Ironically, she craved carbohydrates because her neurotransmitters were low. She was in a downward spiral to a low-neurotransmitter state and this made her seek other avenues to feel good.

Mary: This past Thanksgiving I once again binged on sugar. I was so disappointed in myself because I thought that I was cured from this type of behavior. I had not had any sugar for the previous nine months. I was concerned that I had ruined my whole healing process, but when I woke up the next morning, it was easy to start eating well again. There was no backlash at all.

When Christmas came around, I was worried that I would binge again. Every year at Christmas, Edna, who is like a second mother to me, bakes cookies for my family, something she has done ever since I was a baby. My children leave one of Edna's cookies out for Santa every Christmas Eve. In the past I would wait until all of the presents were wrapped and under the tree, then sit down and eat the cookie they left for Santa and several more. This year I thought long and hard about eating that cookie because I did not know if I could eat just one. I knew that one cookie would not be harmful, but I was worried that one cookie would set off my bingeing. This is always how it had happened before. I really didn't want to risk bingeing, but I was horrified at the thought of giving up this Christmas tradition and throwing the cookie away. I wondered if I would feel more emotionally deprived if I did not eat the cookie, or if I would feel more physically ill if I did and binged. My emotions won, and I sat peacefully by the Christmas tree and enjoyed the cookie. It is hard to express how I felt when I realized I would not eat any more. I felt like it was a miracle.

Dr. Schwarzbein: Mary's "miracle" happened because she was well into her transition process. In the past nine months, Mary had followed the SPII program and her hormones were in much better balance. Because of this, she was able to have just one cookie. You can read more about Mary's transition in chapter 9.

I have seen an immense improvement in Mary's health in the short months that we have been working together. During her initial visit with me and for several subsequent visits, she could not get through a session without breaking down into tears. Now she can talk to me without crying and feels much stronger than she did before. And the good news is that in less than a year she has grown back some bone tissue.

Mary: I used to sleep only five to six hours, but now I get at least eight. I spend a lot more time with my children, and I do things that really matter to me. I am not frazzled and frantic all the time, which is really positive. A lot of people have noticed a change in my behavior. I used to be really wound up and people just sort of tolerated me. Since I have been on the program, people who really love me and know me can pick out the change. That is remarkable. Another positive change is that I don't crave carbohydrates anymore.

When I saw my other doctor, who addressed just the bone loss problem, he wasn't really addressing the whole person. That's what Dr. Schwarzbein's program does, and it is what's so remarkable to me. I've always intuitively believed that drugs are not the answer. It's really about treating the whole person. I just feel blessed that I was able to get on this path somehow.

Are you like Mary? Do you have a high-adrenaline lifestyle? Is it going to take some time for you to heal? Take the high-adrenaline lifestyle quiz (see next page) to determine whether or not you may be an adrenaline addict, or if you have possibly burned out your adrenal glands.

Do You Have a High-Adrenaline Lifestyle?

Check off any of the statements below that apply to you.

☐ Do you skip meals on a regular basis?

☐ Do you count your calories?

☐ Are you dieting and losing weight quickly?

☐ Are you on a very low-carbohydrate diet when you do not need to be on one? You should not be on a low-carbohydrate diet if you *do not have* excessive fat around your midsection associated with one or more of the following: high triglyceride levels, high blood pressure disease or Type II diabetes.

☐ Are you constantly on the go?

☐ Do you find that you do not take any downtime for yourself during the day because you are too busy helping others?

☐ Do you work long hours because it stimulates you?

☐ Do you constantly create your own stress?

☐ Do you deprive yourself of getting enough hours of sleep in the night because you do not have the time, or do you wake up in the middle of the night worrying about anything and everything?

☐ Do you drink more than one caffeinated beverage or take caffeine pills during the day?

☐ Do you smoke cigarettes or use other nicotine products?

☐ Do you take stimulant diet pill products which contain ma huang, ephedra or Dexedrine?

☐ Do you only do cardiovascular exercises such as high-impact aerobics or running?

☐ Do you take low-dose estrogen birth control pills?

☐ Are you menopausal and not taking hormone replacement therapy?

☐ Are you menopausal and taking hormone replacement therapy designed so that you do not have monthly uterine bleeding? This is known as continuous combined hormone replacement therapy. Examples would be Prempro or Premarin and Provera daily, or natural estrogen with high daily doses of progesterone.

☐ Do you take Armour thyroid?

☐ Do you take cytomel in levels that cause your blood T3 to be higher than the normal range?

☐ Do you take any form of thyroid replacement therapy that makes your TSH level below normal range?

☐ Do you take prescription medications including stimulants to treat depression, attention deficit hyperactivity disorder or any other medical conditions?

If you answered yes to any of the above, you are creating higher than normal adrenaline levels in your body. If you answered yes to three or more, you have a high-adrenaline lifestyle and may have already burned out your adrenal glands. If you answered yes to the last question, you have definitely burned out your adrenal glands.

If you have burned out your adrenal glands, do not be afraid to heal. The How To section will describe the best possible way for you to go through your transition.

If you have done any of the above and are not doing them now—congratulations! You are in the healing process or have already healed.

By balancing your lifestyle to balance your adrenaline levels, you will have a better metabolism and live a healthier, happier and longer life. But adrenaline is not the only hormone you need to balance. Chapter 5 is all about insulin. Find out what Arthur did to overproduce insulin throughout his life and why he ended up undergoing open-heart surgery requiring five coronary artery bypass grafts (CABGs).

Summary

- Adrenaline, a major hormone known as the "fight/flight" hormone, is made in the adrenal glands and is being secreted constantly.
- Adrenaline sustains life by keeping your heart beating and allows you to use up your functional and structural biochemicals as well as food so that you can use them to think, move and do all of the activities of daily living such as breathing, eating and having bowel movements. It also signals the turnover of old cells to make room for new ones.
- Chronic oversecretion of adrenaline leads to lifestyle-based endocrine disorders.
- The initial symptom of too much adrenaline is a feeling of well-being as you use up your body's biochemicals and lean body tissues for function and energy. This feeling can be as addictive as any drug.
- If you are an adrenaline addict, you will have a difficult time emotionally and physically going through your transition.
- To be healthy and have strong bones you must keep adrenaline levels balanced.
- To determine if you are an adrenaline addict, or have possibly burned out your adrenal glands, take the high-adrenaline lifestyle quiz.
- By balancing your lifestyle to balance your adrenaline levels, you will heal your metabolism and achieve optimum health.

* * *

Now that you've learned about adrenaline, we are going to take a look at another major hormone in chapter 5: insulin. You will find out what insulin is and how your nutrition and lifestyle habits affect its secretion. You will also learn all about the problems you can develop if your insulin levels remain too high for many years.

Five

The Truth About Insulin

Insulin has received a lot of press in the past few years—most of it bad. You may have read about what happens to your health when insulin levels are chronically high, and you may even have gone on a low-calorie or low-carbohydrate diet to try to lower your insulin levels so that you could prevent disease and/or lose weight. But you need to know that *chronic low insulin levels are just as harmful as chronic high insulin levels.* Since insulin is another one of the major hormones, it is important that you do not try to eliminate it but instead learn to balance your insulin levels.

Why Insulin Is Important

Insulin keeps your body from using up too many of your biochemicals. It is also a major rebuilding hormone. It helps you rebuild all your functional biochemicals such as enzymes, hormones and neurotransmitters; your structural biochemicals such as cells, muscles and bones; and your energy biochemicals, fats and glycogen.

Your long-term survival depends upon your ability not to waste away in times of "famine," as well as your ability to rebuild all your biochemicals. So eating enough of the right foods and balancing your insulin levels are essential for your health.

You Really Are What You Eat

Your body cannot rebuild biochemicals if you do not eat, and the types of foods you eat determine the types of biochemicals you will rebuild. If you eat healthy, balanced meals that include proteins, healthy fats, nonstarchy vegetables and real carbohydrates, you will have the material you need to rebuild your functional and structural biochemicals and glycogen (the storage form of sugar).

When you skip meals, fast or go on an extremely calorie-restricted diet, you are not rebuilding at all.

If you eat a high-carbohydrate/low-fat diet, you cannot rebuild your functional and structural proteins and fats because you are not eating enough healthy proteins and fats to build them. Instead, you will mostly rebuild your energy biochemicals—sugars and fats—that can be used for energy if needed or stored as glycogen or fat if you do not need them for energy.

If you eat a high-protein and vegetable diet, you will not secrete enough insulin and with time you will use yourself up more than you rebuild.

Therefore, if you are not eating well, you will have a mismatch between utilization and rebuilding, which will result in a damaged metabolism.

Glandular-Based Insulin Disorders

When your body stops making insulin, you have Type I diabetes—a glandular-based insulin endocrine disease. The good news is that Type I diabetes is uncommon, and insulin can be replaced. The other glandular-based insulin endocrine disorder is an insulinoma,* a pancreatic tumor that produces and secretes too much insulin. Like most glandular-based endocrine disorders, it is rare.

Lifestyle-Based Insulin Disorders

Lifestyle-based insulin disorders—not glandular-based insulin disorders—are the ones that are most likely to affect us. These problems are caused by the under- or oversecretion of insulin in response to daily poor nutrition and lifestyle habits.

Lifestyle-Based Endocrine Disorders Caused by Low Insulin Levels

One of the causes of low insulin levels is eating too little food. Food is one of the triggers that stimulates the release of insulin from your pancreas. If you do not eat enough food, you will not secrete enough insulin. If your insulin levels are too low, you will use up your biochemicals faster than you will be able to rebuild them. This is the same type of problem that is seen with the oversecretion of adrenaline discussed in chapter 4. All the same lifestyle-based endocrine disorders that are caused by high adrenaline levels can also be caused by low insulin levels. Remember, adrenaline helps your body use up your biochemicals, and insulin helps your body rebuild them. Therefore, high adrenaline levels and low insulin levels have the same effects.

Since you already have learned what these effects are in chapter 4, this chapter focuses on the lifestyle-based, chronic, high-insulin disorders that are caused by years of poor nutrition and lifestyle habits.

---

*There are 12 million people with diabetes. Less than 10 percent have Type I diabetes. Insulinomas occur in one case out of 250,000 patient-years.

Low-Insulin Effect

A low-insulin effect can occur with low insulin levels or with high insulin levels.

When you undersecrete insulin, you end up with low insulin levels, which keep you from rebuilding your biochemicals as fast as you use them up. In other words, your body uses itself up and you "waste away" because your insulin effect is low.

Low insulin levels, however, are not the only cause of a low-insulin effect. You can also have a low insulin effect when your insulin levels are high. Here is how that happens.

When your adrenaline and insulin levels are both high, but your adrenaline levels are higher than your insulin levels, you cannot rebuild your biochemicals as quickly as you use them up. Your insulin effect is still low even though your insulin levels are high. You will waste away, but not as quickly as you would if your insulin levels were low.

It is the ratio between how you use up your biochemicals and your ability to rebuild them that determines your insulin effect. If you use up more than you rebuild, you have a low-insulin effect. If you build up more than you use, you have a high-insulin effect. When utilization matches rebuilding, you have a normal insulin effect, which is the goal.

Whether your insulin levels are low or both insulin and adrenaline are high—and your adrenaline levels are higher than your insulin levels—the low-insulin effect is the same: You waste away. The latter occurs over a longer period of time, and it is more difficult to recognize that you are destroying your metabolism because it occurs more slowly.

Causes of Low-Insulin Effect
Due to Low Insulin Secretion

Very low caloric intake: five hundred calories or less a day
Hypoglycemia (low blood sugar): Your pancreas stops secret-
ing insulin when your blood sugar gets too low.
High-protein/nonstarchy vegetable diet
Starvation

Causes of Low-Insulin Effect
Due to Higher Adrenaline Than Insulin Levels

Everything that causes adrenaline levels to be too high (see
chapter 4). Adrenaline increases the utilization of biochemicals; insulin builds them back up. So if your adrenaline levels
are higher than your insulin levels, your insulin effect is lower.

Arthur's Story: It Was Almost Too Late

As with most lifestyle-based endocrine disorders, the hormone
imbalance is present for years before any diseases are apparent. This
was the case with Arthur. He is a perfect example of a person whose
poor nutrition and lifestyle habits caused chronic high insulin levels
and a high-insulin effect, but he did not even know that he was damaging his metabolism until it was almost too late.

Arthur: Food has always been very central in my life. I learned early on
from my family to eat for comfort, to celebrate, to socialize and to relieve
stress. Eating became my universal response to whatever was going on in
my life.

I specifically recall eating cookies often. I ate cookies to relieve stress or
really for any occasion. I would come home from school and have cookies

and milk. And before I would go to bed I would have cookies and milk. I would also buy a dozen cookies at the store and by the time the day was over, they'd be gone. A bag of donuts never got too far either.

This is how it was in my family. When we had family get-togethers, we always ate. And we ate a lot of carbohydrates. I had a grandmother who was a great cook, and she loved to bake. We always had really good bread and other baked goods like cookies and pies around because we lived about two blocks from her, and she baked all the time.

I ate a lot of sweets, but I wasn't much of a vegetable eater. I thought they were just there to decorate my plate, but that they weren't important. So I would serve myself a small portion of them and then eat mostly potatoes, meat and desserts.

I was fairly active as a kid. I rode my bicycle everywhere I wanted to go, but I never had a regular exercise routine or played any sports. So when I became an adult and got busy with work, I never thought to exercise for my health.

I never had a weight problem until I was in my thirties, so it didn't occur to me to diet until then. Prior to that, I ate what I wanted and never gained an ounce. I've dieted off and on ever since to keep my weight down. I tried all kinds of diets. Low-calorie, low-fat, and high-carbohydrate diets. My attitude about dieting was that as soon as I got through the diet, I would go back to my regular eating habits, but I would cut the volume of it way down. And so I never really made a lifestyle change. It just was a way to lose weight.

After every diet I tried, I would eventually gain back all the weight I lost plus more. When I was in my thirties, I probably had forty pounds or so to lose. But as time went on it became more like sixty to eighty pounds.

Dr. Schwarzbein: I explained to Arthur that breads, grains, cereals, fruits, fruit juices, starchy vegetables, legumes, sugary foods, some milk products and alcohol are part of the food group called carbohydrates. And carbohydrates stimulate the pancreas to release high amounts of insulin. His years of overindulging in meals high in breads, cookies, pies, donuts and potatoes led to his chronic high insulin levels. But because high insulin levels do not cause immediate damage to the metabolism, it took several years before Arthur developed his first symptom—his weight problem.

Carbohydrates: How They Are Digested into Sugar, Cause the Release of Insulin and Are Converted to Fats

For the purpose of simplicity, we are going to consider the actions of insulin as though it is the only hormone in your body telling your cells what to do. But remember—insulin, like all hormones, does not act alone; all the hormones of the body are connected, and they are helping each other regulate all the same biochemical reactions simultaneously.

Let us follow carbohydrates through your system to see how they affect insulin secretion. For this example, we are going to divide your body into two parts: inside and outside the body.

Breaking Down Carbohydrates into Sugar

The intestinal tract is made up of your mouth, esophagus, stomach, small intestine, large intestine (colon) and rectum. It can be thought of as being *outside* of your body since it is in contact with the outside at both ends. It is in the digestive tract from your mouth to your small intestines that the food you eat is digested (broken down) into its smallest possible building blocks.

When you digest carbohydrates, you break them down into sugar. Sugar is small enough that it can pass from the small intestines (*outside* the body), through the intestinal wall and into the blood system (*inside* the body). This process is called absorption; therefore, the purpose of digestion is absorption.

The area of the bloodstream where sugar enters is called the *portal vein*. Though its name is not important, it is important for you to know that the portal vein links your small intestines directly to your liver and not to any other organs or cells. This path is a one-way highway.

Insulin and Sugar

It is at the level of the portal vein that insulin is introduced into the bloodstream proportionate to the amount of incoming sugar. The insulin and sugar travel directly to the liver where the liver cells take up sugar from the bloodstream because insulin tells the liver cells to open up their doors—or receptors—and let the sugar in.

Inside the liver cells, sugar can then be processed through four distinct pathways:

Sugars can be broken down to generate a form of energy called *adenosine triphosphate* (ATP), which is used by the cells to provide fuel for biochemical reactions.

Sugars can be linked back together to form the human carbohydrate known as glycogen, the storage form of sugar.

Sugars can be converted into triglycerides, a type of fat.

Sugars can be converted into cholesterol, another type of fat.

You cannot store ATP because ATP can only be made if it is used immediately by the liver. Since the liver does not need a lot of ATP at any given moment, you are not going to convert most of the sugar from your meal into much ATP production. However, you can store sugar as glycogen. Glycogen stores will be used later on for energy, but in the meantime they are stored in the liver cells. Since there is not much room in the liver for glycogen stores, most of the incoming sugar is diverted to the fat pathways.

Excess Sugars Are Converted into Fats

Your body has systems in place that try to block the damage that happens when too much sugar enters your portal vein at a given moment. The most common process is to convert your excess sugars into two types of fats: triglycerides and cholesterol. This small piece of information—that *excess* sugars are converted into these two types of fats—tells you that sugars are more damaging to the human body than fats are. High fats in your bloodstream are damaging, too, but high levels of sugar in your bloodstream will damage you first. So what you need to do is eliminate refined and excess sugars from your diet so that the amount of sugar entering the portal vein is not overwhelming to your body.

Instead of eating refined (processed) carbohydrates, eat real carbohydrates—such as whole grains, legumes, starchy vegetables and fruits. It is also important to eat the correct amount of carbohydrates for your current metabolism and activity level so that they are not in

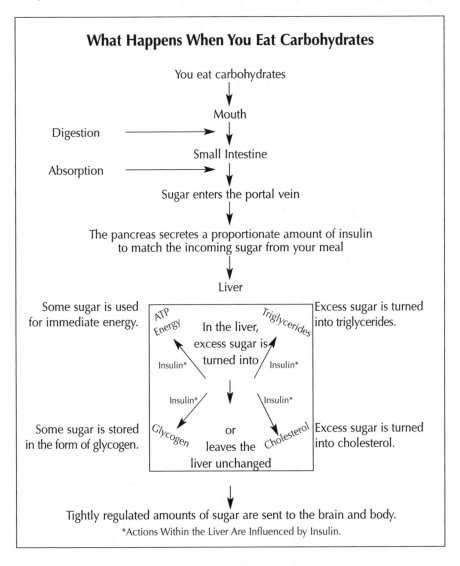

What Happens When You Eat Carbohydrates

You eat carbohydrates

Mouth

Digestion

Small Intestine

Absorption

Sugar enters the portal vein

The pancreas secretes a proportionate amount of insulin to match the incoming sugar from your meal

Liver

Some sugar is used for immediate energy.

In the liver, excess sugar is turned into

ATP Energy

Insulin*

Triglycerides

Insulin*

Glycogen

Insulin*

or

leaves the liver unchanged

Insulin*

Cholesterol

Excess sugar is turned into triglycerides.

Some sugar is stored in the form of glycogen.

Excess sugar is turned into cholesterol.

Tightly regulated amounts of sugar are sent to the brain and body.

*Actions Within the Liver Are Influenced by Insulin.

excess of what your body needs to use for energy. (See chapter 11 for more information about healthy carbohydrates.)

How Fats Travel Through the Body

Where do these fats that are produced in the liver go? Initially, into the bloodstream, and since the bloodstream is mostly made up of water, the fats in the liver must be packaged within a protein coat in order for them to travel through the bloodstream. Fats and water do not mix, but proteins and water do. To visualize this, just think of what happens when you try to mix water and oil. They do not blend together. The oil always rises to the top.

These protein-coated packaged fats are triglyceride and cholesterol carriers called very low-density lipoproteins (VLDLs). VLDLs are secreted out of the liver cells into the bloodstream, where they travel from the liver to the rest of the cells of your body. With the aid of insulin, VLDLs initially unload their triglycerides to the cells. If the cells need energy at that moment, they will use the incoming triglycerides for energy; if not, they will be stored as fat.

When all the triglycerides have been removed from the VLDL, it is left with only cholesterol, and we call this protein-coated cholesterol carrier a low-density lipoprotein (LDL). The LDLs continue to travel through the bloodstream and, with the help of insulin, unload their cholesterol inside the cells. Cholesterol is used for many body functions (see Functions of Cholesterol in the Body, page 94).

Liver Forming VLDLs and Then LDLs

Sugar Enters the Portal Vein

The Pancreas secretes a proportionate amount of Insulin to match the incoming sugar from your meal

LIVER

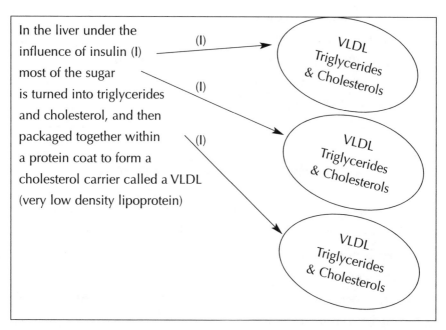

In the liver under the influence of insulin (I) most of the sugar is turned into triglycerides and cholesterol, and then packaged together within a protein coat to form a cholesterol carrier called a VLDL (very low density lipoprotein)

VLDL Triglycerides & Cholesterols

VLDL Triglycerides & Cholesterols

VLDL Triglycerides & Cholesterols

The VLDLs travel through the bloodstream to the cells of the body and with the aid of insulin unload their triglycerides inside your cells. When all the triglycerides are unloaded we call the protein coated cholesterol carrier a LDL (low density lipoprotein).

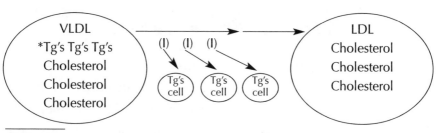

*Triglycerides

Functions of Cholesterol in the Body

- Forms insulation around nerves to keep electrical impulses moving
- Helps maintain a healthy immune system
- Important structure in all cell membranes—those found inside and around the cells
- Keeps cell membranes flexible and permeable
- Keeps moods even by stabilizing neurotransmitters
- Necessary for brain function
- Used to make important hormones

Meanwhile, Back at the Liver . . .

Let's go back to the liver. When sugar and insulin enter the liver from the portal vein, not all the sugar is taken up by the liver cells. The sugar that is not taken up travels through the liver and out the other end of the liver.

Next, the sugar and insulin travel together through the bloodstream and come into contact with the other cells of the body, including the brain cells. Insulin binds to its receptors on the cells, signaling the uptake of the excess sugar by the cells. The sugar that enters the cells can be used immediately for energy, or it can be stored as glycogen or fat for later use.

Sugar, Insulin and the Brain

Unlike most cells, brain cells are not insulin-dependent. This means that they do not depend on insulin binding to the cells in order for sugar to enter inside. How much sugar enters inside the brain cells depends on how much circulating sugar is in your bloodstream at a given moment. If there is a large amount of sugar in your blood-stream, a lot of sugar will enter your brain cells—and this can cause a lot of damage to your brain cells.

One of the most important functions of insulin is to make sure that too much sugar does not enter into your brain cells. This is where the insulin-dependent cells of the body such as the liver, muscle and fat cells step in. Insulin diverts excess sugars after you eat a meal into these various cells to ensure that too much sugar will not enter your brain cells. This is crucial for your survival.

On the other hand, initially, your brain can *only* use sugar—not fats—for the energy it needs to function and stay alive. Ironically, you will not survive for very long if you do not get enough sugar going to your brain. The bottom line is: too much sugar is harmful to the brain; too little sugar is even more harmful. Again, the body demands balance to stay healthy.

How Your Body Uses Energy

Your cells require energy biochemicals to stay alive. Brain cells, red blood cells and specialized cells of your kidneys initially use sugar as their energy biochemical. The rest of your cells can use sugars and fats interchangeably.

The only time that your brain, red blood and kidney cells use fats for energy is when you have not eaten in over seventy-two hours. At that point these cells can switch to using ketones (a breakdown product of fats) for energy.

However, do not think that this is a good thing—it is not. By the time you start to utilize your ketones for energy, you have used up your glycogen stores and have destroyed functional and structural biochemicals while your body has eaten itself up to survive. When you stop this "famine" or fast, your insulin levels will rebound higher than before to help you rebuild. So you will rebuild your functional and structural biochemicals and rebuild more fat stores. Putting your body into ketosis is never a good thing.

Dr. Schwarzbein: When Arthur was younger, before he damaged his metabolism, he was able to process all the excess sugar he ate into triglycerides and cholesterol and not gain weight because his cells would use the triglycerides for energy and the cholesterol for rebuilding functional and structural biochemicals. Even though his insulin levels were high from his poor nutrition and lifestyle habits, his adrenaline levels were higher. Therefore, his insulin effect was low. That is why he initially had normal weight and normal triglyceride and cholesterol blood levels.

However, by the time he was thirty, Arthur's body could no longer process all the excess sugar he ate because his metabolic needs were lower. He continued to overeat carbohydrates and convert all his excess sugar into cholesterol and triglycerides. Since he still had a relatively healthy metabolism, he was able to unload these fats into his cells. Because his cells could no longer process all the cholesterol and triglycerides, they were stored as fat instead. That is why his triglyceride and cholesterol blood levels stayed within normal ranges even though he was gaining weight.

For the first time in his life Arthur was overweight. Though his insulin levels were higher than his adrenaline levels (a high-insulin effect), he had not damaged his metabolism yet. If he had understood how he had gained his fat weight in the first place, instead of believing that calories in equal calories out, he never would have started dieting. But he did diet, and that raised his insulin levels even higher.

The real damage started when he began to diet to get rid of his excess fat stores instead of balancing out his meals and adding in a cross-training exercise program. (See the How To section for more information about how to eat balanced meals and exercise for good health.)

When Arthur dieted by restricting his calories, his insulin effect was lowered. This allowed him to use up his functional and structural biochemicals, as well as his storage biochemicals (sugar and fats) and lose weight. This gave him the false impression that his diet was "working." But because he was not eating well, Arthur was not able to rebuild his functional and structural biochemicals. Using up more than rebuilding his biochemicals damaged his metabolism. Every time he stopped dieting, his insulin levels rebounded higher than before in an attempt to catch up with rebuilding. Since he was not eating well (he always ate too many carbohydrates), he continued to convert the excess sugar he ate into fats.

Because Arthur repeated this process of dieting over and over again, his higher insulin levels over an extended period of time finally caught up to him. Inadvertently, he had turned himself into a fat-producing machine, and his cells had become completely overloaded with triglycerides and cholesterol so that they would not accept any more fats inside.

Now Arthur was overweight and had abnormal blood cholesterol (high triglyceride and cholesterol) levels. But these were not the only health issues he had. He was now also insulin-resistant.

You, like Arthur, need to learn what habits cause high insulin levels so that you stop signaling your body that it needs to turn excess energy into fats. By improving your nutrition and lifestyle habits, you, too, can get your body to stop overproducing fats.

Arthur: I never realized that I had any serious health problems until the week after my sixtieth birthday. I did have some minor surgeries but never any health issues—or so I thought. My cholesterol was high-borderline, but the doctors never seemed to worry about it particularly, so I didn't either.

I went to the doctor because I was having this numbness in my left arm. I would feel it when I'd walk the dog or mow the grass; that arm would hurt so bad that I'd just have to push the mower with my right arm. And I didn't think a whole lot about it because every now and then I'd stop the mower to empty the bag, and the pain would go away. I did not have any chest pain. When I finally went to see the doctor, he said, "You're going into the hospital tonight." And that's when they discovered that I had a 90 percent blockage in one artery and an 80 percent blockage in another; the other three arteries had 75 percent blockages. They did five bypasses on me [coronary artery bypass grafts (CABGs)].

Dr. Schwarzbein: Unbeknownst to Arthur, he had health problems long before the age of sixty. They just were not identified before that fateful day.

Years of high insulin levels resulting in overproduction of cholesterol from excess energy caused Arthur to develop heart disease. The excess cholesterol he made was oxidized (see Oxidation, page 99), and this damaged cholesterol (oxidized cholesterol) ended up as plaque in his arteries.

It is important to understand that the cholesterol in your body that comes from eating cholesterol-rich foods and the cholesterol you make in your liver from excess energy are not the same. It is the overproduction of cholesterol in your liver that leads to the type of cholesterol that is easily oxidized and increases your risk of heart disease.

Symptoms of Heart Disease or Heart Attack

Blocked arteries do not always cause chest pain. In fact, one of the most common symptoms of coronary artery blockage is pain down your left arm during physical exertion that goes away when you stop whatever you are doing. If you experience this type of feeling while you are walking, running, doing housework or mowing the lawn, you need to be evaluated for heart disease. Some other symptoms to watch for are the following:

- Chest pain that feels more like someone sitting on your chest then a stabbing type of pain
- Stabbing chest pain, but this is unusual
- Shortness of breath with exertion or at rest
- Unexplained heartburn
- Pain that goes down your right arm or both of your arms. (This is less common than down your left arm)
- Light-headedness and/or dizziness
- Nausea and vomiting
- A cold, clammy sweat

If you experience any of these symptoms for more than five minutes, particularly crushing chest pain, call 911 immediately. You may be having a heart attack. If you experience any of these symptoms off and on, especially if you have had poor nutrition and lifestyle habits for years, consult your doctor as soon as possible for a heart evaluation. You may have heart disease.

High Levels of Insulin Are
Initially Protective, but Later Lead to Disease

The key to understanding the role of insulin and why it goes up after you eat is to realize that high levels of sugar in the bloodstream are very damaging. If insulin did not communicate to your liver and other body cells that excess sugar is around and needs to be processed or taken up into the cells, the ensuing high blood-sugar levels would cause a lot of tissue damage through oxidation. Therefore, excess sugar must be cleared out of the bloodstream very quickly after a meal, and insulin is the biochemical communicator that makes this happen. High insulin levels in the short term are very protective, but they catch up with you in the long term and increase your risk for the degenerative diseases of aging.

Oxidation

As living, breathing beings we need oxygen to survive. The great irony is that oxygen also contributes to our eventual death. Part of the natural aging process involves oxidation.

Oxidation is a process that forms free radicals in your body. Free radicals are molecules that are missing or have an extra electron. Oxygen or other chemicals can react with other atoms and rob them of an electron, leaving an unpaired electron behind. When this happens, free radicals are formed. Since electrons like to be paired, free radicals roam your body looking to steal an electron from your tissues, a process that damages your tissues.

Since the amount of free radicals in your body at a given moment is usually minimal, your body can normally neutralize them with substances known as antioxidants—before tissue damage ever happens.

It is only when there is an excessive amount of free radicals in your body that your body is overwhelmed and cannot neutralize all the free radicals. This is when major changes to your metabolism occur— leading to a higher risk of the degenerative diseases of aging.

Protecting Your Body Against Free Radicals

Antioxidants are your body's natural defense systems against free radicals. You get antioxidants in the food you eat and in certain herbs, or you make them in your body. The following is a partial list of major antioxidants. Some interfere or are contraindicated with different medications, so be sure to consult your physician or pharmacist before using any of them.

• **Alpha lipoic acid**

This biochemical is produced in the body in small quantities, but it is a very powerful antioxidant. Studies show that it can help people with diabetes decrease the damage from high blood-sugar levels.

• **Bilberry**

This herb keeps your capillaries and red blood cell membranes strong and flexible, and it may enhance vision.

• **Burdock**

This herb has been shown to protect against cancer by controlling cell mutations.

• **Carotenoids**

This class of vitamins is found in red, yellow, green and orange vegetables and fruits. Alpha- and beta-carotenes, lycopene and lutein are the most commonly known. They may help protect you against cancer by reducing oxidative damage to your DNA. It is important to take them together as a complex instead of individually.

• **CoEnzyme Q-10**

This biochemical is made in the body. It is most famously known for its protective effects against heart disease.

• **Curcumin**

Curcumin is found in the spice turmeric. It stops the oxidation of cholesterol, thereby protecting you against plaque formation in your arteries.

• Estradiol

This hormone is the natural human estrogen made by the ovaries. It helps neutralize free radicals.

• Flavonoids

These plant extracts are very potent antioxidants. They are found in fruits, vegetables, spices, seeds, nuts, flowers and bark. They protect your antioxidant vitamins from oxidative damage.

• Garlic

This herb helps prevent fats from being oxidized.

• Ginkgo biloba

This herb is a powerful antioxidant that protects your brain, retina (back of your eye) and cardiovascular system.

• Glutathione

This protein is produced in the liver from the amino acids cysteine, glutamic acid and glycine. It helps defend your body from cigarette smoke, radiation, cancer chemotherapy and toxins such as alcohol. The rate at which we age has been correlated with the amount of glutathione in our system. Glutathione can be taken in supplement form, or its production can be boosted by taking N-acetylcysteine and L-Methionine (see below).

• Grape seed extract

This plant extract is made from the seeds of the wine grape. It can cross the blood-brain barrier and protect your brain and spinal nerves from oxidative damage.

• Green tea

It is the polyphenols in green tea that are protective. They help shield your DNA from free radical damage.

• L-Methionine

This amino acid neutralizes hydroxyl radicals that are formed during strenuous exercise or exposure to high levels of radiation. Hydroxyl radicals damage all cell types.

• Melatonin

This hormone is a potent universal antioxidant. It is one of the few antioxidants that protects your mitochondria (the energy making organelle inside your cells). Do not take this in supplement form. Instead, learn what you need to do to make more of this hormone from its precursor, serotonin (see chapter 6).

• N-acetylcysteine (NAC)

This biochemical is a more stable form of the amino acid cysteine. It can be taken in supplement form. It is used to produce glutathione in your liver. Discuss the use of NAC with your physician if you are diabetic because it may interfere with the action of insulin.

• Nicotinamide adenine dinucleotide hydrogen (NADH)

This biochemical is made in the body and plays a central role in DNA repair and maintenance. It may also prevent the neurotransmitter dopamine from auto-oxidation that may damage sensitive parts of your brain.

• Pycnogenol

This plant extract is produced from the French maritime pine tree. It is in the same class of antioxidants as grape seed extract so it also can cross the blood-brain barrier and protect your brain and spinal nerves from oxidative damage.

• Selenium

This essential trace mineral partners up with vitamin E to protect tissues and cell membranes. *Caution:* Amounts higher than one milligram daily may be toxic.

• Silymarin

This herb is extracted from the seeds of the milk thistle plant. It has been used for years to treat liver disease.

• Superoxide dismutase

This enzyme neutralizes the most common and possibly the most dangerous free radicals—superoxide radicals.

• Vitamin A

This vitamin protects your eyes, lungs and skin.

• Vitamin C

This vitamin is one of your body's first lines of defense against free radicals in your body fluids.

• Vitamin E

This vitamin helps prevent the oxidation of fats. It partners up with selenium to protect your cell membranes. *Caution:* Do not take more than 1,000 IU a day.

• Zinc

This essential trace mineral prevents the oxidation of fats.

Sugars: More Damaging Than Fats or Insulin

Since sugars are more easily oxidized than fats, they are more damaging to your body. Therefore, if you do not secrete enough insulin to clear the excess sugar out of your bloodstream and into your cells, you will have high blood-sugar levels and form higher amounts of free radicals.

High blood-sugar levels are also more damaging to your body than high insulin levels. That is why your body immediately secretes higher amounts of insulin when you consume a high amount of carbohydrates—to protect you. Insulin communicates to your cells that the sugar needs to be "detoxified" into fats, and you have escaped harm, at least for a while.

But nothing is free. High levels of insulin over many years cause health problems. Unfortunately, you cannot feel or see the damage that is occurring from chronic high insulin levels, so it never crosses your mind that you need to change your poor nutrition and lifestyle habits.

In summary, sugars cause more damage in the short term than either fats or insulin do. Therefore, your body will exchange high sugars for higher fats and higher insulin levels to protect you for the moment. But your body cannot protect you forever. If you continue to consume too many carbohydrates, including refined sugars, the higher fats and insulin levels will eventually cause health problems, too. I cannot say it often enough—balance is essential for good health.

Remember:
- Excess sugars are more damaging than excess fats.
- Excess sugars are more damaging than excess insulin.
- Excess fats and insulin are still harmful.

Insulin Sensitivity

You are insulin-sensitive when all the functions of insulin are working. Since insulin sensitivity is normal, your goal is to be and/or stay insulin-sensitive.

The following is what happens when you eat carbohydrates if you are insulin-sensitive:

- Sugar is taken up by your liver.
- Excess sugar in your liver is turned into triglycerides and cholesterol.
- Triglycerides and cholesterol are taken up by various cells of your body.
- Sugar is also taken up by your cells.
- When all the sugar and fats are in your cells, blood-sugar levels start to drop and insulin levels go back down.
- You eat again and the whole process starts all over.

When you are insulin-sensitive, your insulin levels initially rise after a meal and come back down again in between meals. If you eat a balanced meal, you will not notice these fluctuations because they are not very dramatic.

However, you *can* feel these initial insulin fluctuations if you are eating a high-carbohydrate meal, especially if carbohydrates are the only food you ingest. The increased sugar load entering your body causes a high release of insulin, which then tells your liver and cells to process the excess sugar, and there is a rapid inflow of sugar inside all your cells. This leaves less sugar in your bloodstream, and your insulin levels drop dramatically so that you do not become hypoglycemic.

The more your insulin levels fluctuate between high-highs and low-lows, the more likely you are to experience the symptoms or signs of fluctuating insulin levels listed below. You can have none, one, some or all of these symptoms. Every person is different.

Clammy skin	Irritability
Fatigue	Light-headedness
Foggy thinking	Loose bowel movements
Heart palpitations	Panic attacks
Insomnia	Sugar cravings

On Your Way to Becoming Insulin-Resistant

If your poor nutrition and lifestyle habits become chronic, your insulin levels will eventually not fluctuate as much between highs and lows. Instead, they will remain higher than normal in between meals (what is called "partial insulin resistance"). This happens because years of producing fats and sugar from eating excess carbohydrates begins to fill your cells with energy they cannot use. Because your cells are partially filled with energy, they do not respond to insulin as quickly, and your blood-sugar levels do not fluctuate dramatically. Therefore, your insulin levels do not fluctuate rapidly either. Instead of being used for energy, the food you eat is mostly stored as fat. You are not completely insulin-resistant at this point because your fat cells will accept triglycerides and sugar to store, and your blood triglyceride and sugar levels remain normal.

Unfortunately, you usually do not recognize that you are becoming insulin-resistant. Your body's reaction to your habits is on a metabolic continuum. You start off insulin-sensitive and then, because of poor nutrition and lifestyle habits, you become partially insulin-resistant. If these habits continue for many years, you develop full-blown insulin resistance. See chart on page 112.

When you are partially insulin-resistant, you will experience one, some or all of the following symptoms. Every person is different.

Acne
Ankle swelling
Burning feet
Constipation
Decreased memory or
    concentration
Depression
Fatigue
Fluctuating high blood pressure
    readings

Fuzzy brain
Infertility
Irregular menstrual cycles
Irritability
Loose bowel movements alter-
    nating with constipation
Water retention
Weight gain

Full-Blown Insulin Resistance

Eventually, from sustained high levels of insulin, you become completely insulin-resistant. All your cells are completely overfilled with fats and sugar, and they barely respond to the action of insulin. At this point you usually have high triglyceride blood levels. (High triglyceride levels are not indicators of insulin resistance only. Smoking, stress, birth control pills and drinking alcohol can also raise triglyceride levels in your bloodstream, but that does not necessarily mean that you are insulin-resistant. Do not diagnose yourself as insulin-resistant from your triglyceride blood test alone.)

When you are insulin-resistant, you have high fasting insulin levels, you carry your excess fat weight around your midsection, and you have one or more of the following symptoms or diseases.

- **Abnormal cholesterol profiles:** High triglyceride levels with low high-density lipoprotein (HDL) levels and high apolipoprotein B levels.
- **Hypertension:** Sustained high blood pressure.
- **Type II diabetes:** Sustained high levels of sugar in the bloodstream.
- **Coronary atherosclerosis:** Plaques in the heart arteries which may cause a heart attack when they rupture.
- **Cerebral atherosclerosis:** Plaques in the brain which may cause a stroke when they rupture.
- **Cancers:** Abnormal cell growth. Breast, prostate and colon cancers are the most common cancers associated with high insulin levels.
- **Stein-Leventhal syndrome (SLS):** SLS is a female clinical condition of infertility (anovulatory menstrual cycles), fat-weight around the midsection, acne and/or facial hair.

In summary, because high sugar levels are always harmful, your body tries to protect itself by secreting higher levels of insulin. This is a normal response by your body to keep you alive longer. But nothing is free. If you continue to consume too many carbohydrates for your current metabolism and activity levels and thus cause chronic high levels of insulin, you will damage your metabolism. This will lead to inefficient regeneration, to insulin resistance and to a higher risk for the degenerative diseases of aging.

Arthur: After my surgery, my doctor put me on a low-fat diet and I got fatter. I didn't eat any fat on that diet, but I ate a lot of bread and low-fat snacks. This included all the low-fat cookies I wanted. I got really frustrated because what they asked me to do didn't work. I wasn't losing any fat weight, and I'd go to rehab, and they would hassle me all the time. They'd say, "You're not losing any weight." And I'd say, "Well, I'm doing what you told me to."

Dr. Schwarzbein: Arthur continued to gain weight because he was told to follow the exact poor eating habits that caused him to have trouble in the first place. It is very disturbing to note that the medical profession is still misdiagnosing and prescribing the wrong program for people with heart disease and high insulin levels.

Arthur: The reason I got myself into this mess to begin with is that I never liked the way I looked when I was fat. Since I never connected my weight issues with my health, I just dieted to look good—I wanted my clothes to fit me. I thought it was related to calories in versus calories out. So I wasn't concerned with my health at that point because I never had to be. However, I do remember that I always heard that you were healthier if you were thinner.

Dr. Schwarzbein: Arthur, like many people, believed that being thin is all that matters. But doing all the wrong things to maintain a particular weight is one of the worst things you can do to your metabolism. A list of myths and truths about metabolism appears below. How many myths have you accepted as truths?

Myths and Truths About Metabolism

Myth: Weight (body composition) is related to caloric input versus caloric output.
Truth: Calories do not determine your body composition; your hormones do. This is because your hormones determine your current metabolism. Restricting your calories to lose weight leads to a low-insulin effect that will eventually destroy your metabolism. Do not make the mistake of counting calories. Eat balanced meals to keep your hormones balanced and your metabolism working efficiently.

Myth: Eating fat makes you fat because there are nine calories in a gram of fat.
Truth: Not all fats are fattening. Healthy fats are used as the material to rebuild cells and certain hormones. Therefore, when you eat healthy fats and make functional and structural fats from

them, you do not store them as fat. Also, since fats are more satiating than carbohydrates, it is harder to overeat them because your body regulates their intake.

Myth: If you are losing weight, you must be doing something right.

Truth: Not all weight loss is healthy. Just because you are losing weight does not mean that you are doing something that is good for you. If you are on a diet and losing weight too quickly, you are losing your functional and structural biochemicals as well as storage fat. The loss of these biochemicals will destroy your metabolism. You need to be healthy first to lose your fat weight, not lose weight to become healthy.

Myth: Food is the only factor in achieving and maintaining your ideal body composition.

Truth: Eating well is not enough. You need to be aware that your stress levels, the toxic chemicals you ingest, the amount of exercise you do, your hormone levels and the food you eat all work together to determine your body composition. If you spend your entire life counting calories to keep your weight down, instead of improving these other areas of your life, you will destroy your metabolism and never achieve your ideal body composition.

Myth: Fat-free foods help you lose fat.

Truth: Fat-free foods may make you fatter. Most fat-free foods are filled with extra sugar to make them taste better, and eating excess sugar makes your body store fat. Read the labels and stay away from processed fat-free foods.

Myth: It does not matter what you eat as long as it is low in calories.

Truth: What you eat does matter. It is important that you eat the foods that you are made of. You rebuild from proteins, healthy fats, nonstarchy vegetables and real carbohydrates. You do not rebuild when you eat junk food, even if it is low in calories.

Myth: Some people would be fatter if they did not diet.
Truth: Dieting makes you fat. Restrictive diets destroy your metabolism by causing you to use up your biochemicals faster than you can rebuild them. Most people who are overweight got there by yo-yo dieting.

Myth: Unlucky people are born with a damaged metabolism.
Truth: Luck has nothing to do with a damaged metabolism. While it is true that some people are born with a damaged metabolism, most people are born with a healthy one. You determine your current metabolism by what you do and eat on a day-to-day basis—because your current metabolism is acquired, not genetic.

Myth: If I am gaining weight, I must be doing all the wrong things.
Truth: Sometimes you have to gain weight to lose weight. If you begin with a damaged metabolism and then make the nec-essary improvements to your nutrition and lifestyle habits, you can expect to gain weight as you heal. Once your metabolism is healed, you are ready to achieve your ideal body composition.

Myth: If I am thin, I must be healthy.
Truth: Thin people are not always healthy. You can be too thin for all the wrong reasons. You are not healthy if you are thin and have a damaged metabolism.

> **Myth:** Once your metabolism is destroyed you can never repair it.
> **Truth:** It is never too late to heal your metabolism. The good news is that by following the SPII program, your metabolism can be repaired. But you will not heal overnight.

Arthur: My bypass surgery disrupted my complacency a little. Once I read *The Schwarzbein Principle* and started working with Dr. Schwarzbein, things have been different. Until that time I had never found a program that made sense to me. After my first visit with her, I just knew that this was the way to go and that it was going to make a difference.

With time I will be able to eat a few more carbohydrates, but I'm not going to be eating them like I used to. The thing that really made her program simple was when she explained the PFVC acronym.

Dr. Schwarzbein: Eating a PFVC meal means eating a healthy **p**rotein, a healthy **f**at, a nonstarchy **v**egetable and a real **c**arbohydrate at every meal.

Arthur: I'm now thinking about proteins, healthy fats, vegetables and real carbohydrates and how to create that balance, rather than thinking about where I can get the best desserts. I'm also doing a lot of cooking because I figure if I'm going to try to heal myself, I will do all the meal planning and cooking so that I can fix what I need. And that has helped.

So, I'm pretty much making more of a commitment to this as a way of life, rather than just a diet program.

I feel pretty good for being sixty-four. When I compare myself to other people my age, I think I am doing well. My energy is good, and I can work as much now as I could when I was younger. I would like to be thirty and know what I know now, but I don't feel like it's too late for me.

Oh, and by the way, I have been able to lose about twenty-five pounds and two pants sizes without cutting back my calories!

Dr. Schwarzbein: By improving his eating habits, Arthur has begun to heal his metabolism and is on his way to good health and improved body composition.

Insulin Sensitive to Full-Blown Insulin-Resistant: A Metabolic Continuum

———————————————— ➤ TIME ————————————————➤

	Insulin Sensitive	Partial Insulin Resistance	Full-Blown Insulin Resistance
Insulin levels	Fluctuate appropriately. Are low after a 12-hour fast and in between meals.	Fluctuate, but not as high or as low. However are still low after a 12-hour fast and in between meals.	Do not fluctuate normally. Insulin levels remain inappropriately high after a 12-hour fast and in between meals.
Symptoms of hypoglycemia	Can occur especially after eating a meal high in refined carbohydrates.	Does not usually occur. You get symptoms of hypoglycemia when you are insulin sensitive.	Does not occur because of insulin resistance.
Weight gain	You can gain weight if you eat poorly but not usually a rapid fat weight gain.	It is easier to gain fat weight now.	You already have fat weight around your midsection and are less likely to put on weight very quickly now.
Triglyceride levels	Triglyceride levels are normal after a 12-hour fast.	Triglyceride levels are normal after a 12-hour fast.	Triglyceride levels are high after a 12-hour fast.

Everyone starts off insulin-sensitive and then, because of poor nutrition and lifestyle habits over time, becomes partially insulin resistant. It is not until the cumulative effect of years of poor habits catches up to us that full-blown insulin resistance occurs. An exception to this pattern is seen in adolescence when children are going through puberty. Changes in growth hormones during this time put children at a higher risk of becoming full-blown insulin-resistant at an earlier age. There is an epidemic of insulin resistance in children now and it can be mostly attributed to the worsening of nutrition habits—increased caffeine and refined sugar consumption—in the countries in which this epidemic is found.

As Arthur said, the SPII program is not a diet. It is a way of life that will ensure proper balancing of all your hormones. If your hormones are balanced, you will regenerate efficiently, which leads to an improved metabolism and a lower risk for the degenerative diseases of aging. The good news is that the SPII program also works if damage has already occurred, as seen in Arthur's case. He cannot undo the fact that he had coronary bypass surgery, but he can prevent needing another surgery by taking better care of himself. It is never too late!

In summary, insulin is a major hormone that ensures we will continue to rebuild and not waste away. Unfortunately, if we secrete too much insulin over many years due to poor eating habits, like Arthur, we eventually rebuild too much, acquire insulin resistance and cause a higher risk for the degenerative diseases of aging.

The good news is that by improving your nutrition and lifestyle habits and balancing your insulin levels, you can prevent this from happening—or treat it, if it has already happened.

You have seen that both insulin and adrenaline imbalances can lead to lifestyle-based endocrine disorders. The same is true for cortisol imbalances. Annie's story in chapter 6 is all about cortisol.

Summary

- Insulin, a major hormone, prevents you from using up your biochemicals too much if you do not eat enough food.
- Insulin helps rebuild your enzymes, hormones, neurotransmitters, cells, and other functional and structural biochemicals.
- Your long-term survival depends upon your ability not to waste away in times of famine, as well as your ability to rebuild all of your biochemicals.
- It is important to eat the correct amount of carbohydrates for your current metabolism and activity level to avoid the over- or undersecretion of insulin.
- A low-insulin effect can occur with both high and low insulin levels and causes the same problems as too much adrenaline.

- When you digest carbohydrates, you break them down into sugar, and insulin is secreted in response to sugar entering the bloodstream.
- Excess sugars in the bloodstream are converted into two types of fats: triglycerides and cholesterol.
- Excess sugars in the bloodstream are more damaging to the human body than excess fats or excess insulin because excess sugars cause more free radical formation.
- Oxidation occurs when free radicals steal an electron from your tissues, thereby damaging your tissues.
- Antioxidants are your body's natural defense against free radical formation.
- Your goal is to be and/or stay insulin-sensitive. You are insulin-sensitive when all of the functions of insulin are working.
- Sustained high levels of insulin eventually lead to insulin resistance.
- High insulin levels can cause blocked arteries. You may have blocked arteries and not know it because they do not always cause chest pain.
- A list of myths and truths about your metabolism were listed in chapter 5. How many myths have you accepted as truths?
- Insulin resistance is an indicator of a damaged metabolism and increases the risk that you will develop the degenerative diseases of aging.
- By improving your nutrition and lifestyle habits and balancing your insulin levels, you can reverse or prevent insulin resistance.

* * *

You have now learned about two of the major hormones that affect how successfully you age: adrenaline and insulin. In chapter 6 we will take a look at cortisol, a major hormone that is not as well known as adrenaline and insulin. You may be surprised to learn what a big part cortisol plays in our high-stress lifestyles and how it can affect your health.

Six

Cortisol—
The Forgotten Hormone

M any of my patients have heard of both insulin and adrenaline, but when I ask them if they have heard of cortisol, the answer is usually no.

Cortisol, like adrenaline and insulin, is a major hormone. Along with adrenaline, cortisol is continuously being made and secreted by your adrenal glands and is one of the stress hormones of the body.

Functions of Cortisol

As you read about cortisol, keep in mind that for the purpose of simplicity we are going to consider the actions of cortisol as though it is the only hormone in your body telling your cells what to do. But remember—cortisol, like all hormones, never acts alone. All the hormones of the body are connected, and they help each other regulate all the same bodily functions.

Here are some of the things that happen when cortisol binds to its cell receptor sites.

Cortisol and Blood Pressure

One of cortisol's main functions is to keep your blood pressure from going too low. This helps your body sustain enough blood flow to the brain, heart and other organs. So cortisol is instrumental in keeping you alive. Cortisol makes sure your blood pressure does not get too low by regulating the firmness and stiffness of your arteries. Stiffer arteries maintain a higher pressure. Cortisol also plays a role in water regulation. The more water in your bloodstream, the higher the pressure.

Cortisol and Blood Sugar

Another important function of cortisol is that it helps the liver to store glycogen and increase new sugar production. This prevents severe hypoglycemia (low blood sugar).

Cortisol and Your Brain

Cortisol is one of the hormones responsible for mobilizing energy for your brain. Your brain requires sugar twenty-four hours a day to function, and it gets its sugar from the sugar in your bloodstream that is either supplied from food or from sugar made by your liver. If your blood-sugar levels start to drop, your body goes on emergency alert and secretes more cortisol. Cortisol directs your cells to break down your structural and functional proteins that are then converted by the liver into sugar for the brain. Cortisol also blocks the uptake of sugar into your muscle cells, which keeps more sugar in your bloodstream and makes it more available for brain fuel.

Another way that cortisol ensures that your brain gets a constant supply of sugar is to cause the breakdown of fats into glycerol and fatty acids. The glycerol can be converted into sugar for brain fuel, and the fatty acids fuel the conversion.

Finally, cortisol protects your brain by making sure your brain fats are not used up for fuel. Your brain is made up of 90 percent cholesterol and other fatty acids. When your body needs fuel and you do not eat, you want to make sure that your body does not eat your brain for energy. Cortisol protects your brain by mobilizing peripheral proteins and fats, instead of brain fats, to be used as energy.

Cortisol Helps Fight Inflammation

Cortisol also tells your body not to overdo inflammation. Inflammation is critical in the processes that fight off bacteria, viruses and other foreign proteins. Inflammation is also critical to healing injuries. However, too much inflammation can cause destruction of your own cells as well. By reducing the inflammatory response, cortisol helps you minimize cellular damage.

Cortisol—One of the Stress Hormones

The actions of cortisol occur in your body day in and day out whether or not you are stressed. But during acute stress, cortisol is secreted in much higher amounts.

When you experience acute stress, cortisol is oversecreted for many reasons. Besides raising your blood pressure, cortisol mobilizes your energy for movement and warmth and keeps your brain fed. Cortisol also helps your body fight off potential infections and inhibits the amount of inflammation in your body that might occur from an injury. You may never need all these functions of cortisol, but your body is prepared for them nonetheless.

When Cortisol Levels Are Too High or Too Low

There are many glandular-based endocrine causes of both low- and high-cortisol states. (See Tables 6.1 and 6.2.)

If cortisol production or levels are low, you may need to take cortisol hormone replacement therapy or stop taking the drugs that are causing the low cortisol state.

If cortisol production or levels are high, you need to have surgery, take medication to correct the high-cortisol problem or stop the steroid drugs that are causing the problem.

Do not be overly concerned about these types of cortisol endocrine disorders—except for the use of the glucocorticoid steroids—since they occur so infrequently. But if you do have one of these problems, you need to seek the help of an endocrinologist.

Table 6.1: Some Causes of Low Cortisol Levels

Addison's disease	An autoimmune destruction of the adrenal glands. Fortunately, this is a rare disease and most people will make adequate amounts of cortisol throughout their lifetimes so that they will not need to take cortisol hormone replacement therapy.
Secondary adrenal insufficiency	The adrenal glands are regulated by the pituitary through the production of a hormone called adrenocorticotropic hormone (ACTH). If the pituitary gland does not make adequate amounts of ACTH, the adrenal glands do not make adequate amounts of cortisol.
Congenital adrenal hypoplasia	A rare genetic condition where the adrenal glands are not fully formed.
Congenital adrenal hyperplasia	A rare genetic condition where there is an enzyme defect in the production of cortisol.
Surgical intervention	Surgical removal of the adrenal glands.

Adrenal gland destruction	Destruction caused by metastatic cancer, hemorrhage, lymphoma, or infections such as tuberculosis or fungal diseases.
Trauma	Damage to the adrenal glands caused by blunt or sharp trauma.
Drugs that have an effect on the production or action of cortisol	Ketoconizole (anti-fungal), Dilantin (anti-seizure), phenobarbital (antiseizure) and rifampin (antituberculosis drug) are some of the drugs that decrease cortisol levels by affecting enzymes that are involved in cortisol metabolism. The new abortion drug, mifepristone (RU 486), decreases the action of cortisol by blocking the binding of cortisol to its receptor site.

Table 6.2: Some Causes of High Cortisol Levels

Benign tumors	Benign tumors of the pituitary gland (overproduce ACTH) or adrenal glands (overproduce cortisol).
Cancer	Some cancers secrete high levels of ACTH, the hormone that directs the adrenal glands to produce more cortisol.
Hyperplasia	A bilateral enlargement of the adrenal glands.
Glucocorticoid steroids	These medications are used as anti-inflammatory agents in the treatment of asthma, arthritis, autoimmune disorders, allergic reactions and inflammation. Taking them chronically is one of the most common reasons for too much cortisol in the body.

Daily Cortisol Fluctuations—Annie's Story

The daily fluctuations in cortisol levels that occur in response to your nutrition and lifestyle habits can lead to lifestyle-based endocrine disorders. Therefore, what you do on a day-to-day basis is going to determine your cortisol levels and thus your quality and quantity of life.

If you have or have had poor nutrition and lifestyle habits that cause high-cortisol levels like Annie's (below), you need to learn what effect this has had on your body and how you can change your daily habits to find your way back to health.

If Annie had realized what her habits were doing to her metabolism and health, she would have changed them.

Annie: I grew up in a high-stress household. My mom and dad did not get along well, and I remember being very nervous about their relationship. I became the one who tried to hold things together, but I also looked for ways to get out of the house.

As an adolescent I took piano lessons and dance lessons, or I would go home with my friends after school. In high school I was on the swim team and student council, and I was a member of numerous clubs. I loved being busy because if I was busy doing something, I didn't have to be at home and deal with my family life.

I started puberty when I was ten years old. I began putting on weight and heard all sorts of comments about, "What a pretty face she has—what a shame." I wasn't obese by any means, but I wasn't a "skinny Minnie" either.

My mom took me to my family doctor when I was twelve because of my weight. He put me on diet pills and a nine-hundred-calorie-a-day diet. I lost the weight quickly, but it didn't stay off and I began a cycle of crash diets that lasted for a long time.

In my twenties I became a chemical "junkie" of sorts. I did not feel alert and alive without several cups of strong coffee and diet colas every day, and I would drink them instead of eating. I would drink strong coffee all day long for energy, and I would drink alcohol at night to relax.

I drank alcohol often at parties, after work with friends or at social gatherings. If I drank I didn't eat. I was basically living on coffee, diet colas and alcohol, and a little food because I did not want to gain weight.

As I got older, it became harder to diet and harder to take off weight. It always came back on, and I'd usually gain even more weight. I began to feel terrible about myself. I thought that everyone was staring at me and thinking I was so ugly and fat. I was wearing a size 10!

And what was worse was that I couldn't get that stimulant high anymore. No matter how many meals I skipped or how many stimulants I used, I couldn't maintain a sense of well-being.

Dr. Schwarzbein: Annie, like many women who come to see me, realized years later that wearing a size 10 is perfectly healthy and normal. Looking back, they all wonder what made them think otherwise, because today they would be very happy wearing a size 10. The pressure to wear a certain size of clothes—which leads to unhealthy dieting and stimulant use—is a leading cause of accelerated metabolic aging leading to the degenerative diseases of aging.

Annie's high-cortisol lifestyle habits caused her to use up her biochemicals faster than she could rebuild them, and she ended up with a badly damaged metabolism.

Stress and Cortisol

Stresses can be emotional, nutritional, chemical, physiological or hormonal. Your body responds identically to all these stresses because it cannot distinguish the differences between them. Stress responses are like reflexes—you get the same response no matter what the stimulus.

Cortisol was designed for survival stresses, not for self-induced ones caused by poor nutrition and lifestyle choices. If you encounter a life-threatening stress, higher cortisol levels will benefit you and help keep you alive. If the stress is self-induced, however, higher cortisol levels will damage you further. Since you live in the twenty-first century, you are living longer anyway because of cultural and scientific advances. Unfortunately, the stress responses of the body are designed more for prehistoric times than for modern ones. Therefore, cortisol's actions of trying to keep you alive longer from a stressful situation are not as beneficial as they once were.

The following are examples of life-threatening versus self-induced stresses. It is the self-induced stresses you have control over and need to address in order to stay healthy.

Emotional Stress

Life-threatening

When you secrete cortisol in response to emotional stress, your body does not know if you have encountered a modern-day equivalent of a saber-toothed tiger or a personal or work-related stress. No matter the cause of your emotional stress, whether it is life-threatening or not, your adrenal glands will secrete more cortisol.

If you need to mobilize energy and increase your blood pressure to send more blood to your cells so that you can run away from a "saber-toothed tiger," then this response is life-giving. Using up your biochemicals so you can run away will keep you alive longer.

Self-induced

However, if you are seated at your desk and upset with all the work you have piled up in front of you, then secreting more cortisol will raise your blood pressure and use up your energy reserves without much benefit to you. Using up your biochemicals in this situation will not keep you alive longer because there is no immediate threat to your life.

This chronic use of your biochemicals in response to emotional stresses causes you to age faster—it does not prolong your life. Therefore, the risk/benefit ratio of secreting more cortisol while you are seated at your desk becomes high.

Nutritional Stress

Life-threatening

Another time that cortisol is advantageous is in time of true famine. When there is not enough food available, your body mobilizes its functional, structural and energy biochemicals to be used as brain food as well as fuel for other vital functions of your body. Breaking down and using up your biochemicals to feed your brain will keep you alive longer. In other words, you are "eating yourself up to stay alive."

At the same time, your body begins shutting down nonessential functions such as your ability to get pregnant and to build nonessential tissues such as hair, skin and nails in order to survive. Your body understands that a famine is not the time to look good and attract a mate to have a baby. It is just trying to keep you alive.

Self-induced

However, if you diet or restrict calories, skip meals or eat junk food on purpose, your body perceives this as a famine, too—and you can shut down the same nonessential body functions. Using up your biochemicals and shutting down nonessential functions in this situation are not going to prolong your life because in today's world your life expectancy is already greater than a short-term famine.

In fact, this type of behavior will shorten your life. Again, the risks of excess cortisol outweigh the benefits. There is not a real famine, but your body cannot differentiate between the real and the artificial stresses. Therefore, you are using up your biochemicals unnecessarily, and you will age faster.

Chemical Stress

Life-threatening

Exposure to a poison is a chemical stress, and your body will respond to it with an outpouring of cortisol because it is one of the only defenses you have. Even though the likelihood that you will survive this type of stress is very low, your body will die trying. Since you are probably going to die anyway, secreting cortisol in this situation is not going to harm you in the long term.

Self-induced

In contrast, drinking too much alcohol is an example of self-poisoning, a forced chemical stress. Your body secretes cortisol to overcome the toxic effects of alcohol just as it would a lethal poison.

Too much alcohol blocks your liver from breaking down glycogen into sugar for brain energy, and cortisol helps your body bypass this blockage by breaking down your biochemicals to be used to make new sugar. This response is helpful so that you do not die from hypoglycemia (low blood sugar). But this is a self-induced artificial stress, and using up your biochemicals for this purpose will damage your metabolism. Therefore, drinking too much alcohol will age you faster.

Physiological Stress

Life-threatening

Exposure to extreme cold weather is an example of a physiological stress where the secretion of cortisol is lifesaving. Your ability to use up your biochemicals to stay warm is crucial to your survival.

Self-induced

Overexercising is also a physiological stress. Excessive movement may give you a feeling of well-being, but it uses up functional and structural biochemicals and ages you faster. This is probably why most elite athletes are not long-lived individuals.

Hormonal Stress

Life-threatening

The loss of any hormone is a stress to your body because all hormone systems are connected; if one hormone system is out of balance, they are all out of balance. If you stopped producing a major hormone, you would die rather quickly. But if you stopped producing a minor hormone, one of the major hormones such as cortisol would have to be secreted in higher quantities to try to take the place of the minor one. This would work for a short time to keep you feeling and functioning better, but the increased utilization of biochemicals that occurs over the long term would age you faster.

Self-induced

We now have the ability to replace many missing hormones. Choosing *not* to take hormone replacement therapy when it is needed is a stress to your body.

* * *

In summary, what all these stress responses have in common is that they are lifesaving in the short term and damaging in the long run. When we used to die at a younger age due to environmental stresses such as exposure, famine or accidents, the oversecretion of cortisol was life-giving because it protected us in stressful situations; we did not live long enough for it to harm us. But now that we are living longer, chronic high levels of cortisol as a result of poor nutrition and lifestyle choices are causing us to use up our biochemicals faster, which shortens our potential life span.

Why the Body Secretes Cortisol in Higher Levels

Stresses, including

Depression, mental stresses or other mental concerns (e.g., worrying about upcoming surgery)—to mobilize energy to keep your brain fed

Doing too many things or keeping busy all day long—to mobilize energy to keep your brain fed

Exposure to cold—to fight off infections and mobilize energy for warmth

Fever, illness or infection—to reduce inflammation and fight off infections

Fright—to mobilize energy and keep your blood pressure higher for sudden movement, and to reduce potential inflammation

Pain—to reduce inflammation

Severe burns, surgery and trauma—to reduce inflammation and fight off infections

Poor nutrition, including

Low blood-sugar levels, hypoglycemia or not enough carbohydrates in a meal—to mobilize energy to keep your brain fed

Low caloric intake or skipping meals—to mobilize energy to keep your brain fed

Certain chemicals, including

Alcohol—to mobilize energy to keep your brain fed

Marijuana—to mobilize energy to keep your brain fed

Exercise problems, including

Anticipation of an athletic competition—to mobilize energy to keep your brain fed and to mobilize energy and keep your blood pressure higher for sudden movement

Overexercising, especially cardiovascular exercises—to mobilize energy and keep your blood pressure higher for excessive movement, to mobilize energy to keep your brain fed and to reduce inflammation

Hormonal response

In response to adrenaline and insulin—to help your body balance the actions of these other major hormones.

The Effects of Too Much Cortisol

Most initial responses to acute stresses are lifesaving because your body is trying to keep you alive in response to the stressful situation. Short bursts of cortisol are good for you. However, chronic oversecretion of cortisol leads to excessive using up of structural and functional biochemicals. This causes depletion states such as a weakened immune system, infertility, a decrease in bone and muscle mass, loss of hair, thinning of skin, inability to grow nails, and a decrease in concentration and memory.

Below is a listing of some of the other disorders and symptoms of chronic high cortisol levels. As you read more about the damage caused by chronic oversecretion of cortisol, keep in mind that you are not trying to eliminate this hormone—you are trying to keep it balanced. Low levels of cortisol are more damaging in the short term than high levels are because cortisol is a life-giving hormone.

- Protein deficiency state—If you continuously convert your proteins into sugars, you will develop a protein deficiency state. This is manifested as symptoms or health problems such as depression, loss of memory and concentration, loss of lean body tissues—such as muscles and bone, or increased susceptibility to injuries.
- Type II diabetes
- High cholesterol and triglyceride levels
- Redistribution of your body fat from your arms and legs to your midsection. This type of midsection fat gain, known as the "apple shape" body, is a sign for increased risk of stroke, cancers, Type II diabetes and heart attacks.
- High blood pressure
- Weakened immune system
- Burned-out adrenal glands and more instead of less inflammation

Annie: In my thirties I decided it was time to get serious about my health. I began to exercise obsessively and eat a low-fat, high-carbohydrate diet. I taught aerobics, took up running, lifted weights and exercised hard about two hours a day. I continued to drink lots of coffee and diet colas because I honestly did not know that they were bad for me since they helped curb my appetite. I thought that anything that kept me from overeating was a good thing. They also helped keep me going during the day. I was miserable trying to keep up my workout schedule and eat this low-fat diet, but my goal was to be thin and healthy.

For the first time in my life my carbohydrate cravings were off the chart. I mostly ate carbohydrates such as low-fat cookies, nonfat ice cream and, especially, breads and cereals. I was surprised by these cravings because they were so strong. After an aerobics class I would run two miles to a restaurant and eat waffles with syrup—no butter, of course.

The USDA had just released their new food guidelines, the food pyramid. So I thought that I was supposed to be eating a lot of carbohydrates—and I would exercise harder to balance out my calorie consumption. I'd exercise more before and after I ate because I was afraid of gaining weight.

Dr. Schwarzbein: Annie's low-calorie, low-fat, high-carbohydrate diet and overexercising kept her cortisol levels high. She initially felt healthier because of her habits, but the chronic oversecretion of cortisol caused her to use up more functional and structural biochemicals than she could rebuild. She ended up with severe carbohydrate cravings and fatigue from the depletion of her serotonin levels. A low-serotonin state leads to an increase in carbohydrate cravings and a need for an energy boost around 3 to 4 P.M. daily. This is why she ate carbohydrates all day and drank caffeinated beverages.

Life Is Anti-Serotonin

From the moment you are born to the moment you die, you constantly use your brain to observe, create, think, multitask, memorize, worry, read and invent things. And these are just some of the many brain functions that occur on a daily basis. The more you do in a day, the more brain biochemicals you use in order to perform all your tasks. These brain biochemicals are called *neurotransmitters.* It is easy to use up our neurotransmitters because we are so busy nowadays.

Once you use up your neurotransmitters, you need to rebuild them. Efficient rebuilding of neurotransmitters is controlled by your hormones and requires that you eat balanced meals and get the right vitamins and minerals. Unfortunately, as we age and want to do more, we find ourselves limited by our declining ability to rebuild used up neurotransmitters. You experience this dilemma when you find yourself overwhelmed by daily tasks or when you are searching for words to complete a thought or sentence.

One of these neurotransmitters is called *serotonin.* Serotonin keeps you feeling calm and happy. If serotonin levels are low—and you do not feel calm and happy— it is harder to eat well, avoid ingesting toxic chemicals, manage stress and get the right amount of exercise.

Rebuilding Serotonin

Since how you think and feel depends on your serotonin levels, it is important to learn what you can do to help your body rebuild this neurotransmitter.

The analogy I like to use when I teach someone how serotonin is regenerated is to have them imagine a sink full of fluid with a brain submerged in it. The fluid in the sink is serotonin and when the sink is filled with serotonin, the brain is happy and functioning at its optimum. I use the image of the faucet flowing (at increased or decreased levels) as analogous to new serotonin production, and the image of the drain (plugged or unplugged) as analogous to serotonin utilization.

You can end up with low serotonin levels in three ways: production may be down (faucet flow is decreased), or utilization may be high (the drain is unplugged), or both production and utilization are off at the same time.

Signs and Symptoms of
Intermittent Low Serotonin Levels

If you have intermittent low serotonin levels, you may experience any or all of the following signs and symptoms:

- Body aches and pains
- Cravings for sugar, alcohol, caffeine, nicotine and/or recreational drugs
- Fatigue
- Headaches
- Insomnia
- Intestinal bloating
- Irritability
- Low memory and/or concentration
- Low mood

Syndromes and Disorders
Caused by Chronic Low Serotonin Levels

If your serotonin levels are chronically low, you may develop one or more of the following syndromes or disorders:

- Attention deficit disorder (ADD) or attention deficit/hyperactivity disorder (ADHD)
- Chronic fatigue syndrome
- Depression
- Fibromyalgia
- Irritable bowel syndrome
- Migraine headaches
- Premenstrual syndrome
- Seasonal affective disorder (SAD)

In order to correct your low-serotonin state, you need to increase your faucet flow and plug your drain.

Increasing faucet flow—or the production of serotonin—involves both making more serotonin and then secreting it as needed.

You make serotonin from tryptophan, an essential amino acid. You also make and secrete more serotonin in the summer and the daylight than in the winter and the darkness. Additionally, you secrete more serotonin in the presence of cortisol and adrenaline.

So to turn up your faucet flow you need to eat balanced meals, get enough exposure to sunlight and have healthy adrenal glands.

You increase your *utilization* of serotonin anytime cortisol and adrenaline levels get too high—that is, when you are awake, stressed, when you ingest alcohol and/or other stimulants such as refined sugar, nicotine and caffeine, or when your estradiol levels get too low.

Therefore, plugging your drain—or slowing down the utilization of serotonin—involves getting enough sleep, stress management, avoiding or tapering off toxic chemicals, and taking HRT, if needed.

Causes of Decreased Faucet Flow

- Artificial sugars; these damage the cells that make serotonin
- Burned-out adrenal glands
- Dieting
- Hypoglycemia
- Hypothyroidism
- Lack of sunshine
- Skipping meals
- Not eating enough proteins or healthy fats
- Not eating foods that contain tryptophan (see box, page 133)

Causes of "Unplugged" Drain

- Anger/hostility
- Being busy all day long
- Birth control pills
- Ingestion of refined sugars, caffeine and/or alcohol
- Low-estradiol levels caused by menopause/stress/malnutrition/genetic reasons
- Overexercising
- Stimulants
- Street drugs
- Stress
- Tobacco/nicotine
- Too much thyroid hormone or the use of Armour thyroid

Increasing Your Faucet Flow

Since serotonin is made from an essential amino acid called *tryptophan* that your body cannot make, you need to eat foods that contain tryptophan (see box) or take a tryptophan supplement in order to have the material you need to rebuild serotonin. (See Table 6.3.)

For the tryptophan that you eat or ingest to become serotonin, it has to cross the blood-brain barrier to get inside your brain, and this requires insulin. So it is important that you do not skip meals and that you eat enough carbohydrates for your current metabolism and activity level or else you will become hypoglycemic, which lowers the amount of insulin in your bloodstream.

Once inside the brain, tryptophan will first be converted into 5-hydroxy-tryptophan (5-HTP) and then 5-HTP becomes serotonin. These biochemical pathways require the minerals calcium and magnesium, essential fatty acids, C and B vitamins and many hormones, including insulin and thyroid.

Serotonin becomes melatonin when your environment is dark.

When it is night, winter, raining or foggy, or you just stay in a dark room, your body will convert more serotonin to melatonin, and this can lead to a low-serotonin state. Therefore, one way to increase your faucet flow is to get adequate light.

Additionally, if you eat balanced meals you will have all the materials you need to increase your faucet flow. But if you only eat carbohydrates, you will end up serotonin-depleted.

Restoring your serotonin levels is not as simple, however, as just eating balanced meals and getting adequate light. The rate at which you can make serotonin decreases as you get older—think of this as a decreased faucet flow. Therefore, it is also important as you get older to work on plugging your drain.

Tryptophan-Rich Foods

almonds	shellfish
cottage cheese	soy foods (tofu, tempeh, etc.)
oatmeal	tuna
peanut butter	turkey
peanuts	

Plugging Your Drain

Once your sink is half-full, increasing your faucet flow *without* plugging the drain will only keep your sink half-full. If you produce and use serotonin at the same rate, you will not restore your serotonin levels—you will only maintain them.

Here are some ways to plug your drain and increase serotonin levels.

Get some downtime. Downtime includes anything that puts your brain at rest, such as sleep, meditation, play, laughter, joy, reading and massage.

You can also rest your brain with exercise—if you do an exercise that you like and one that keeps you from thinking about anything else. For example, if you are making lists or figuring out your schedule while you are exercising, you are not getting downtime. Likewise, try to stay away from competitive sports if you get angry when you lose. Getting angry lowers your serotonin levels further and defeats the purpose of exercising for downtime.

Make sure you are eating enough to match your current metabolism and activity level or else you will become hypoglycemic. Also, be careful not to overexercise (see chapter 14), because overexercising unplugs your drain.

Using HRT to Plug Your Drain

If you are a woman, another plug for your drain is the hormone estradiol. It works to keep serotonin levels up by decreasing your brain's ability to eliminate serotonin. Your body loses its ability to produce estradiol during menopause, and you may experience depression or mood swings when this happens. Hormone replacement therapy (HRT) should improve serotonin levels in this situation. Most birth control pills block your estradiol action. This is why you should not take them for a long time, if at all.

Using Antidepressants to Plug Your Drain

Antidepressants known as selective serotonin reuptake inhibitors (SSRIs) also plug your drain by blocking the reuptake of serotonin into brain cells. Ideally, you would like to balance and restore your serotonin levels without needing these drugs. However, if your adrenal glands are burned out, if you are severely depressed or have been suicidal, do not quit taking your medication. Work on your nutrition and lifestyle habits first, and when your metabolism has improved, you can work with your physician to taper off your medication.

As long as you are working on your nutrition and lifestyle habits to heal your metabolism, taking an antidepressant drug is not the worst thing you can do to your health. It is when you use these types of medicines to make yourself feel better, but ignore your nutrition and lifestyle habits, that you will get worse over time by using them. However, they can have side effects, so make sure you work with a physician who is well-versed in these medications and their potential side effects.

Table 6.3: Natural Substances
to Help Increase Faucet Flow or Plug the Drain

Vitamin C	Increases flow
B vitamins	Increases flow
Omega-3 fatty acids	Increases flow
Tryptophan	Increases flow
5-hydroxy tryptophan (5-HTP)*	Increases flow
Calcium	Increases flow
Magnesium	Increases flow
Omega-6 fatty acids	Increases flow
S-adenosyl-methionine (SAMe)	Plugs the drain
St. John's wort	Plugs the drain

*New research suggests that long-term use of 5-HTP, a serotonin precursor supplement, may be harmful. Some brain cells are not designed to make serotonin. They cannot make serotonin because they cannot make 5-HTP. But given 5-HTP, these cells can make serotonin when they should not be doing so—and this is not good for you. If you need to be on a serotonin precursor on a daily basis for longer than one year, talk to your doctor about getting a prescription for tryptophan. The short-term or intermittent use of 5-HTP should be fine, but never take it with an antidepressant and never take more than 200 mg at bedtime without medical supervision. If you get anxiety, heart palpitations or bizarre sleep-disrupting dreams when you take either tryptophan or 5-HTP, reduce your dose or stop taking them altogether.

Yes, You *Do* Have Low Serotonin

Many people have a low-serotonin state but do not realize it because they do not feel depressed. But you can have low serotonin levels and not feel depressed if you are skipping meals or self-medicating with refined sugar, caffeine and/or alcohol all day long. These poor nutrition and lifestyle habits stimulate your body to recycle more serotonin into your brain—making you feel better temporarily. So if you were suddenly to eat regular meals and/or stop your self-medication, you might feel depressed because your low-serotonin state would be revealed.

If this happens to you, your adrenal glands are probably burned out, and you need to improve your nutrition and lifestyle habits in order to heal them and restore your serotonin levels. This takes time because your body is not capable of increasing serotonin production immediately. Be patient. The sink will fill up again. But while it is filling up, you may have to continue using caffeine (which keeps adrenaline effects higher) to keep your faucet flowing and/or an SSRI drug to plug the drain.

Remember, you are not healed until you have gone through a healing process. Improving your nutrition and lifestyle habits will start you through your transition, but it will take time to complete your transition.

How Addictions Develop

Stimulants and other toxic chemicals are addicting because they initially cause the release of a lot of serotonin into your brain, making you feel calm and happy. This is a feeling that people strive for every day. The irony is that these same toxic chemicals that give you an immediate release of serotonin cause you to use up more serotonin— or they damage the cells that make serotonin.

When serotonin levels are low, your body craves anything that will make serotonin levels rise, even if it is only temporary. Most people eat too many carbohydrates and/or refined sugars or they self-medicate all day long with caffeinated beverages such as coffee, tea, iced tea or sodas. Or they may smoke cigarettes, drink alcohol and/or use recreational drugs to keep their serotonin levels higher. This is how addictions get started and are maintained.

The American Lifestyle: A High-Cortisol Lifestyle

In the 1990s, Americans already had high-stress lifestyles that included television, telephones, fax machines and radio communications. But that stress was nothing compared with the amount of stress we are experiencing today. With the rising popularity of home computers and the availability of video games, e-mail and the Internet, new dimensions have been added to our already busy schedules. We are constantly bombarded with information, and we are in instant communication with everyone.

Hormonally, this means that our bodies secrete more cortisol. Our bodies break down as we use up biochemicals in order to process all this information and communication. And to make matters worse, we no longer have the time to take care of ourselves. We do not eat as well, sleep as much or exercise enough. Or we *over*exercise. The end result is that we are using up biochemicals more than we are rebuilding them. This leads to a hormonal imbalance that initially causes us to seek comfort behaviors.

Some people relieve their stress by overeating carbohydrates (comfort eating), some by drinking alcohol to relax (comfort drinking), others by excessive cardiovascular exercises and some by doing all of these things.

These behaviors may make you feel better in the short term. But since they do not lower your cortisol levels, and in some cases even raise your cortisol levels, you may develop the signs and symptoms of high cortisol levels (see box, page 138). Like Annie, you can have one, two, several or all of these conditions.

Signs and Symptoms of High Cortisol Levels

Acne, oily skin
Ankle swelling
Anxiety, panic attacks
Cataracts
Decreased energy
Decreased libido
Decreased memory and concentration
Depression
Easy bruising
Emotional lability (abrupt mood changes)
Fatigue
Hair loss
Headaches
High blood pressure
Higher levels of cholesterol
Increased appetite
Increased blood-sugar levels
Increased craving for sugar, nicotine and alcohol
Increased facial hair
Increased thirst
Insomnia
Impotence
Irritability
Loss of lean body tissue
Loss of bone mass
Lower back problems
Muscle weakness, especially in upper arms and thighs
Round or moon face with or without a ruddy complexion
Thinning head hair
Weight gain around the midsection

Lifestyle-Based Cortisol Disorders Can Lead to Disease

If you have a high-cortisol lifestyle, you will first experience the signs and symptoms of high cortisol levels listed on page 138. Over time, however, you will develop a degenerative disease of aging. The degenerative diseases most commonly associated with prolonged high cortisol levels are Type II diabetes, hypertension, stroke, osteoporosis, cholesterol abnormalities, depression and heart attacks. Although Annie had many health problems associated with a high-cortisol lifestyle, she changed her habits before she developed a degenerative disease of aging.

Annie: When I was thirty-five years old I ruptured three discs in my lower back after I took a bad fall, and my doctor gave me cortisone shots and pain pills. I continued to work for a year even though I was in pain. Finally he prescribed bedrest for a month and then I went through physical therapy to learn to live with my injury. But I did not learn how to slow down.

My hectic life resumed as soon as I could leave the house. I was on the go from the time I got up in the morning until I went to bed at night. I couldn't exercise like I had before because of my pain, and I immediately started gaining weight at an alarming rate.

As I gained weight, I tried new diets. I did Nutri-System, Jenny Craig and Weight Watchers. They would work for a while, but as soon as I went back to eating a normal diet, I gained weight again. I felt like a failure.

And if weight gain wasn't enough, I started to fall apart physically and emotionally. I couldn't sleep through the night anymore, I had new aches and pains, I couldn't exercise because I was injured, and my emotions were up and down. I was a mess. So I started drinking more frequently again. I'd have a glass or two of wine after work to unwind.

Dr. Schwarzbein: If you are like Annie and eating a normal diet makes you gain weight, you have a damaged metabolism. You will need to heal your metabolism first before you can lose weight. Stop trying to lose weight to be healthy. This does not work. You are only destroying your metabolism further if you continue to diet.

Alcohol and Cortisol

If you drink alcohol chronically, cortisol is secreted. In susceptible individuals this leads to alcoholism because cortisol initially gives you a feeling of well-being as you secrete neurotransmitters into your brain. Annie never became an alcoholic, but she did use alcohol to make herself feel better. She also used alcohol as a diet aid since drinking alcohol causes you to use up your biochemicals and may suppress your appetite.

High cortisol also causes redistribution of your body fat. It signals your body to take fat from your arms and legs and store it around your midsection. This is where the term "beer belly" comes from. However, some people do not drink alcohol and still have this body type (big belly, skinny arms and legs) from chronic stress. Either way, this is a sure sign of chronically high cortisol levels that are associated with an increased risk of all the degenerative diseases of aging.

Depression and High Cortisol Levels

Depression is also associated with higher levels of cortisol secretion. And higher levels of cortisol secretion can *cause* depression. This is a vicious cycle, but not everyone with chronic high cortisol levels will become depressed. Annie never did.

Steroids Are Cortisol Derivatives

One of the treatments for bulging or ruptured discs is the use of glucocorticoid steroids, such as prednisone, cortisone and medrol. Glucocorticoid steroids are drug derivatives of cortisol. They have the same action as your own cortisol but are much stronger. In Annie's case, these drugs were used for their anti-inflammatory property. The irony is that these types of drugs give immediate relief from inflammation, but the continual use of them will cause more tissue damage with time because, just like cortisol, they cause your body to break down structural biochemicals.

Taking steroid drugs for a long period of time also damages your metabolism. In fact, next to poor nutrition and lifestyle choices, steroid drugs are the biggest reasons for lifestyle-based causes of cortisol disturbances.

In certain circumstances, the use of glucocorticoid drugs will save your life. If you have a life-threatening situation, such as an asthma attack, and need to use these steroids, use them. You can recover from their side effects and heal the damage that they cause after you are better.

Your Bad Habits Will Catch Up with You!

Stopping exercise will only cause weight gain if you already have a damaged metabolism. Annie had destroyed her metabolism from poor nutrition and lifestyle habits long before she stopped exercising. Her rapid weight gain was just one more sign that her chronic high-cortisol lifestyle had caught up with her.

Annie: I ended up in Dr. Schwarzbein's office five years ago for hormone replacement therapy (HRT) after I had a hysterectomy at age forty-four. I was losing my hair, I was weepy and irritable, and I couldn't sleep at night. I was fat besides.

I developed allergies, and I would break out in hives for no reason. I even had asthma one winter, and I had never had asthma before in my life. Prior to seeing her I had been tested for diabetes, cancer, and thyroid disease. Nothing showed up on those tests, so I was very surprised when she told me that I had more wrong with me than just the need for estrogen hormone replacement therapy. I thought that estrogen alone would solve everything.

After starting HRT and beginning to improve my lifestyle, I freaked out when I began to gain weight. There were times I actually thought about throwing my hormones out the window and dumping the eating plan for a nine-hundred-calorie diet. I fought the program for the first two years. I had a hard time believing that this plan could be good for me because I was getting fatter and I was still craving sweets. But I knew deep down inside that what Dr. Schwarzbein was telling me was the answer. I'd spent almost three decades living a crash-diet lifestyle, and it obviously didn't work. I trusted Dr. Schwarzbein and decided to stick with it even when I was very discouraged. She kept telling me to hang in there, that it would take time to heal because of all the years of damage that I had done to my body.

Dr. Schwarzbein: When I first met Annie I was not sure if all her problems were related to her lack of estrogen or not since I was not aware of her whole life history. Annie and I worked together for months to get her menopause HRT perfected, and some of her symptoms such as lack of energy, hair loss, irritability and sense of well-being improved. Her weepiness went away completely. It only became clear that something else was wrong when her blood tests showed that her estrogen hormones were balanced but she continued to complain of weight gain and insomnia.

One Hormone Problem Can Mimic Another

When more than one hormone system is out of balance, it is sometimes difficult to recognize which hormone is causing problems. The first hormone system that must be addressed is the one that is obviously missing. If HRT of that system does not improve all of your symptoms, the loss of that hormone is not the cause of all of your problems. It is time to look elsewhere.

High cortisol levels due to poor nutrition and lifestyle habits mimic many other hormonal problems. Most people with high cortisol levels feel that their thyroid levels are low, or they are insulin-resistant: All three of these hormonal problems cause weight gain and the inability to lose weight despite dieting. If you have many of the signs and symptoms of a high-cortisol lifestyle (see box, page 138), and have had your thyroid, insulin or other hormone systems checked with normal results, then, like Annie, you may have a lifestyle-based endocrine imbalance that involves too much cortisol. Alternatively, you may have a lifestyle-based endocrine imbalance that involves too *little* cortisol.

Cortisol—Too Much or Too Little?

Since all hormones are connected, there is a great overlap between the symptoms and signs of low- or high-hormone states. High cortisol levels make you gain fat weight around your midsection; low cortisol levels make it impossible for you to burn off fat weight. The symptom looks to be one and the same to you—you are overweight! The only way to distinguish between low or high cortisol is to test your adrenal gland function. In the December 2001 issue of the medical journal the *Endocrinologist*,* Swedish researchers tested the reliability of saliva cortisol levels and found them to be accurate. They also classified different degrees of adrenal gland function (from healthy function to adrenal gland burnout) based on these studies. Ask your physician to test your adrenal glands or visit my Web site at *www.SchwarzbeinPrinciple.com* to find out how you can be tested.

High Cortisol or High Insulin?

When you have too much cortisol, you will have a lot of the same symptoms and signs as when you have too much insulin—you over-build fats, have high blood pressure and can develop Type II diabetes. Since cortisol is one of the anti-insulin hormones (it blocks the action of sugar uptake in the muscle cells), high cortisol levels is one of the major causes of insulin resistance. You can see how confusing this all can become, but let me try to simplify this by saying that you need to measure your hormone levels to determine which hormone(s) is causing the problems. If it looks like high insulin, it may be high cortisol instead. Have your fasting insulin levels tested by a reputable lab, and have your cortisol levels tested through saliva testing.

Roland Rosmond, M.D., Ph.D., et al. The Endrocinologist Vol. 11, #6, "Alterations in the hypothalamic pituitary adrenal axis in metabolic syndromes," 12/01 pgs. 491–497.

Low-Cortisol, Lifestyle-Based Endocrine Disorders

Because low-cortisol, lifestyle-based endocrine disorders cause the same type of problems and diseases that low-adrenaline, lifestyle-based endocrine disorders do, they will not be discussed here. (See chapter 4 for the problems and diseases associated with low-adrenaline [low-cortisol], lifestyle-based endocrine disorders.)

Gaining Weight: Do Not Give Up!

Like many of my patients, Annie was unhappy and ready to throw in the towel when she began to gain weight. It is very difficult psychologically to believe in a program that causes you to gain weight initially, even when you know intellectually that you are improving your habits. But there is no other way to heal.

If you are hormonally out of balance, your current weight does not reflect your true metabolism. You may think that you have a better metabolism than you really do because you have learned to equate how good your metabolism is with how much you weigh. But remember, your hormones, *not* your weight, determine your metabolism.

Even if you are overweight to begin with, you may still weigh less than you would have if your cortisol levels had not been high. Chronic high-cortisol levels decrease your lean body tissue and make you weigh less because your body is using up your functional and structural proteins and fats.

In the process of rebalancing your hormones, you will first unmask your true physiology. Before you can burn off the fat that has been stored, you have to rebuild your functional and structural biochemicals. As you rebuild your biochemicals, you will also store some fat. Therefore, you have to gain weight to heal your metabolism so that you can achieve your ideal body composition. As Annie, Arthur and I had to find out the hard way, there are no shortcuts.

Annie: Dr. Schwarzbein suspected my cortisol levels were too high and were probably working against the healing program. She began to question me about the stresses in my life. She found out I worked at least two jobs all the time and that when things slowed down in my life, I either went looking for something to create a little excitement or life handed me something new to deal with. I got married, we built a house, a relative was sick, my husband's job was in jeopardy, I started my second master's degree—she was always amazed when I went in to her office and told her how things were going. It seemed my life was always in turmoil or a state of high excitement. I thrived on stress, but I didn't realize that was what I was doing. As she began to explain the effects of high cortisol to me, it was as if she were reading me the shortened version of my life story. Her message finally got through to me.

For the past three years I have made a big effort to eat better and exercise consistently, but it wasn't until six months ago (September 2001)—when I finally started to work on stress management—that I began to feel better than I've felt in a long time. I now work only one job, and I've learned what I can control and change to eliminate unneeded stress. I'm learning to pamper myself. I guard my free time, I stop saying yes to everyone who asks, I get pedicures and I enjoy being with my husband.

I haven't healed completely from my high-stress lifestyle, but I'm on my way. I have a strong belief in God and know I don't need to control every single element of my life. I'm calmer and more content than I've ever been.

My waistline is coming back and I can see my body composition starting to change. I've learned that it isn't my looks that matter but my health. I know that my weight will continue to drop and that this time it will stay off because I'm not on a diet. I've made eating and habit changes for life.

Dr. Schwarzbein: The SPII program is a five-step program. You can improve your quality of life by addressing a few of these steps. However, if you want to completely heal your metabolism and achieve your ideal body composition, you have to address all of the program's five areas. Even though Annie had made great strides in improving her health by changing her eating habits, exercising and taking HRT, she did not start to see changes in her waistline until she tapered off caffeine and worked on managing her stress. But as I told Annie, she was right on track. Even the most well-intentioned person cannot make all the necessary changes in nutrition and lifestyle habits at one time. This program is a process; it is not a diet.

It Is Never Too Late to Heal

Annie felt like a failure when dieting and overexercising did not keep her thin and healthy because she did not know what else to do. The more she tried, the worse she got. Are you in this situation? If your story is like Annie's, do not despair. It is never too late to heal. If, like Annie, you have a lifestyle-based endocrine disorder from a cortisol imbalance, now is the time to take charge and reverse your hormone imbalance before you get a degenerative disease of aging. Or if you already have a degenerative disease, it is time to heal. But like Annie, you, too, will have to go through a transition of healing by changing your nutrition and lifestyle habits so that you can achieve optimum health.

Summary

- Cortisol, a major hormone, is made and secreted by the adrenal glands.
- Cortisol's life-sustaining functions are to keep blood pressure and blood sugar from going too low.
- Cortisol is secreted in times of emotional, nutritional, chemical, physiological or hormonal stress.
- Stress responses are like reflexes—you get the same response no matter what the stimulus.
- During acute stress, cortisol helps raise blood pressure, mobilize energy for movement and warmth, and keep your brain fed. It also inhibits inflammation and helps your body fight infections.

- Over time, the daily fluctuations in your cortisol levels caused by poor nutrition and lifestyle habits can lead to lifestyle-based cortisol disorders.
- The American lifestyle is a high-cortisol lifestyle.
- Chronic oversecretion of cortisol leads to excessive using up of biochemicals, leaving you with depletion states such as a weakened immune system, infertility, a decrease in lean body mass, hair loss, thinning skin, inability to grow nails, and a decrease in concentration and memory.
- Chronic oversecretion of cortisol can lead to a serotonin-depleted state.
- Since how you think and feel is dependent on serotonin, it is crucial to make sure that you have enough serotonin. In order to correct your low-serotonin state, you need to increase its production and decrease its utilization.
- Short-term use of glucocorticoid steroids (cortisol derivatives) helps inflammation, but long-term use will cause tissue damage.
- High cortisol levels caused by poor nutrition and lifestyle habits mimic other hormonal problems.
- Low cortisol, lifestyle-based endocrine disorders cause the same types of problems and diseases that low-adrenaline, lifestyle-based endocrine disorders do.
- A chronic high-cortisol lifestyle will lead to one or more of the degenerative diseases of aging.
- It is never too late to prevent or treat a lifestyle-based cortisol endocrine disorder.

* * *

By now you are beginning to understand how the individual major hormones regulate the different functions of your body and affect your health and longevity. But as I have said all along, all the hormones of the body are connected—they help each other regulate all the same bodily functions. In chapter 7, we will put all the major hormones together and also take a look at some of the minor hormones that affect your aging process.

Seven

Putting It All Together

It is now time to put together all the information you have learned so far and determine what you need to do to improve or heal your metabolism so that you can slow down or reverse your aging process.

So far we have looked at adrenaline, insulin and cortisol as separate hormones that direct which functions your cells will carry out. By now you have probably noticed that the symptoms and problems associated with imbalances in adrenaline, cortisol and insulin overlap. As stated in previous chapters, none of these hormones acts alone. This is because all hormones are connected, and they are helping each other regulate all the same biochemical reactions at the same time. It is time to learn how they all interact with each other and how they affect your aging process. But first, let's review what you have learned.

Slowing Down/Reversing the Aging Process

As discussed earlier, slowing down or reversing your aging process depends on improving your metabolism. A healthy metabolism depends on your body's ability to regenerate efficiently. Your body's ability to regenerate efficiently depends on your hormones. *You* control your hormones because nutrition and lifestyle habits determine which hormone(s) will be secreted and in what quantity. Therefore, by keeping your hormones balanced through healthy nutrition and lifestyle habits, you determine your health and your aging process.

Remember, regeneration is the combination of using up and rebuilding your body's biochemicals. You use up your biochemicals as you go about your daily routine and then rebuild new biochemicals to use again when your body is resting—after you eat and while you sleep.

The ideal is to have all your regeneration reactions in balance— what you use up, you rebuild. Since your hormones determine how your body regenerates, you need to balance the hormones that use up your biochemicals and the hormones that rebuild your biochemicals to keep these reactions in balance. Each type of hormone needs to balance out the other so that you are not using up your biochemicals more than rebuilding them, or rebuilding them more than using them up.

Major and Minor Hormones: Balance Is the Key

The major hormones keep you currently alive because they are responsible for maintaining life-sustaining functions. The minor hormones also play a role in your body's health, but their role is not as obvious. Most of the growth hormones of the body are minor hormones. Their main role is to help you rebuild—something you can neither feel nor see while it is happening. Both types of hormones play a role in the quality of your life.

In general, when your body is out of balance, it is because your major-hormone levels have been too high for too long, leading to, among other problems, a decrease in your minor-hormone levels, and possibly even your major-hormone levels as well.

As stated throughout this book, you do not want to get rid of your major hormones. If your major-hormone levels are too high or too low, what you want to do is change your nutrition and lifestyle habits to bring them back into balance. You also do not want too many or too few minor growth hormones either. Balance is the key.

Balancing Your Hormones: It's Easier Than You Think!

The good news is that your hormones are connected. If you improve your nutrition and lifestyle habits, you will be able to balance all your hormones, unless your body can no longer make a specific hormone. If that is the case, you need hormone replacement therapy (HRT).

Since all your hormones communicate with one another, what balances one hormone will balance the others. With this in mind, you are going to learn how to balance all your hormones by balancing just a few of them.

Adrenaline, Cortisol and Insulin Are Always Present

In chapter 4 you read that adrenaline helps you access all the different biochemicals of your body. Therefore, it is one of the "using up" hormones. In chapter 5 you read that insulin helps you rebuild your biochemicals *and* slows down your ability to use up your biochemicals; therefore, insulin is a "rebuilding" hormone. Chapter 6 explained how cortisol helps you use up proteins, fats and sugar biochemicals, but if your cortisol levels stay too high for too long, you will store fat around your midsection. For the sake of simplicity, you should still consider cortisol a "using up" hormone.

But none of these hormones is present in your body by itself. They are all there together, and the amounts of each of these hormones in your bloodstream determines the functions of your cells. That is why balance is so important. Any and all chronic imbalances between your major hormones will damage your metabolism.

Adrenaline and Cortisol

If adrenaline levels and cortisol levels are high, but adrenaline levels are higher than cortisol levels, you are using up *all* your biochemicals faster than you can rebuild them.

If both hormone levels are high, but adrenaline levels are lower than cortisol levels, you use up proteins and sugars faster, but not necessarily your fats.

Adrenaline and Insulin

If both adrenaline and insulin levels are high, and your adrenaline levels are higher than insulin levels, you are using up *all* your biochemicals faster than you can rebuild them. But not as fast as when your insulin levels are low.

If both hormone levels are high, and your insulin is higher than adrenaline, you are rebuilding *all* your biochemicals faster than you can use them up. But you are not rebuilding as fast as you would be if your adrenaline levels were low instead of high.

Insulin and Cortisol

If both cortisol and insulin levels are high, but cortisol is higher than insulin, you use up your proteins and sugars but store more fat weight around your midsection. You would store less fat weight and use up more proteins and sugars if your insulin levels were normal or low.

If both hormone levels are high, but insulin is higher than cortisol, you will rebuild more proteins and sugars and store weight around your midsection. You would rebuild more proteins and sugars and store less weight if your cortisol levels were normal or low.

Adrenaline/Cortisol and Insulin

If the ratio of your adrenaline/cortisol levels is higher than your insulin levels, you will use up your biochemicals faster than you can rebuild them, especially if your insulin levels are low or normal.

If the ratio of your adrenaline/cortisol levels is lower than your insulin levels, you will rebuild your biochemicals faster than you can use them, especially if your adrenaline/cortisol levels are low or normal.

Caution: Do Not Use Up Your Biochemicals Faster Than You Can Rebuild

How much you do on a daily basis determines your need for biochemicals. The more you do, the more you need. The more you use up your biochemicals, the more you need to rebuild them. If you use up your biochemicals faster than your body can rebuild them, you are destroying your metabolism and accelerating your aging process. Therefore, you do not want to use up your biochemicals more than you can rebuild them for too long.

If you chronically diet, overexercise, ingest too many stimulants and are under too much stress, you will use up your functional, structural and energy (including storage) biochemicals faster than you can rebuild them. If this were to go on unchecked, you would not survive. Since your body wants to keep you alive while you are engaging in these habits, it will secrete more insulin to try to slow down the damage. Since you will not be able to maintain this high-adrenaline/ cortisol lifestyle forever, when you stop your dieting, overexercising or using stimulants, or you manage your stress better, your body initially will secrete a large amount of insulin. This excessive insulin release is the only way your body has to repair itself. Higher insulin levels help your body rebuild all the functional, structural and energy biochemicals it lost during the stress but what you rebuild is dependent on what you eat. You will rebuild all these biochemicals plus more fat as long as you are eating healthy, balanced meals. If you are eating junk food or too many carbohydrates, you will rebuild mostly fat biochemicals.

Table 7.1 summarizes the activity of the major hormones—adrenaline, insulin and cortisol—and the minor growth hormones—DHEA, human growth hormone (HGH) and thyroid. Each major hormone is listed separately to emphasize that your body responds differently to each of these hormones. The minor growth hormones are grouped together because they all basically act in the same way.

By understanding the triggers and actions of these six hormones, you can make necessary changes in your nutrition and lifestyle habits that fit your individual needs.

Table 7.1: Major and Minor Hormones: Triggers and Actions

Hormone/Type	Triggers	Actions
Adrenaline* Using up Hormone**	Acute stress, being busy, skipping meals, stimulants, diets, lack of sleep, low-carb intake, low estrogen, most BCPs, high progestogens, high androgens (DHEA or testosterone), overdoing cardiovascular exercises, refined sugars, high-protein intake	Keeps heart beating Uses up proteins Uses up fats Uses up glycogen/sugar
Insulin* Rebuilding Hormone**	Carbohydrates: If you eat only carbohydrates, you will mostly rebuild glycogen or fat. These fats are used as energy or stored. Meals: If you eat balanced meals from the SPII program, that is, follow the PFVC plan***, you rebuild proteins, fats and glycogen. These fats are used for structure or energy, or they can be stored. Any habit that increases adrenaline and/or cortisol levels triggers insulin.	Prevents wasting away Keeps you rebuilding Builds proteins if you eat proteins Builds fats if you eat carbs or fats Builds glycogen if you eat carbs

*Major hormone; **Using up or rebuilding hormone (a hormone is considered to be a using up hormone if it uses up proteins; a rebuilding hormone if it builds up proteins); ***PFVC stands for protein, healthy fat, nonstarchy vegetable and real carbohydrate; ****Minor hormones

Cortisol* Using up** Hormone	Chronic stress, skipping meals, low-carb intake, overdoing any type of exercise, diets, chronic lack of sleep, alcohol, glucocorticoid steroids	Helps maintain blood pressure Uses up proteins Uses or builds fats Uses up glycogen
Growth Hormones****: HGH, DHEA, and Thyroid Rebuilding Hormones**	Balanced adrenaline, cortisol and insulin, REM sleep, balanced meals, resistance-training exercises, adequate sex steroids, serotonin. Each requires adequate levels of the other growth hormones.	Build proteins Use up fats Use up glycogen/sugar

*Major hormone; **Using up or rebuilding hormone (a hormone is considered to be a using up hormone if it uses up proteins; a rebuilding hormone if it builds up proteins); ***PFVC stands for protein, healthy fat, non-starchy vegetable and real carbohydrate; ****Minor hormones

Major Hormones

Remember, all of your major hormones work together, but it is easier for you to determine the lifestyle changes you need to make by considering their actions alone again. Let's briefly review the actions and triggers of each major hormone individually.

Adrenaline

Half of a healthy metabolism is the ability to use up your biochemicals, and adrenaline is one of the hormones that lets your body do this. Adrenaline helps you access and use your biochemicals for all of your daily activities, and it helps you access and use your food for energy so that your body can perform all its functions. It also signals the breakdown of old cells to make room for new ones, keeping your cells younger and functioning better.

Below is a list of items that trigger adrenaline. As you read this list, you will realize that you cannot stop your daily activities—and you should not; you are not trying to eliminate everything that triggers adrenaline. Remember, this hormone keeps your heart beating. However, you *do* want to make changes in the habits that continuously keep your daily adrenaline levels too high. If your adrenaline levels are too high, you will use up your biochemicals too quickly and age faster.

Check off all the adrenaline triggers that pertain to you. The step number that follows each trigger corresponds to one of the five steps in the SPII program and should be used as a guide to help you make the necessary changes to your nutrition and lifestyle habits.

To refresh your memory, the five steps of the SPII program are:

Step 1 (chapter 11): Healthy nutrition, including supplementation
Step 2 (chapter 12): Stress management, including getting enough sleep
Step 3 (chapter 13): Tapering off/avoiding toxic chemicals
Step 4 (chapter 14): Cross-training exercises
Step 5 (chapter 15): Hormone replacement therapy (HRT), if needed

Adrenaline Triggers

☐ **Skipping meals** Food is the material you use for energy and to rebuild, so make it a priority to never skip a meal again. This is a very easy way to help keep adrenaline levels from going too high. Learn why skipping meals destroys your metabolism. **(Step 1)**

☐ **Dieting** Restrictive diets cause your body to use up biochemicals faster than it can rebuild them. Since dieting destroys your metabolism, it is important that you never go on a fad diet again. Learn to eat balanced meals. **(Step 1)**

☐ **Low carbohydrate intake** Eating too few carbohydrates is just as damaging as consuming too many. Learn to eat the right amount of carbohydrates for your current metabolism type and activity level. **(Step 1)**

☐ **High protein intake** Consuming too much protein is just as harmful as not eating enough protein. Learn the signs and symptoms of consuming too much protein. **(Step 1)**

☐ **Acute stress** You will not be able to completely avoid stress throughout your life, but you can learn how to manage and respond to it better. **(Step 2)**

☐ **Being busy** The more you do, the more biochemicals you use up. Decide what is really important to you. Instead of prioritizing your schedule, learn to schedule your priorities. **(Step 2)**

☐ **Lack of sleep** Your body does most of its rebuilding during the time it is in REM (dream) sleep, so if you do not get enough REM sleep you age faster. Learn what you need to do to get enough REM sleep. **(Step 2)**

☐ **Refined sugars** Because your body cannot use refined sugars to rebuild, eating excessive amounts of refined sugars destroys your metabolism. Learn how to successfully taper off refined sugars. **(Step 3)**

☐ **Using stimulants** The use of stimulants is usually a form of self-medication and indicates a hormonal imbalance. Learn which stimulants are the worst for your body and how to successfully taper off them. **(Step 3)**

☐ **Birth control pills (BCPs)** Birth control pills destroy your metabolism. Learn how dangerous these drugs really are. **(Step 3)**

☐ **Overdoing cardiovascular exercises** You *can* overexercise, which causes your body to use up biochemicals faster than it can rebuild them. Learn how to cross train to keep your hormones balanced. **(Step 4)**

☐ **Low estrogen levels** If your estrogen levels are too low you are not rebuilding effectively. Learn the nutrition and lifestyle changes you need to make to produce estrogen more efficiently. **(Steps 1 through 4)**

☐ **Menopause** If you are in menopause, learn the four rules to ensure you take HRT correctly. **(Step 5)**

☐ **High progestogens** Both progesterone and Provera are progestogens. Progesterone is the natural or bioidentical progestogen. This means it is the hormone made in your body.

Contrary to popular belief, you can get too much progesterone. Too much of any hormone is just as harmful as too
little. Provera is a man-made progestogen—a drug not found
in nature—and is not bioidentical to any hormone found in
your body. Any amount of unnatural progestogen is bad for
you. Learn why it is important to take the bioidentical hormone that used to be made in your body. **(Step 5)**

❏ **High androgens (DHEA or testosterone)** Have your DHEA-S (a
metabolic breakdown product of DHEA) levels evaluated if
you are taking DHEA. If this level is high, you are taking too
much DHEA. Have your free testosterone and luteinizing hormone (LH) levels evaluated if you are taking real testosterone
replacement therapy. LH is the pituitary hormone that determines if you have too much or too little testosterone. If LH is
high, you have too little testosterone; if LH is low, you have too
much testosterone. If you take a synthetic testosterone such as
methyl-testosterone, discuss changing to a bioidentical form
with your physician. Learn why it is important to measure your
hormone levels when you are taking HRT. **(Step 5)**

Insulin

Insulin counters the actions of adrenaline and cortisol and is your
universal rebuilding hormone. Insulin is important because it keeps
you from using up more than rebuilding your biochemicals. Insulin
tells the body to rebuild functional, structural and energy biochemicals from the proteins, fats and carbohydrates that you eat.

You can only rebuild if you eat, however, and what you rebuild depends
on what you eat. Proteins are made from other proteins. Healthy fats can
be made into structural and functional fats such as cell membranes and
hormones. Sugar may be used for energy, biochemically combined with
other sugars to build the human carbohydrate glycogen, or it may be converted into fats to be stored for later energy needs (storage fats).

Eating a high-carbohydrate, low-fat diet leads to more rebuilding of carbohydrates and storage fats—and much less rebuilding of functional and structural proteins and fats.

Eating the SPII program way—using the PFVC formula*—supplies your body with what it needs to rebuild efficiently. What you eat determines what you rebuild on a day-to-day basis. This is something over which you have complete control and can learn to do well.

Any habit that triggers the release of adrenaline and/or cortisol also causes a release of insulin to prevent your body from using up its biochemicals completely and to signal the need for rebuilding. This is a good thing. If you did not have a means of communicating to your body that it needed to stop using up its biochemicals quickly, or that it needed to rebuild, you would only use them up, and you would not survive for very long. The way to balance high insulin levels, in this case, is to work on the habit that triggered one of the using-up hormones.

Check off all the insulin triggers that pertain to you. The step number that follows each trigger corresponds to one of the five steps in the SPII program and should be used as a guide to help you make the necessary changes to your nutrition and lifestyle habits. See page 156 for the five steps.

Insulin Triggers

- ☐ **Eating too many carbohydrates** Learn to eat the amount of carbohydrates that you require for your current metabolism and activity level. **(Step 1)**
- ☐ **Eating unbalanced meals** Balanced meals consist of healthy proteins, healthy fats, nonstarchy vegetables and the right amount of real carbohydrates for your current metabolism type and activity level. If you already eat balanced meals, you do not need to work on this step. However, if you do not eat balanced meals, learn about the four food groups. **(Step 1)**
- ☐ **Any habit that increases adrenaline and/or cortisol levels** Work on balancing your nutrition and lifestyle habits so that

*A PFVC meal includes healthy proteins, healthy fats, nonstarchy vegetables and real carbohydrates.

you can keep your body from using up too many functional and structural biochemicals and overbuilding storage fats. **(Steps 1 through 5)**

Cortisol

Like adrenaline and insulin, cortisol is also a major hormone. It helps your body maintain your blood pressure, use proteins for function and energy, and use glycogen for energy. It also helps your body mobilize fats to be used in times of real stress, but these fats will be stored in times of chronic artificial stress. It is an important hormone to maintain good health, but as with all hormones, too much cortisol over long periods of time will destroy your metabolism.

However, you do not want to eliminate cortisol completely. This hormone keeps you alive. For example, being overly busy is a stress that triggers your body to release more cortisol, and you do not want to completely stop everything that you are doing to keep from secreting any cortisol. Instead, learn to manage your daily activities better to balance your cortisol.

You will notice that the triggers for cortisol and adrenaline overlap. They are both stress hormones and are secreted together in times of stress. The big difference between their triggers is that alcohol, a depressant, raises cortisol levels, while stimulants increase adrenaline effects.

Check off all the cortisol triggers that pertain to you. The step number that follows each trigger corresponds to one of the five steps in the SPII program and should be used as a guide to help you make the necessary changes to your nutrition and lifestyle habits. See page 156 for the five steps.

Cortisol Triggers

☐ **Low carbohydrate intake** If you do not eat enough carbohydrates, your body will use its proteins for brain fuel and this will destroy your metabolism. Learn how to balance your meals. **(Step 1)**

☐ **Skipping meals** Your body perceives skipping meals as a stress. If you never skip a meal again, you will be eliminating one of the unnecessary triggers of cortisol. Learn how many times to eat during a day. **(Step 1)**

☐ **Dieting** There is nothing good about losing weight quickly. Quick weight loss from dieting uses up your functional and structural biochemicals as well as your energy biochemicals and destroys your metabolism. Learn how good nutrition leads to good health. **(Step 1)**

☐ **Chronic stress** Stress triggers the release of cortisol and adrenaline together. If the stress is acute, adrenaline levels are higher than cortisol levels. If the stress is chronic, cortisol becomes the main hormone released. Though you will not be able to completely avoid stress throughout your life, you can avoid self-imposed stress. Learn how to include downtime in your daily schedule. **(Step 2)**

☐ **Chronic lack of sleep** You will never achieve hormonal balance if you are not sleeping enough. Learn how many hours of sleep are needed for optimum health. **(Step 2)**

☐ **Alcohol** Alcohol is a toxin, so it is best to avoid it completely. But if you must drink it, drink wine or beer only and keep your consumption to a minimum. Learn how to taper down or off alcohol completely. **(Step 3)**

☐ **Glucocorticoid steroids** These synthetic hormones are used in some situations to save your life. However, the risk-to-benefit ratio is not worth it in non-life-threatening situations. Discuss your need for these drugs with your physician, and if you do not need them, learn how to taper off them. **(Step 3)**

☐ **Overdoing exercise** Working out excessively is not good for you. Learn how to exercise "smarter" not "harder." **(Step 4)**

The Minor Growth Hormones

Human growth hormone (HGH), DHEA and thyroid are some of the minor hormones that signal your body to rebuild proteins and break down fats and glycogen.

These hormones have been promoted as the keys to antiaging throughout the past decade, and they are still getting much media attention today. This claim is partly true. The loss of any one of these three hormones does lead to accelerated aging. However, any one of the major hormones—adrenaline, cortisol or insulin—plays a larger role in antiaging. In fact, one of the biggest factors that causes a decrease in these minor hormones is the over- or undersecretion of any of the major hormones.

Understanding that the major hormones play a greater role in anti-aging and that the minor hormones play a lesser role helps to put these hormones into perspective. The most important thing you can do is balance out your major hormones. Once you have achieved this, your body has the chance to improve its production of your minor hormones. Give your body time to heal before you consider taking HRT. *An exception to this rule is when your body can no longer make a hormone; then HRT is appropriate.* Just make sure you really need it, and that you do not get more than you need.

It is normal for the production of your minor hormones to decrease as you grow older. When this happens, you do not rebuild as well as you once did. Signs of this include loss of skin and muscle tone, loss of bone tissue, decrease in memory and concentration, decrease in flexibility and movement, and many other bodily signs associated with aging.

Turning Back the Clock

It is reasonable to want to turn back the clock and get rid of all the signs of aging by taking the minor hormones. But having too much of these hormones is worse than losing the ability to make them at peak levels. This means you have to be very careful if you are going to take HRT for the natural decline of any of your minor hormones. I believe it is more important to change your habits to get your body to produce more of these hormones than it is to take HRT. By increasing your own production of these hormones, you can achieve the results you are after.

When you take a hormone that your body can still make, your body loses its ability to regulate it. The regulation of hormones by communication between them is vital to your health and well-being. You can actually age yourself faster by taking a hormone that your body can still make. The irony is that taking a minor hormone only for anti-aging purposes can age you faster.

If you are taking a minor hormone, make sure that you are working with a medical professional who understands how to prescribe and adjust the dose of the hormone for your individual needs. This includes having your hormone levels tested regularly.

Producing Minor Growth Hormones When You Are Young

When you are young, your body rebuilds itself better because it is able to readily produce growth hormones. During this time of your life, you often develop bad habits because your body's ability to rebuild well may fool you into believing you are "getting away" with your poor nutrition and lifestyle habits.

Most people do not want to harm themselves intentionally. They truly believe that they are doing the right things because they are thin and do not yet have any of the signs and symptoms of hormonal imbalances.

But when your ability to produce minor hormones decreases, you can no longer compensate for your poor habits. When you start experiencing the symptoms of this hormonal decrease, you do not realize that your poor habits are the cause because you have been doing them for years without problems.

However, now you know that how you feel is not always the true indicator of what is happening inside your body.

Check off your lifestyle habits and hormone problems. The step number that follows each habit or problem corresponds to one of the five steps in the SPII program and should be used as a guide to help you make the necessary changes to your nutrition and lifestyle habits. Refer to page 156 for the five Schwarzbein Principle II steps.

Minor Hormone Triggers

☐ **Imbalance of your adrenaline, cortisol and insulin hormones** Your minor hormones can never be in balance unless your major hormones are in balance. Learn how to balance all your hormones by following the Schwarzbein Principle II program. **(Steps 1 through 5)**

☐ **Unbalanced meals** You make your minor hormones more efficiently by eating proteins, healthy fats, nonstarchy vegetables and real carbohydrates at every meal. Learn about these different food groups. **(Step 1)**

☐ **Insomnia/lack of sleep** By getting adequate amounts of REM sleep, your body will be able to make your minor hormones more efficiently. Learn about REM sleep. **(Step 2)**

☐ **Low serotonin** Serotonin converts into melatonin, a very important sleep hormone. If you do not sleep well, you cannot make adequate amounts of your minor hormones. Learn why sleep is restorative. **(Step 2)**

☐ **Not doing enough resistance-training exercises** Your body secretes more of your minor hormones when you are doing resistance exercises. Learn about resistance exercises. **(Step 4)**

☐ **The loss of sex steroids** Estradiol and testosterone influence the production of HGH, DHEA and thyroid. If you are missing these sex hormones, you need HRT. Learn about the best way to take HRT. **(Step 5)**

☐ **The loss of a minor hormone** HGH, DHEA and thyroid need each other. Each of these growth hormones requires the other two in order to be produced efficiently. If your body can no longer make any one of these hormones, it is appropriate for you to take the missing hormone. Learn how to take HRT to mimic normal physiology. **(Step 5)**

Recognizing Poor Nutrition and Lifestyle Habits

Many people cannot tell that their poor nutrition and lifestyle habits are causing them to age faster. Below are some real-life scenarios of people whose poor nutrition and lifestyle habits have led to more using up than rebuilding of functional, structural and energy biochemicals. Do you recognize yourself among this group?

Do you have so many commitments that you skip meals or eat fast food and do not take the time to sleep enough?

Jim, a thirty-five-year-old father of four children under the age of four and the president of his own company, loves to socialize and do cardiovascular exercises. He only sleeps six hours a night so that he can fit everything in. He is tired, but he drinks caffeinated beverages all day to keep him going. His high-adrenaline lifestyle also keeps him going. Overall, he still feels and looks good, and therefore he is not aware that his habits will lead to a major "crash" one day.

Do you only eat high-carbohydrate, low-fat meals and overdo cardiovascular exercises?

Gordon, a fifty-four-year-old tennis instructor, stayed "in top shape" on this type of program until the age of forty-five. One day he woke up to find himself with increased weight around his midsection and a negative outlook on life. Since he had been eating and exercising this way for years, his conclusion was that he was getting older and there was nothing he could do about his situation. He did not realize that his poor lifestyle habits had caught up with him. His adrenaline/cortisol levels were initially higher than his insulin levels; therefore, he did not gain weight until his metabolism had been damaged.

Are you overworked and underfed?

Dorothy, a forty-five-year-old high-powered executive, releases her stress by overexercising. She does not eat much proteins, fats or carbohydrates because food robs her of her energy. But she thinks she is healthy because she does eat a lot of nonstarchy vegetables and salads. She also drinks many caffeinated beverages to keep her going throughout the day, and she has two hard-alcohol drinks at night to relax. She is very underweight and already is experiencing bone loss. Dorothy is still not convinced, however, that her habits are a problem because she is thin and she feels good. She is a "crash" waiting to happen.

Have you been eating a lot of candy and ice cream instead of meals, and still stayed thin most of your life?

Sally, a forty-nine-year-old, was doing "well" until the age of forty-eight when she went into menopause. She never considered changing her eating habits before then because she had had good energy and she was thin. It wasn't until menopause that her past caught up with her. When she began eating real foods and taking HRT, she put on twenty pounds immediately because she started healing her damaged metabolism by rebuilding her structural, functional and energy biochemicals. When you first start to heal, you do not have a healthy metabolism—and this leads to rapid weight gain. Your body is over-building to repair the damage. There is no other way to heal.

Do you thrive on stress so that you are constantly on the go and require sugar, caffeine, alcohol and exercise to keep you feeling well?

Martin, a forty-four-year-old professor, loves his job so much that he often stays up all night running chemical experiments. After a night of no sleep, he drinks a lot of coffee in the morning to keep going throughout the day. He also likes to socialize with friends and drink alcohol to relax. He does understand the importance of balancing his meals. Knowing this keeps him from "crashing" all together. He is still able to ride his bike and swim as fast as always, so he does not feel the need to change his high-adrenaline and high-cortisol lifestyle. Because he is only forty-four years old, Martin's body is still able to compensate for his poor nutrition and lifestyle habits. But his ability to rebuild quickly will not last forever.

Do you smoke cigarettes to stay thin and feel good?

Valerie, a fifty-eight-year-old retired teacher, continues to smoke even though she is fully aware that smoking is not good for her. Every time she tries to quit, she gains weight and feels tired. She is not interested at this time in going through nicotine withdrawal. She continues to use up her biochemicals and probably will not quit smoking until she has a life-threatening illness.

Are you eating a low-carbohydrate diet to keep your insulin levels low?

Tom is a forty-six-year-old Type I diabetic. After he learned that high-insulin levels are harmful, he tried to stay on a very low-carbohydrate diet to keep his insulin dose low. He ended up not taking enough insulin, which put his body into ketosis. Ketosis is the breakdown of your fats into chemicals called ketones that occurs when your insulin levels are too low. However, after I explained to Tom that too little insulin was more damaging than too much, he corrected this problem by increasing his daily total insulin dose and increasing his carbohydrate intake to match his current metabolism type and activity levels.

Are you addicted to chocolate?

Amy, a forty-four-year-old physician, thinks chocolate is better than sex. She gets into cycles of eating it every day until her skin breaks out and she gets overly anxious. She then tries to stop eating chocolate cold turkey and manages to avoid it for about five to six weeks until her cravings get the best of her. She does not understand that she is addicted to chocolate because her stressful lifestyle has resulted in a lower serotonin state. Until she heals her low-serotonin state, she will stay "addicted."

Do you binge eat?

Linda, a forty-one-year-old, has been binge eating sweets for most of her life. She has tried to keep her weight down by not eating meals after a binge, but this has only resulted in increased bingeing. Now Linda is eating three balanced meals and two snacks a day to try to rebalance her hormones and repair her metabolism. She has learned that she still needs to eat balanced meals even if she binges. This will help decrease her impulse to binge.

Do you overdo it?

Jacob, a seventy-one-year-old aerospace engineer, came out of retirement in order to work on a very exciting project that he had finally convinced a big company to fund. He spent fourteen hours a day working on mathematical equations to support his theories, and because he was so excited by this opportunity he ate and slept very little. Six months into the project, the funding money ran out and Jacob went home dejected. He became mentally and physically exhausted as he found himself with nothing to do all day long. By overdoing and overworking all those months, Jacob had burned out his adrenal glands. He now had to take time to heal again.

As you can imagine, there are many different reasons for hormonal imbalances. The good news is that you can follow one program, the SPII program, to balance your hormones. If you incorporate the program's five steps into your daily lifestyle, you will achieve successful aging. You will live well and live longer, and be as healthy as possible. It does not get much better than that.

The Transition to Healing

So far you have learned about the importance of keeping your hormones balanced in order to achieve a healthy metabolism and an ideal body composition. For those of you who must heal your metabolism, part II describes what you will experience. As you begin your journey to optimum health, you will go through a *transition* process that will enable your body to heal from your previous poor nutrition and lifestyle habits. You will learn what to expect during your transition, so that you can continue the healthy habits that will ensure your success.

Summary

- Because all hormones are connected, the health problems associated with imbalances in adrenaline, cortisol and insulin overlap.
- To slow down or reverse the aging process, you must improve your metabolism. A healthy metabolism depends on your body's ability to regenerate efficiently, and your hormones control regeneration.
- If your major hormone levels have been high for too long, the systems of your body will be out of balance. Among other problems, this imbalance will lead to a decrease in your minor hormone levels and possibly even your major ones.
- All the hormones of the body are connected, and they are helping each other regulate all the same biochemical reactions simultaneously.
- By understanding the triggers and actions of adrenaline, insulin, cortisol, HGH, DHEA and thyroid, you can change your nutrition and lifestyle habits to balance all your hormones.
- If your body cannot make a hormone, it is time for hormone replacement therapy (HRT).
- A decrease in minor hormone production is normal as you grow older. This decrease is manifested in a loss of skin and muscle tone, a loss of bone tissue, decrease in memory and concentration, and decrease in flexibility and movement.
- When you are young, your body is able to make growth hormones and rebuild itself. This is often when you develop bad habits—because it seems you can "get away" with them.
- When your body's ability to produce minor hormones decreases, you start to experience the symptoms of your poor nutrition and lifestyle habits. You don't see your poor habits as the reason for these health problems because you have been doing them for years without any ill effects.

- Following the SPII program will help you balance all of your hormones, heal your metabolism, regenerate efficiently and achieve optimum health.

* * *

Now you understand how hormones work together and how balanced hormone levels are the key to successful aging. But what will happen as you begin to improve the habits that are damaging your metabolism? Part II explains what you will experience during your transition to optimum health.

PART II

The Transition

Eight

The Transition

E veryone goes through what I call the *transition* to restore their metabolism, achieve an ideal body composition and obtain optimum health. The transition is a journey of healing. You can only *be* in your transition if you are improving your nutrition and lifestyle habits.

During your transition your hormones will change in response to the nutrition and lifestyle changes you make, and this allows you to heal. However, you will not have balanced hormones immediately—balanced hormones do not occur overnight. There are sequential steps of healing that everyone must take.

When you initiate your transition process by improving your habits, your body will begin to rebalance its hormones. Your body will also rebuild all its functional and structural biochemicals that were not made efficiently during your previous poor habits. The more damaged your current metabolism, the longer it will take for this process to be completed.

By taking the time to follow the necessary steps in the SPII program to balance your hormones, you will heal your metabolism. When you have healed your metabolism, you are primed to lose fat weight, if needed. Once you have lost all your stored fat, you are through your transition.

The Four Transition Stages

For most people, the transition to a healthy metabolism and optimal health consists of four main stages:

- Initial starting point
- Healing phase
- Fat-burning phase
- Healed state

Here is what to expect as you journey through your transition to health. You begin at your initial starting point and then enter a healing phase that may consist of a self-medicating phase. Then you enter a fat-burning phase—if you need to burn fat before you finally reach a healed state.

Depending on your current metabolism, your body may skip the healing and/or fat-burning phases.

Let's look at each stage in more detail.

1. The Initial Starting Point

The initial starting point is your current metabolism type and age when you start improving your habits and begin entering your transition. Listed below are the four metabolism types an individual can have:

1. Insulin-sensitive with healthy adrenal glands
2. Insulin-resistant with healthy adrenal glands
3. Insulin-sensitive with burned-out adrenal glands
4. Insulin-resistant with burned-out adrenal glands

These metabolism types are not genetic but acquired. Everyone begins life insulin-sensitive with healthy adrenal glands.* It is only after years of poor nutrition and lifestyle habits that you may become insulin-resistant or have burned-out adrenal glands—or have both conditions.

Your age and how long you have had your current metabolism affect the duration of your transition. The older you are and the longer your metabolism has been damaged, the longer it will take for you to complete your transition.

Your Goal

Your goal is to stay or become insulin-sensitive and to have healthy adrenal glands or to heal them. Therefore, the goal is to have a metabolism where you are insulin-sensitive with healthy adrenal glands.

If you are starting out with this metabolism, your transition to healing requires improving your daily habits to keep from damaging your metabolism.

If you start out insulin-resistant with healthy adrenal glands, your goal is to become insulin-sensitive and keep your adrenal glands healthy.

If your current metabolism is insulin-sensitive with burned-out adrenal glands, your goal is to stay insulin-sensitive and heal your adrenal glands.

If you are insulin-resistant with burned-out adrenal glands, you must heal both sides of your metabolism to reach your goal of insulin-sensitive with healthy adrenal glands.

Insulin-Sensitive

You are insulin-sensitive if your body responds to all the actions of insulin, including the ability to make and store fats. Refer to chapter 5 for an expanded explanation of what insulin does. Note, however, that

---

The rare exception is the person born with a genetic error of metabolism.

just as with insulin resistance, you can gain fat weight around your midsection when you are insulin-sensitive. Therefore, do not confuse having excess fat weight around your midsection with being insulin-resistant (see below).

Insulin-Resistant

You are insulin-resistant if you have an elevated fasting insulin level with one or more of the following signs/disorders: excess fat weight around your midsection, high triglyceride levels and low HDL levels, high blood pressure, Type II diabetes, and/or coronary artery disease. You will probably need to ask your physician to order a fasting insulin and cholesterol profile in order to determine if you are insulin-resistant or not. Or visit my Web site at: *www.SchwarzbeinPrinciple.com,* to find out how you can be tested.

There are three paths that lead to insulin resistance:

- Years of high insulin levels due to poor nutrition and lifestyle habits.
- Years of high adrenaline and/or cortisol levels due to poor nutrition and lifestyle habits.
- Years of high insulin, adrenaline and cortisol levels due to poor nutrition and lifestyle habits.

If you recognize that you are on any of these paths, *now* is the time to change your habits!

Are you insulin-sensitive, insulin-resistant or on the way to becoming insulin-resistant? Identify yourself here (check one):

___I am insulin-sensitive.

___I am insulin-sensitive on the way to insulin-resistant.

___I am insulin-resistant.

___I am not sure, so I will ask my physician to order blood tests.

Are Your Adrenal Glands Healthy or Burned Out?

Your adrenal glands make both adrenaline and cortisol. Years of oversecreting these two hormones can burn out your adrenal glands. If you have burned out your adrenal glands, you need to restore their function before you can achieve optimum health.

You have healthy adrenal glands if you can stop all your high-adrenaline and/or cortisol habits cold turkey without experiencing withdrawal symptoms and completely falling apart emotionally and/or physically.

If you are addicted to white sugar, caffeine, nicotine, diet pills, alcohol, overexercising and/or street drugs, or if you are always tired, have a "fuzzy" brain or cannot handle stressful situations, your adrenal glands are probably burned out.

Your adrenal glands are burned out if your adrenal saliva test shows low cortisol levels throughout the day. Ask your physician to test your adrenal glands or visit my Web site, *www.SchwarzbeinPrinciple.com,* to find out how you can be tested.

Do you have healthy or burned-out adrenal glands? Are you on the path to burning them out? Identify yourself here (check one):

____I have healthy adrenal glands.

____I have healthy adrenal glands, but I am on the path to burning them out.

____I have burned-out adrenal glands.

____I am not sure, so I will ask my physician to test my adrenal gland function through saliva testing.

Now, put together your insulin status and your adrenal gland state to identify your current metabolism type (check one):

____I am insulin-sensitive and have healthy adrenal glands.

____I am insulin-resistant and have healthy adrenal glands.

_____I am insulin-sensitive and have burned-out adrenal glands.
_____I am insulin-resistant and have burned-out adrenal glands.

Note: If you are not sure what your current type is and you want to start this program before your laboratory tests are back, consider yourself insulin-sensitive with burned-out adrenal glands.

2. The Healing Phase

In the healing phase your body will repair itself from the damage caused by years of poor nutrition and lifestyle habits. You always have higher insulin than adrenaline/cortisol levels during this phase because this is a rebuilding time.

It may seem as if you are in suspended animation during this phase because though you are healing, it doesn't feel or seem that way. As you improve your habits, you are rebuilding your biochemicals at a much higher rate than you are using them up, and this causes you to feel tired and to gain fat weight.

Your Current Metabolism Is Revealed During the Healing Phase

During the healing phase you expose your current metabolism because your hormones will react to your new and improved nutrition and lifestyle habits and reflect their true state.

If you are insulin-sensitive, your insulin levels will fluctuate appropriately with your carbohydrate intake; if you are insulin-resistant, your insulin levels will stay high while you are healing.

For example, if you are insulin-sensitive, your fasting insulin levels are within normal ranges, and when you eat carbohydrates, your levels rise to match your carbohydrate intake so your body can process the food. Once you process your food, your insulin levels come back down to normal.

But if you are insulin-resistant, your fasting insulin levels are already higher than normal, and they will stay high, even if you improve your eating habits, until you have become insulin-sensitive again.

If your adrenal glands are healthy, your adrenaline/cortisol levels will respond appropriately to your habits; if your adrenal glands are burned out, your adrenaline/cortisol levels will stay low until your glands have had a chance to heal. You have worn them out and depleted their ability to respond as they would under normal circumstances.

What Happens to Your Hormones During the Healing Phase

Here is what happens to your hormones during your healing phase—depending upon your current metabolism.

If you are insulin-sensitive with healthy adrenal glands, your hormones will immediately become balanced when you improve your habits; therefore, you are instantly through your healing phase.

If you are insulin-resistant with healthy adrenal glands, your insulin levels will remain high despite your improved habits until your body has a chance to heal and you become insulin-sensitive again. However, your adrenaline/cortisol levels will normalize immediately.

If you are insulin-sensitive with burned-out adrenal glands, your insulin levels will respond appropriately to your improved habits, but your adrenaline and cortisol levels will stay low while your adrenal glands heal; they will normalize when you have completely healed.

If you are insulin-resistant with burned-out adrenal glands, your insulin levels will remain high, and your adrenaline/cortisol levels will remain low. As you heal, your insulin and adrenaline/cortisol levels will slowly normalize.

How Your Body Heals

Unfortunately, your body will not start working efficiently the moment you improve your habits. As previously stated, you did not damage your metabolism overnight, and you will not heal it overnight.

During the healing phase, you are still hormonally out of balance. As your body begins to correct this imbalance, you may experience any number of disturbing symptoms.

For example, as your adrenaline/cortisol levels drop, you may feel withdrawal symptoms such as fatigue, irritability and depression. As your insulin levels rise, you may gain fat weight and/or experience salt and water retention.

The more damaged your current metabolism is, the longer you will need to stay in the healing phase and the more fat your body produces. In fact, as your ratio of insulin to adrenaline/cortisol increases, your symptoms will worsen.

As awful as this may sound, this is your body's only way to heal. So do not be put off by the healing phase—it is simply a reflection of the damage that came before it.

Since insulin is a rebuilding hormone and adrenaline and cortisol are using-up hormones, you can only heal from years of using up your biochemicals by rebuilding them—this means higher insulin-to-adrenaline/cortisol levels. Unfortunately, even though you begin to improve your habits, the damage has already been done by your previous poor habits. Therefore, you will not instantly reap the rewards of your better habits.

For example, when people stop smoking, they may gain a lot of fat weight and feel tired and listless. They usually tell me they never should have stopped smoking because now they feel lousy and are fat besides.

What they don't realize is that the only way their bodies can heal is by raising their insulin levels higher than their adrenaline levels, so they will gain fat weight as their bodies heal from years of smoking. The damage occurred while they were smoking, not after they stopped. The only way to avoid having to heal from smoking is to never smoke in the first place.

If you are a smoker, the best thing you can do for your health is to quit and begin healing from years of using up your biochemicals more than rebuilding them due to nicotine use.

There is a subpart to the healing phase: the self-medicating phase. The self-medicating phase occurs whenever you do anything that raises your adrenaline/cortisol levels closer to your insulin levels.

The Self-Medicating Phase

Since your insulin levels must be higher than your adrenaline/cortisol levels for your body to heal, it does not always feel very good to be in the healing phase of your transition. It is during this time that the self-medicating phase becomes important in keeping you on the path to restoring your metabolism.

In this phase you use one or more of the following to make yourself feel good enough to continue your healing process: small amounts of stimulants, alcohol and refined sugars. Overexercising is also a form of self-medication. Self-medicating makes you feel better in the short-term because using up your biochemicals always feels better than rebuilding them.

In the self-medicating phase you still have higher insulin than adrenaline/cortisol levels, but you narrow the gap between your rate of rebuilding and using up. Your self-medicating habits raise your adrenaline/cortisol levels closer to your insulin levels, and you prolong your transition because self-medicating keeps you closer to your current metabolism than to your goal metabolism.

It is sometimes necessary to self-medicate to get through your transition, especially if you begin with burned-out adrenal glands. The How To section outlines the best ways to self-medicate if you need to.

Do not make the mistake of thinking you are self-medicating if you have not changed any of your habits! You cannot "be good" part of the time and revert to your poor habits the rest of the time. If you over-self-medicate and your adrenaline/cortisol levels get higher than your insulin levels, you will no longer be in your transition process, and you will continue to damage your metabolism.

3. The Fat-Burning Phase

The fat-burning phase of the transition occurs after your body has done all its rebuilding in the healing phase. The main changes to your body composition during the healing phase is an increase in lean body tissue, such as muscles and bones rather than a decrease in fat weight per se. However, do not get discouraged, you will have started to burn off some of your excess fat-weight during the healing phase and are now ready to burn off the rest.

You begin your fat-burning phase only after your hormones are completely normalized and your metabolism is healed. Only then is your body ready to burn off the rest of your stored fat if it needs to. All your symptoms of fluctuating adrenaline, cortisol and/or insulin levels will be gone, and you will feel great. During this phase you will be rebuilding and using up your functional and structural bio-chemicals again at an equal rate.

4. The Healed State

The healed state is when all of your hormones are balanced, your metabolism has healed and you have achieved your ideal body composition. You are now through your transition and have achieved the ideal current metabolism type. You are insulin-sensitive and have healthy adrenal glands. When you are in this state, you are rebuilding as many biochemicals as you are using up and have the lowest risk for the degenerative diseases of aging. Your goal now is to keep your hormones balanced so that you do not damage your metabolism again.

Timing Is Everything

The time it takes to go through the transition is different for everyone. The transition to a healthy metabolism can occur very quickly, or it can take months or years to complete.

If you have a healthy metabolism, you will be able to complete your transition quickly once you change your nutrition and lifestyle habits.

If you begin with a badly damaged metabolism, however, it may take you years to completely heal. But you *can* heal. It is never too late. You are closer than you think.

Why You Do Not Lose Weight Right Away

During the transition from a damaged metabolism to a healed one, you will become healthier—but you will not have the body composition you want right away. Why? Because you first need to heal your metabolism before you can achieve your ideal body composition. *You need to be healthy to lose weight, not lose weight to be healthy.* It is only when you have completely healed your metabolism that you are primed for losing all your excess storage fat.

Do not confuse losing weight according to the bathroom scale with losing excess fat weight. If you quickly lose weight while your metabolism is still damaged you are not just losing storage fat—you are also losing your functional and structural proteins and fats and causing further damage to your metabolism. And since protein weighs more than fat, you may think that the lower number on the scale is a good thing when it is not.

The key to becoming and staying healthy is to burn off your storage fats while retaining your functional and structural proteins and fats.

It Takes Time to Heal

The time it takes to heal your metabolism is normal and *unavoidable.* You may as well start to heal now; there is no alternative. The sooner you start your transition, the sooner you will get through it and obtain optimum health.

For those of you who are starting off with a damaged metabolism, you cannot escape the time it takes to heal, but you will have the advantage of knowing what you need to do to shorten your transition time. My transition took a long time because I began with a badly damaged metabolism, and I did not know what I needed to do to heal myself.

Dr. Schwarzbein's Transition

My transition was not a typical one. I spent seven years healing my metabolism because I did not have a specific plan to follow. This was during the late '70s and early '80s when the recommended food plan was a higher carbohydrate diet. Because I switched from eating refined sugars to eating complex carbohydrates and unbalanced meals, I became insulin-resistant while I was still in the process of healing my adrenal glands.

As I healed, I went from insulin-sensitive with burned-out adrenal glands to insulin-resistant with burned-out adrenal glands, then to insulin-resistant with healthy adrenal glands and finally to insulin-sensitive with healthy adrenal glands. Because I did not know what I needed to do to heal, I took many unnecessary detours and ended up with all the different current metabolism types. Along the way I tried different eating programs until I finally hit upon the balanced food program that enabled me to heal completely.

I am going to explain my complicated transition by describing the changes in my major hormones and how they affected me throughout the different stages of my healing. Sometimes adrenaline and cortisol are not linked to each other, but in my case they still were; so if adrenaline went up, cortisol did, too. When adrenaline went down, so did cortisol.

Therefore, to simplify, I will discuss what happened to me in terms of adrenaline versus insulin only. But remember, all my hormones were involved.

My own nutrition and lifestyle habits—eating lots of refined sugary foods and overdoing cardiovascular exercise—initially stimulated the release of large amounts of adrenaline. This is why I was so thin; adrenaline causes your body to use up its biochemicals. However, these same habits also made me very unhealthy. From years of using up more than rebuilding my biochemicals, my body was used up, too.

I thought that I had the best metabolism in the world. I could and did eat thousands of calories of refined sugar a day, and I did not gain an ounce. But in reality I had already badly damaged my metabolism. I was not eating enough of the right foods for my body to rebuild. Accessing and using up your biochemicals is only half of what it takes to have a healthy metabolism; the other half is eating well and rebuilding. Because I was using up my biochemicals at a rapid rate and barely rebuilding, I did not have a healthy metabolism even though I stayed thin.

My body was also secreting high amounts of insulin in response to my high-adrenaline levels to prevent me from completely wasting away. This was a good thing. When adrenaline/cortisol levels rise, insulin levels also rise to modify the amount of using up of your biochemicals that is occurring in your body. If your body were to continue to use up its biochemicals because of high adrenaline/cortisol levels, and you did not have this insulin stopgap, you would die. So your body secretes more insulin in an attempt to keep you alive longer. An example of this built-in survival mechanism is when you go on a diet and eat fewer calories. You initially lose weight rapidly, but the longer you restrict your food intake, the slower your rate of weight loss. In fact, you may even stop losing weight. In this case, your body senses it is using itself up too quickly, so it secretes more insulin to counteract rapid weight loss. This is a very powerful survival instinct and is what kept me alive despite my poor eating habits.

The amount of refined sugar that I ate raised both my adrenaline and insulin levels, but my adrenaline levels rose higher than my insulin levels. However, because refined sugar cannot be turned into functional or structural biochemicals, the higher amounts of insulin I secreted could only keep me from using up all my biochemicals completely—it could not help me rebuild. I was using up faster than I could rebuild.

My Initial Starting Point

When I was sixteen, I was all skin and bones. I was five-foot-eleven, weighed 125 pounds and was very underweight and unhealthy. I had very little muscle and no fat on my body at all. I had asthma, chronic bronchitis, irritable bowel syndrome and cystic acne. I was hormonally out of balance with both high adrenaline and high insulin levels.

Because I did not think that I would live a long time if I continued to be this unhealthy, I began to look for some solutions to my health problems. This was the initial starting point of my transition.

I was insulin-sensitive with burned-out adrenal glands, but my hormones did not reflect this until I entered the healing phase, which exposed my underlying physiology.

Entering My Transition

I began to improve my eating habits in an attempt to improve my health. When I began adding other foods to my diet besides refined sugar, my body perceived that the "starvation" crisis was over and it was time to rebuild.

I had entered my healing phase and my body began rebuilding more than using up. But because I was eating a high complex-carbohydrate diet, I mostly rebuilt storage fats and not functional or structural proteins and fats.

In terms of my hormones, my adrenaline levels came crashing down and dipped even lower than normal, and my insulin levels rose even higher because I was eating so many complex carbohydrates. I was addicted to refined white sugars, and this meant that my adrenal glands were already burned out. If they hadn't been burned out, my adrenaline levels would not have dipped so low.

The fact that my insulin levels stayed high was initially a reflection of my high-carbohydrate intake. If I had been eating a balanced diet, my insulin levels would have normalized. As it was, my insulin levels were very high and my adrenaline levels were very low.

I developed insulin-resistance over the next few years because I was eating too many complex carbohydrates and not enough proteins. I started off insulin-sensitive with burned-out adrenal glands, and then I became insulin-resistant with burned-out adrenal glands, but I did not have this type of current metabolism for very long. My adrenal glands were already in the process of healing because I had stopped eating refined sugars, which was the main reason my adrenal glands had burned out to begin with.

Because I had badly damaged my metabolism for many years before I improved my habits, and because I ate large amounts of complex carbohydrates, I gained a lot of fat weight throughout my midsection. I also experienced significant water retention with bloating and ankle swelling.

I had learned that you can only hold onto water if you have salt in your body, so I went on a two-gram salt diet to lessen my swelling. This did help, but it did not treat the real reason I was retaining fluids—high insulin levels.

I was very unhappy about gaining fat weight, but what really made my healing phase difficult was that I was always fatigued. I did not know that running on high adrenaline for all those years was one of the reasons I was so tired now.

Because my adrenal glands were burned out, nonvital functions such as a sense of well-being and fertility shut down. My body kept me alive, but feeling good was not its priority and neither was making a baby.

The other thing that made me so fatigued was all the complex carbohydrates I was eating. The combination of higher insulin levels, from eating too many carbohydrates, and very low adrenaline levels, from burned-out adrenal glands, made me extremely tired.

Despite my fatigue and weight gain, I recognized that I felt slightly better. I was much calmer, and my nervous edge was gone; I knew deep down that I was doing the right thing by trying to eat better foods.

This does not mean that I did not think of going back to my old ways. I had many thoughts about going back to eating cotton candy, Pixi-Stix and my own milky, sugary oatmeal so that I could have energy—even nervous energy—and be thin again. But something kept me from doing this. I believe that I did not go back to my old ways because I realized that I had been killing myself by eating so poorly.

It may sound as if I easily intellectualized my healing phase, but it was an ongoing internal battle. I did give in many times to the "noise" in my head that demanded sugar for energy. Each time I did, however, I felt so much worse afterwards that after a while all that negative reinforcement made it easier to resist my cravings.

By experimenting with different meal plans, I noticed that I felt better and was less bloated when I ate balanced meals. I started to eat this way consistently about four years into my transition. A year later I had completely healed my adrenal glands, but I was still insulin-resistant.

Self-Medicating Phase

I struggled during my healing phase because I had no idea what was happening to me. I was eating better, but I was gaining weight and feeling tired all the time. This was the opposite of what I expected to happen.

I began to notice that the only time I felt well was when I was exercising. Even though I had been exercising before, I now got to the point where I was spending three to four hours a day doing cardiovascular exercises just so I could feel normal.

Because my adrenal glands were healed at this point, I was able to feel better by increasing my exercise, but I did not know that I was slowing down my own healing process because exercise raises adrenaline levels. In fact, I felt just the opposite. I thought that more exercise would help me lose the fat weight I had put on and would be healthy for me. But I was forcing my body to use up my biochemicals again—through exercise this time, not by eating excessive amounts of refined sugars. This was my self-medicating phase.

Luckily, because I was still improving my nutrition habits throughout my self-medicating phase, I did not go back to my initial starting point of higher adrenaline than insulin levels. Therefore, I was still building more than using up my biochemicals, but at a much slower rate.

When I was not exercising, I felt tired. I was not a caffeine or alcohol person and did not add to my self-medicating by also using these toxic chemicals in order to feel better. I just accepted the fatigue because I could not exercise all day long.

If I had used a lot of caffeine or alcohol early on and increased my exercise to self-medicate, my adrenaline levels would probably have risen higher than my insulin levels again—and I would have returned to my initial starting point.

The Fat-Burning Phase and the Healed State

Fortunately, I had to decrease my daily exercise routine because I was in my third year of medical school and no longer had the time to exercise three to four hours a day. Inadvertently, I stopped self-medicating.

At this point, two and one-half years had passed since I had begun eating balanced meals. Six and one-half years had passed since I had begun to improve my nutrition and lifestyle habits, and my metabolism had completely healed. I was insulin-sensitive with healthy adrenal glands. My hormone levels were normal, and I began the fat-burning phase of my transition.

During this phase, I felt completely better and had all the energy I needed—but I still carried excess fat weight around my middle. As I continued through the fat-burning phase, I kept my muscle mass and burned off all my stored fat. Seven years after starting my transition my hormones were all balanced, my metabolism was healed, and I had achieved my ideal body composition. I was through my transition.

I know now that if I had been following the SPII program, I would have been able to shorten the time it took for me to heal because I would not have become insulin-resistant. But it took me years to find the right nutrition program and to stumble upon all the necessary lifestyle changes I needed to make. It still would have taken years for me to heal—because I started off with such a badly damaged metabolism—but it would have been fewer than seven years.

I finished my transition seventeen years ago. I still have a healthy metabolism, and I have maintained my ideal body composition because I adopted my lifestyle changes for good.

Each of you will experience something similar to what I went through during my transition—though of course your transition won't be identical. Your initial starting point—your current metabolism—and the habits that got you there will be different from mine. How easy it is for you to incorporate the SPII program into your life will also determine the nature of your transition.

As you begin your healing journey, remember these points:

- You *can* heal.
- It is never too late.
- There are no shortcuts.
- You need to take the time to heal.
- This is the time to rearrange your priorities.
- If not now, when?

Summary

- You will have to go through a transition to heal your metabolism, achieve an ideal body composition and obtain optimum health.
- You must improve your habits to enter and stay in your transition.
- The transition consists of an initial starting point; a healing phase (that may or may not include a self-medicating phase); a fat-burning phase (if you need to burn off excess fat); and a healed state. You may or may not experience a healing phase and/or a fat-burning phase depending on your current metabolism.
- The initial starting point is your current metabolism and age when you begin improving your habits and enter your transition.
- You may be insulin-sensitive or insulin-resistant.
- You may have healthy or burned-out adrenal glands.
- The goal metabolism is insulin-sensitive with healthy adrenal glands.
- In the healing phase your body will repair itself from the damage caused by previous years of poor nutrition and lifestyle habits.
- In the healing phase you always have higher insulin than adrenaline/cortisol levels because this is the only way your body has to heal.
- The self-medicating phase is used to keep you feeling better so that you can complete your transition.
- The fat-burning phase occurs after your hormones return to baseline and your metabolism is healed. Your body is ready to burn off stored fat if needed.
- You reach the healed state when all your hormones are balanced, your metabolism has healed and you have achieved your ideal body composition.
- The time it will take to go through the transition is different for everyone.
- You need to be healthy to lose weight, not lose weight to be healthy.

- The key to becoming and staying healthy is to burn off your excess energy biochemicals while retaining your functional and structural biochemicals.
- The time it takes to heal your metabolism is *normal* and *unavoidable.*

* * *

Now you have an idea of what you can expect during your transition, but not everyone's transition will be the same as mine was. In chapter 9 we'll take a look at the transitions of Kelley, Mary, Annie and Arthur, who had different initial starting points and different journeys along their paths to optimum health. You will probably see yourself in one of their stories. You will also read about Liz's success story.

Nine

There Are No Shortcuts

As stated in chapter 8, the path your transition takes will depend upon your initial starting point and how easy it is for you to incorporate the SPII program into your life. Remember that this program is a process, and you will not be able to heal a damaged metabolism overnight, nor will you be able to make all the necessary changes in your nutrition and lifestyle habits at once.

By educating yourself about what you can expect, you should be able to keep yourself on your journey to optimum health.

What to Expect: Insulin-Sensitive with Healthy Adrenal Glands

If you are starting with a good metabolism but have poor nutrition and lifestyle habits, you still have to go through a transition process. However, your transition will be much easier for you than for other metabolism types because you will not experience a healing phase. If you do not carry excess fat weight, you will go directly into your healed state after you improve your nutrition and lifestyle habits.

Since you do not have to feel worse before you feel better, it should be easier for you to make the necessary permanent changes in your habits to ensure you maintain a good metabolism and your ideal body composition.

A word of caution: If you are following the SPII program with a friend or loved one and you breeze through the transition, remember not to sabotage those people who are having a more difficult time. Just because you were able to change your habits immediately and lose fat weight easily, do not think that they are eating too much or eating the wrong things just because they are gaining fat weight.

Their transition will be different from yours because they are starting from a different initial starting point. Because they will be having a more difficult time than you did, be sure to encourage them. Do not discourage them—it may cause them to quit.

Kelley's Transition

Initial Starting Point

Before Kelley changed her habits (see chapter 3), she had widely fluctuating levels of adrenaline, insulin and cortisol throughout the day because she was stressed, using BCPs, eating too few calories or too many carbohydrates, and drinking alcohol and caffeine. Overexercising was also a problem for her.

Healing Phase

In spite of her poor habits, Kelley did not damage her metabolism, so she never had to experience a healing phase. Her initial starting point was insulin-sensitive with healthy adrenal glands. When she changed her nutrition and lifestyle habits and started taking HRT, she immediately went into her fat-burning phase, and her hormones instantly became balanced.

On the Road to Healing

Kelley is still in the fat-burning phase and has not reached her healed state yet because she has only been on the SPII program for a few months. But she is well on her way to being completely healed. Now all she has to do is be consistent, and she will obtain optimum health.

Summary: Insulin-Sensitive with Healthy Adrenal Glands

If you are insulin-sensitive with healthy adrenal glands, the following summarizes your initial starting point and what you may expect:

The Goal
You already have the best metabolism type. However, if you have poor nutrition and lifestyle habits, you may be in the process of damaging it.

The Ability to Regenerate
With this metabolism type you can still use up and rebuild your functional and structural biochemicals at the same rate.

Body Composition
You may or may not be overweight depending on your habits.

Weight Changes
You are already primed to lose fat weight by improving your habits.

Habits
If your nutrition and lifestyle habits cause your insulin levels to be higher than your adrenaline/cortisol levels, you will gain weight. If your adrenal/cortisol levels are higher than your insulin levels, you will lose weight. If all three hormone levels are equally high or low, you will stay the same weight. None of these scenarios is healthy. You may have a healthy metabolism now, but if any one of the hormonal imbalances just mentioned continues over time, your metabolism will become damaged.

Symptoms

The fluctuations of your hormones in response to your poor habits may be causing a myriad of symptoms. (Refer to chapters 4, 5 and 6 for symptoms related to fluctuating hormones.)

Transition Phases

You will not experience a healing phase because you do not have to heal your metabolism. As you begin following the SPII program, you will immediately enter the fat-burning phase or healed state, and all your symptoms will go away.

Transition Time

Your transition will take the least amount of time of any of the current metabolism types because you do not have to repair a damaged metabolism. You only have to change your habits to balance your hormones.

What to Expect: Insulin-Sensitive with Burned-Out Adrenal Glands

Because you are starting with a damaged metabolism, you will have to go through a transition process. You will need to heal your adrenal glands and therefore will experience a healing phase. Since you can experience withdrawal symptoms from tapering off your high adrenaline and/or cortisol habits, you may need to self-medicate. However, if you do not carry excess fat weight, you will go directly into your healed state after you have healed your metabolism. Since you probably will feel worse before you feel better, it will take time for you to make the necessary permanent changes to ensure that you heal your metabolism and achieve your ideal body composition. Do not get discouraged—this is the only way your body knows how to heal.

Mary's Transition

Initial Starting Point

Mary's transition (see chapter 4) was not as easy as Kelley's was because Mary started in worse shape. Her initial starting point was insulin-sensitive with burned-out adrenal glands, but her adrenaline and cortisol levels were higher than her insulin levels because she was overexercising, undereating and consuming too much refined sugar. She was also under-weight, agitated and depressed for the very same reasons.

Healing/Self-Medicating Phases

Mary's story illustrates a different type of transition. She did not experience as severe withdrawal symptoms as she could have during her healing phase because she was taking a prescription antidepressant. If necessary, you can use this form of self-medication to get through a difficult healing phase.

When Mary improved her habits, she went from a higher adrenaline/cortisol than insulin state to a lower adrenaline/cortisol than insulin state. She did not experience any of the symptoms of a higher insulin state such as rapid fat-weight gain and salt and water retention because she ate balanced meals from the time she started the program. But she still had a rough time because her lower adrenaline and cortisol levels made her tired and short of breath with exercise and took her "edge" away. It was in this phase that she considered going back to her old ways, but with encouragement, she stuck it out.

The antidepressant medication helped Mary resist her sugar and stimulant cravings because it kept her serotonin levels higher than they would have been without medication.

As Mary heals her burned-out adrenal glands, she has more energy and is much less emotional. If she continues taking her antidepressant until her adrenal glands have healed, she will avoid any more adrenaline/cortisol withdrawal symptoms. She has made it through the hard part of her transition. She is now in the end of her healing phase.

Fat-Burning Phase

When Mary completes her healing phase, she may have a few pounds of excess fat weight to lose, but not many because she has been very consistent with her improved habits.

Almost Healed

It will probably take Mary another six months to a year to complete her transition and have balanced levels of her major hormones. When this happens, she will be completely healed.

Note: Not everyone with burned-out adrenal glands will require antidepressants to heal, but if you do need them, take them to help you through your transition. In general, I do not recommend the use of antidepressants, but I will prescribe them if someone is having an extremely difficult transition. However, I will only recommend their use until the individual's metabolism is healed.

The Metabolic "Hole"

If it becomes difficult for you to follow your healing program, remember that there was a reason you thought you needed to change your habits in the first place. Don't get stuck with a hormonal imbalance because it feels better in the short term.

Going back to your old ways—the ones that raise your adrenaline and cortisol levels higher than insulin levels—will destroy your metabolism even more. Your body will not be able to maintain this higher adrenaline and cortisol state, and you will end up with a lower adrenaline/cortisol than insulin state.

This will make you feel the same way you did when you tried to improve your habits in the first place. You will be tired, overweight and depressed. Your adrenal glands will be burned out even more extensively, and you may become insulin-resistant.

You will end up with the same hormonal imbalances you would have had in the healing phase, but you will not be in the healing phase because you will not be healing. In fact, you will have dug yourself into a metabolic hole and are now worse off than before.

What to Do When You Are in the "Hole"

Once you are in the hole, you have a choice to make. You can climb out, or you can dig yourself deeper into the hole.

If you continue to search for ways to make yourself feel better instantly, you will dig a deeper hole. If you begin to improve your nutrition and lifestyle habits, you will be able to heal and climb out of the hole. It's up to you.

The SPII program is designed to help you climb out of the metabolic hole you've dug for yourself.

Annie's Transition

Initial Starting Point

By the time I started working with Annie to heal her metabolism (see chapter 6), she was insulin-sensitive with severely burned-out adrenal glands.

She had dug herself deep into a metabolic hole from years of dieting and other poor lifestyle habits. She was already overweight and was hoping that by improving her nutrition habits, adopting a routine exercise program and balancing out her estradiol levels, she would obtain optimum health very quickly.

Healing and Self-Medicating Phases

When Annie improved her habits, her insulin levels were higher than her adrenaline and cortisol levels, and she went right into the healing phase. By improving some of her habits, such as following the nutrition program exactly, getting her estradiol levels balanced, and tapering off caffeine and alcohol, she began healing. But because her stress was still high, Annie's cortisol levels stayed up while her adrenaline levels came down. This kept her in the self-medicating phase longer. It also caused her to start having uncontrollable carbohydrate cravings. The combination of chronic high cortisol levels and a higher carbohydrate intake led to more weight gain.

Annie did not feel as well as she had when her adrenaline and cortisol levels had been higher than her insulin levels, and she decided that this program did not work for her because she immediately gained weight. However, because she had already tried and failed every fad diet in the past, she was intellectually willing to stick it out.

Fat-Burning Phase

Annie stayed in the healing phases longer than she needed to, though, because she did not change her high-stress lifestyle. In fact, she didn't even recognize that it was a problem. I finally got through to her about needing to minimize her stress, and because she finally did something about it, she is no longer in the self-medicating phase. Annie is now primed for fat loss and feels better every day.

Summary: Insulin-Sensitive with Burned-Out Adrenal Glands

If you are insulin-sensitive with burned-out adrenal glands, the following summarizes your initial starting point and what you may expect:

The Goal
Your poor habits have burned out your adrenal glands; therefore, your goal is to heal your adrenal glands without becoming insulin-resistant.

The Ability to Regenerate
You are not using your functional and structural biochemicals efficiently.

Body Composition
You may or may not be overweight depending on your nutrition and lifestyle habits. But whether you are thin or not, you do have a damaged metabolism.

Weight Changes
You are in the group that is most likely to gain fat weight as you heal, especially if your adrenal glands are extremely damaged.

Habits
Either you are using toxic chemicals or an antidepressant to keep you going and feeling better, or you are constantly tired and have "fuzzy" thinking because you do not use them.

Symptoms
As you taper off your high-adrenaline and/or high-cortisol habits,

you may experience withdrawal symptoms such as fatigue, irritability, headaches and/or depression.

Transition Phases

You will experience a healing phase that will probably require you to self-medicate. You may or may not have a fat-burning phase.

Transition Time

Your transition time will be proportional to the amount of time you spend in the healing and fat-burning phases. On the average, it should take you somewhere between one and two years to complete your transition.

What to Expect: Insulin-Resistant with Healthy Adrenal Glands

Because you are starting with a damaged metabolism, you will have to go through a transition process. Since you probably will feel worse before you feel better, it will take time for you to make the necessary permanent changes to ensure that you heal your metabolism and achieve your ideal body composition. Do not get discouraged—this is the only way your body knows how to heal.

You will need to become insulin-sensitive again, and you will therefore experience a healing phase. As you are healing, if you are extremely insulin-resistant—that is, despite better habits your insulin levels still stay very high—you may feel sluggish, bloated, and irritable, and may retain excess salt and water, which can cause ankle swelling and/or higher blood pressure. Because of this you will want or need to self-medicate. Once you have healed you will be primed to burn off excess fat weight. You will then be in your healed state.

I was the only one to experience this current metabolism type. Refer back to my story in chapter 8 for an example of this transition process.

Summary: Insulin-Resistant with Healthy Adrenal Glands

If you are insulin-resistant with healthy adrenal glands, the following summarizes your initial starting point and what you may expect.

The Goal

Your poor habits have caused you to become insulin-resistant; therefore, your goal is to become insulin-sensitive again without burning out your adrenal glands.

The Ability to Regenerate

You are storing more fat than you are using up, and you usually are not building your functional and structural biochemicals efficiently.

Body Composition

You are probably overweight and carry most of your fat weight throughout your midsection.

Weight Change

You can minimize gaining more fat weight as long as you are eating correctly. But you may show a weight gain on the scale from rebuilding your structural biochemicals (mostly muscle and bones).

Habits

You usually believe you must be overeating or underexercising because you are overweight. You usually diet and/or increase your cardiovascular exercises to try to feel better and lose weight. You are in a group that has to be very careful because you feel better when you do not eat enough carbohydrates or food, and this will cause your body to use up your biochemicals instead of rebuild them. But remember, you have a damaged metabolism that needs to heal before you can achieve your ideal body composition. If you do not continue to eat properly, you will delay your healing.

Symptoms
During your healing phase you can feel better, but if you are extremely insulin-resistant, you may feel sluggish, bloated, and irritable, and you may retain excess salt and water, which can cause ankle swelling and/or higher blood pressure.

Transition Phases
You will experience both a healing and fat-burning phase. You may also need to self-medicate to keep you feeling well through your transition, especially if you are extremely insulin-resistant.

Transition Time
It may take a few years for your body to become insulin-sensitive again.

What to Expect: Insulin-Resistant with Burned-Out Adrenal Glands

Because you are starting with a badly damaged metabolism, you will have to go through a lengthy transition process. Since you probably will feel worse before you feel better, it will take time for you to make the necessary permanent changes to ensure that you heal your metabolism and achieve your ideal body composition. Do not get discouraged—this is the only way your body knows how to heal.

You will need to become insulin-sensitive again and to heal your adrenal glands. You will therefore experience a healing phase. As you are healing, if you are extremely insulin-resistant—that is, despite better habits your insulin levels still stay very high—you may feel sluggish, bloated, and irritable, and you may retain excess salt and water, which can cause ankle swelling and/or higher blood pressure. If you taper off your high-adrenaline and/or high-cortisol habits too quickly, you may experience withdrawal symptoms. Because of this you will want or need to self-medicate. Once you have healed you will be primed to burn off excess fat weight. You will then be in your healed state.

Arthur's Transition

Initial Starting Point

Arthur's story (see chapter 5) is a good example of someone who really dug himself deep into a metabolic hole. When I met Arthur, he was insulin-resistant with burned-out adrenal glands. This is the worst metabolism anyone can have. He already had a premature degenerative disease of aging: blocked coronary arteries.

Digging a Deeper Hole

Arthur had unintentionally started through the transition many times in the past by improving his eating habits in between his diets. But he sabotaged his healing because each time he was in the healing phase and gained weight, he did not like the way he looked and felt. He would immediately start a different fad diet program that would raise his adrenaline/cortisol levels higher again so that he could lose weight and feel better.

As Arthur kept yo-yo dieting, he dug himself into a deeper metabolic hole. This is why his adrenal glands eventually burned out. But only part of his adrenal glands stopped functioning well because he was still able to produce a good deal of cortisol.

The combination of chronically high cortisol and insulin levels was the cause of the premature plaque build-up that developed in Arthur's heart arteries. These two hormones also caused a lot of fat gain around his midsection. By the time he had his emergency heart bypass surgery, Arthur weighed more than he ever had before.

He is the perfect example of what may happen to you if you wait too long to change your poor nutrition and lifestyle habits and never heal your metabolism.

Healing Phases

After his heart surgery, it finally dawned on Arthur that what he ate did matter. He has been following the SPII program for the last two years, and he is making progress. He started out with the worst current metabolism, so it will take him some more time to complete his transition. He is still in his healing phase because he is insulin-resistant. And although his adrenal glands are healing, they are still burned-out.

If you are insulin-resistant or have burned-out adrenal glands, you will be in the healing phase of the program longer than people who are insulin-sensitive or who have healthy adrenal glands. Arthur is well on his way to climbing completely out of his acquired metabolic hole.

Summary: Insulin-Resistant with Burned-Out Adrenal Glands

If you are insulin-resistant with burned-out adrenal glands, the following summarizes your initial starting point and what you may expect.

The Goal

You are starting with the worst metabolism type. Your goal is to become insulin-sensitive again and to heal your adrenal glands.

The Ability to Regenerate

You are neither using nor rebuilding your functional and structural biochemicals efficiently.

Body Composition

You are overweight and carry your excess fat weight around your midsection.

Weight Changes

You will probably gain weight before you lose your excess fat weight.

Habits

Either you are using toxic chemicals or an antidepressant to keep you going and feeling better, or you are constantly tired and have "fuzzy" thinking because you do not use them. You usually diet and/or increase your cardiovascular exercises to try to feel better and lose weight. You are in a group that has to be very careful because you feel better when you do not eat enough carbohydrates or food, and this will cause your body to use up your biochemicals instead of rebuild them. But remember, you have a damaged metabolism that needs to heal before you can achieve your ideal body composition. If you do not eat properly, you will delay your healing.

Symptoms

As you improve your habits, you will probably experience the signs and symptoms of adrenaline/cortisol withdrawal and high insulin levels. You may feel sluggish, bloated, depressed and irritable, and/or you may retain excess salt and water, which can cause ankle swelling and/or higher blood pressure.

Transition Phases

You will definitely have to go through an extensive healing/self-medicating phase and a fat-burning phase.

Transition Time

You will take the longest time to heal, but you can still improve your metabolism and your health.

Everyone Is Different

Kelley, Mary, Arthur, Annie and I all went through slightly different transitions because we all had different beginning current metabolisms, and we were all different ages when we began the healing process. The older you are, the longer it may take you to heal.

Kelley started with the best metabolism. She was insulin-sensitive and her adrenal glands were healthy, so it took her the least amount of time to balance out her hormones.

Mary was insulin-sensitive with burned-out adrenal glands. She is still healing, but it will not take her much longer to go through her transition because she is now in the later stages of her healing phase. She also has been able to follow the SPII program consistently for the past nine months, and this has helped her through her transition.

I started out insulin-sensitive with burned-out adrenal glands. During my transition, I experienced every current metabolism type there is because I did not have a program to follow. It took me longer to heal because I did not know what I was doing. I stumbled across a balanced meal program by experimenting with different ways of eating. When I finally did eat well, I was on my way to complete healing. I know that I still would have taken longer to heal than Kelley and Mary because I started out with a worse metabolism, but it should not have taken me seven years.

Annie's initial starting point was insulin-sensitive with burned-out adrenal glands, but she unintentionally extended her transition because she continued her high-stress lifestyle as a means of self-medication. Once she addressed her stress, she was into her fat-burning phase. She now feels better than she has in years and is primed for fat-weight loss.

Arthur started off in the worst shape because he maintained his poor nutrition and lifestyle habits the longest, dug himself into a deep metabolic hole and developed a premature degenerative disease of aging. He was insulin-resistant with burned-out adrenal glands for a very long time before he started his transition. He has the most healing to do. But Arthur has been in his healing program for two years and has made significant progress. He is healthier now than he would have been if he had not started his transition.

All the people you have read about in this chapter so far are still going through their transitions. Now read about Liz who has successfully completed her transition.

Liz's Transition: A Success Story

Liz destroyed her metabolism by following conventi[onal] wisdom—eating a high-carb, low-fat diet and overexercising. L[iz,] like Mary, was insulin-sensitive with burned-out adrenal glands wh[en] she began her transition. But she experienced more fatigue, carb[ohyd]rate cravings, water retention and weight gain than Mary did becaus[e sh]e was not taking an antidepressant—she was not depressed.

Liz completely healed her metabolism and regaine[d h]er energy and vitality after following the SPII program for two years[. Sh]e has achieved her ideal body composition and optimum health.

Her story illustrates that if you stick with this program [yo]u will succeed.

Liz: Sweets were always an issue for me. When I [was] a child I can remember making chocolate-chip cookies and eating t[he d]ough without ever baking the cookies. I thought I would grow out [of i]t one day, but instead my cravings got worse, especially after I star[ted] competing in bodybuilding contests at the age of twenty-one.

I would diet for six months on a no-fat diet to get re[ady] to compete. I ate high-protein meals and some carbohydrates, but I d[id n]ot eat any fat at all. I thought I was doing something healthy for myse[lf.]

When I dieted for my first competition, I had an [easy] time—foods weren't tempting to me. I'd just have a sweet tooth [no]w and again. Overall, it was a good experience.

But after that first competition I started having a har[d ti]me disciplining myself to eat properly—sweets became more of an [issu]e for me. My cravings got worse. I wanted sweet stuff more and more.

I kept competing. I went on the same type of diet eac[h ti]me, but I had to diet for a longer period. I also increased my cardio[vasc]ular exercises from one hour to four hours a day because I was eating [mo]re sugar.

I fell into a routine: I'd set a date for my next show [and] go through months of just torturous dieting. I would find myself figh[tin]g the diet the whole way. It was very uncomfortable, but that is w[hat] I had to go through in order to be lean enough to compete.

I took a break from competing for about two and a half years because during that time my obsession with food and sugar got worse. I couldn't discipline myself enough to keep my body fat at 8 percent; it went up to 24 percent. I was feeling fat and uncomfortable all the time. Then I had a baby, and postpregnancy, I got my sugar cravings back under control. I was ready to compete again.

When I was about thirty-two, things just started to fall apart. I was depressed. I had no sex drive. I was getting injuries for the first time. My skin changed. I was itchy all over. I was losing my hair, and I was just miserable. What made things worse was that I could not sleep. I'd fall asleep at 11 or 12 o'clock at night and be up at 3 o'clock in the morning. If I was lucky, I would get eighteen hours of sleep over a week's time.

Sugar became the only thing I ate. I was like an addict. I would be out gardening and I would look around to see if anyone was watching me. When the coast was clear, I would sneak inside away from my family and eat ice cream. After work, I would go to the market, buy a half-gallon of ice cream and eat the whole thing. It progressively got to the point where ice cream was all I ate because I got so nauseated and sick from eating the ice cream that I couldn't look at real food.

In the meantime, I was disgusted with myself because I was gaining fat and I hated working out—and working out is something I'd done and liked my whole life up until that time. After all, I own a gym, and I work as a trainer. Here I was teaching and counseling people about how to eat and exercise properly, and I was feeling like a total hypocrite because I was supposed to set a certain example. But I wasn't even able to follow my own advice.

About the same time, a client of mine brought me Dr. Schwarzbein's first book and asked me to read it to see what I thought. After reading it I knew I had to go see Dr. Schwarzbein no matter where she was in the world. Luckily, she was close by in Santa Barbara. That was three years ago.

Before my first visit with Dr. Schwarzbein, I started incorporating her program on my own by following the recommendations she made in her book. Then I went on a cruise and actually lost a percent of body fat—and on a cruise! This is where people usually say they gain fat. But it felt so easy to eat the right way. It was only easy for the first six weeks, though, and then the sugar cravings came back. This is when I went to see

Dr. Schwarzbein. She helped me fine-tune my program.

During the next year I continued to struggle with my sugar cravings. They would go away for about six weeks and then come back with a vengeance. It felt like I had a bungee cord wrapped around my waist. It kept pulling me back to the sugar, so I would just give in to it. I went through these cravings' cycles—up and down, up and down, up and down—for about six months before I asked Dr. Schwarzbein to add in some hormones. I felt like we should be seeing more progress. But she told me that I did not have a hormone-deficiency state and therefore I could not take HRT. She told me, "You know what? You are closer than you think you are." She just told me it would take more time.

In the meantime, I was seeing some victories. My mood, my energy, my enthusiasm all came back. My sleep improved, but not completely. However, I was still miserable because I was still eating a lot of ice cream. I was also gaining weight.

Dr. Schwarzbein: Even though Liz was also insulin-sensitive with burned-out adrenal glands, she had a harder time with her transition than Mary did because she could not follow her eating plan immediately. Her serotonin levels were low enough to cause carbohydrate cravings but not low enough to cause depression. She was self-medicating each time she gave in to her cravings. But she was always closer to getting through the healing phase than she thought.

Liz: About nine months later I just gave up because I couldn't beat the sugar anymore. I threw up my hands. I gave up my serotonin supplements. I gave up my vitamin-B supplements. I gave up my food, and I was back on my sugar cycle. This lasted for about six months, and then I went back to see Dr. Schwarzbein.

The thing that actually got me back to Dr. Schwarzbein was that my hair was falling out at a rapid rate. I thought that if I didn't see a doctor soon, I wouldn't have any hair! At my appointment I told Dr. Schwarzbein that this program wasn't working for me. I believed in it, but I did not feel it was working for me. I asked her how to take care of the hair issue within her philosophy.

She just said, "Liz, you are closer than you think." She told me to resume three things: eating consistently, taking the serotonin supplements she had prescribed for me and taking stress doses of vitamin B.

Dr. Schwarzbein: Liz did self-medicate with refined sugar, but she did not do so consistently. Therefore, she went back and forth between self-medicating and not self-medicating. She, too, needed a lot of encouragement, but she was always closer than she thought.

When the Program Doesn't "Work" for You

People who have an initial starting point of insulin-sensitive or insulin-resistant with burned-out adrenal glands do not always make it through the healing phases of their transition. As they adopt healthier habits, their adrenaline/cortisol levels get lower and their insulin levels get higher. They never make it past the beginning of the healing phase because they panic when they put on fat weight. They also do not feel as well as they did before, so they think they must be doing something wrong. They have symptoms such as water retention, "fuzzy" thinking, irritability, depression and fatigue, as well as food, sugar, alcohol and/or stimulant cravings.

Giving Up Is Not the Answer

People who have a tough time with the initial healing phase of the program often think, "This program is not working for me." So they go back to their old ways—the ones that raised their adrenaline/cortisol levels higher than their insulin levels in the first place. Or they adopt new habits to raise their adrenaline/cortisol levels higher again. By going back to a higher adrenaline/cortisol state to feel better, they are preventing their healing. Worse than that, this high adrenaline/cortisol state will cause more damage over time.

If you yo-yo back-and-forth between a higher adrenaline/cortisol state and a lower adrenaline/cortisol state, you will have to start your healing process all over again. You *must* go through the lower adrenaline/cortisol state in order to reach the balanced adrenaline/cortisol state. There are no shortcuts.

You May Feel Worse Before You Feel Better

If you begin your program with burned-out adrenal glands, no matter if you are thin or overweight, you will probably gain some fat weight before you are primed to lose *all* your fat weight. This is normal. Feeling worse before you completely heal is also normal. Do not equate gaining fat weight and feeling tired with "this program does not work" or "this program is not right for me." You cannot have a good metabolism until you have healed your adrenal glands, and you cannot repair your adrenal glands if you avoid the healing phases. You have to go through the healing phases because the damage has already been done—you cannot change your past, only your future.

The good news is that once you go through your transition, by permanently changing your nutrition and lifestyle habits, you should never have to go through it again.

The How To section of this book explains how to self-medicate appropriately so you can make it through your healing phase with a minimum of side effects such as fat-weight gain and fatigue.

Liz: Within two weeks of seeing Dr. Schwarzbein again, I was in a whole different place in my life—one I had never been in before. It was miraculous. I had a new feeling of being even and satisfied—and not just satisfied with food, but satisfied and easy with life. I was calm. And the sugar cravings went away; they just disappeared. That had never happened before in my life. I've been able to discipline myself, but I can't remember when I didn't crave sugar. It was just so revolutionary. It had taken me almost fifteen months of working with Dr. Schwarzbein to get to this place. That was about two years ago.

It's amazing. Dr. Schwarzbein told me that by following the

Schwarzbein Principle program my body would get to its natural proportions by itself. This is true. Now I'm leaner than I ever have been off-season. I do not compete anymore, but I am lean and perfectly satisfied.

Food used to control my life, but now it is not an issue. I don't have any inkling of a craving for sugar at all. This last Thanksgiving everyone was eating pie, and I didn't even want any. It wasn't as if I was exerting any willpower; I didn't want even want a taste.

I remember when I was seeing Dr. Schwarzbein and she would tell me that this would eventually happen. I just could not fathom that because I had never experienced anything like that before. But it is the truth; it finally did happen. Everything she told me would eventually happen did happen. Now I can see what she was trying to say. It isn't about self-discipline; you just don't want sugar. So now I preach that.

I have sent about twelve people, including Mary, to Dr. Schwarzbein because her program is the only one that works. I've been in this business for thirteen years and hers is the only book I recommend to people because I really feel it's the key.

So it's been an awesome time for me. My energy and vitality are back. Although I'm going through a hard time in my life right now—I'm going through a separation—I feel energetic and okay. I feel like I can do this. So not only did Dr. Schwarzbein's program change me physically, it also changed me mentally. I can do and take on things that I couldn't before. I am a whole new person.

Now when I teach and counsel people at the gym, I no longer feel like a hypocrite. I usually share my story with the people I train because I know that they are undereating and overexercising like I was, and I want them to change their habits. I also share with them that a person does not have to have many vices to end up where I was. I think that people need to know that you do not have to smoke or drink caffeinated beverages or alcohol in order to harm your metabolism. You can harm your metabolism by living "pretty clean." They think, "Oh, that can't be me." But it can be.

I also tell people they just have to hang in there no matter how hard or hopeless it seems. I tell them that they are closer than they think.

I'm thirty-five, and I feel like a success story. It's awesome. And I'm an evangelist now.

Dr. Schwarzbein: I couldn't have said it better myself. You are closer than you think.

Summary

- If you need to heal your metabolism, you will not be successful unless you go through the healing phase as part of your transition.
- Habits that raise adrenaline and cortisol levels can be used correctly in the healing phase as a way to self-medicate when you find yourself tired and depressed. But if you use them extensively, they will keep you from ever recovering fully.
- If you are insulin-sensitive with healthy adrenal glands, you still can use and rebuild your functional and structural proteins and fats at the same rate.
- If you are insulin-sensitive with burned-out adrenal glands, you cannot use your functional proteins and fats efficiently.
- If you are insulin-resistant with healthy adrenal glands, you are storing more fats than you are using up.
- If you are insulin-resistant with burned-out adrenal glands, you will take the longest time to heal.
- If you are starting with an efficient metabolism, but have poor nutrition and lifestyle habits, you still have to go through a transition. You will not experience a healing phase. If you do not carry excess fat weight, you will go directly into your healed state when you begin to improve your nutrition and lifestyle habits.
- People with burned-out adrenal glands do not always make it through the healing phases of their transition because they panic when their fat weight goes up. They also feel worse and think that they must be doing something wrong.
- You cannot have a good metabolism until you have healed your adrenal glands, and you cannot repair your adrenal glands if you avoid the healing phase.

- Going back to your old ways will damage your metabolism even more.
- Trying to make yourself feel better instantly will put you in a deeper metabolic hole.
- If you begin to improve your nutrition and lifestyle habits, you will be able to heal and climb out of the hole.
- The SPII program is designed to help you climb out of your hole and help you achieve optimum health.
- Once you go through your transition, you should never have to go through it again.

It Is Time to Begin Your Transition

Your body is designed to keep you alive through stressful times—and it will compromise your health and well-being in order to do so. Therefore, it is up to you to avoid the poor nutritional and lifestyle habits that signal your body that it is in stressful times. You can take control of your habits and ensure that you feel good, stay healthy and age successfully. There is no better time to address your nutrition and lifestyle habits than now. The How To section will guide you through your transition.

PART III

How To

Ten

The Schwarzbein Principle II Program: Introduction

Congratulations! You are now ready to begin the Schwarzbein Principle II Program (SPII) and enter your transition. The SPII program is divided into two parts: the general SPII program and the individual programs for your current metabolism type. To avoid confusion, read only the general program and the individual program for your current metabolism type.

The five steps of the SPII regeneration program are:

1. Healthy nutrition, including supplementation with vitamins, antioxidants, minerals, and amino and fatty acids, if needed

2. Stress management, including getting enough sleep

3. Tapering off of toxic chemicals or avoiding them completely

4. Cross-training exercises

5. Hormone replacement therapy (HRT), if needed

If you have not read the Why To and the Transition sections, I highly recommend that you go back and read them before you begin this section of the book. It's important that you understand how the body works and how it heals itself so that you will be able to make informed nutrition and lifestyle choices. Parts I and II explain how you acquired your current metabolism, guide you in the steps you need to concentrate on the most during your transition and also describe what you may experience as you heal.

It is important to note that the SPII program is a lifestyle change and not a fad diet. The goal is to become or stay healthy. Losing weight to become healthy is a myth. You will achieve your ideal body composition only if you become and remain healthy first.

Though making any improvements in your habits will benefit you, this program is a process, and it may take you time to make all the changes necessary for you to heal. If you remain consistent with your new nutrition and lifestyle habits, you will regenerate and heal your metabolism, achieve your ideal body composition and obtain optimum health.

Identifying Your Personal Physiology and Individual Program

Before you begin incorporating this program into your life, you need to identify your current metabolism type. Understanding your beginning physiology will help you choose the correct meal plans; identify your need for stress-management techniques; determine the necessity of *tapering* off refined sugars, stimulants and other toxic chemicals; make changes to your exercise program; and determine how to start taking HRT, if needed.

Check your current metabolism type and remember that your goal is to become insulin-sensitive with healthy adrenal glands—and to remain that way by improving your nutrition and lifestyle habits. If you do not remember your type, refer back to chapter 8.

_____I am insulin-sensitive and have healthy adrenal glands.

_____I am insulin-resistant and have healthy adrenal glands.

_____I am insulin-sensitive and have burned-out adrenal glands.

_____I am insulin-resistant and have burned-out adrenal glands.

The Importance of Knowing If You Are Insulin-Sensitive or Insulin-Resistant

It is important to know whether you are insulin-sensitive or insulin-resistant so that you do not follow the wrong eating program. Eating the correct amount of real carbohydrates and healthy food for your current metabolism and activity level is necessary for healing and for achieving optimum health. Keep the following guidelines in mind:

If you are insulin-sensitive and do not eat enough carbohydrates or food for your current activity level, you will raise your adrenaline and cortisol levels too high, causing you to use up your biochemicals more than rebuild them. Though you may lose weight in the short term, this type of weight loss will never make you healthy because you will be destroying your metabolism.

If you are insulin-resistant and do not eat enough carbohydrates or food, you will also raise your adrenaline and cortisol levels too high and become more insulin-resistant.

If you are insulin-sensitive and eat too many carbohydrates and too much food, your insulin levels will rise too high and you may become insulin-resistant over time.

If you are insulin-resistant, you need to make sure that you do not eat too many carbohydrates or too much food. Too many carbohydrates or too much food increases your insulin levels and will only make your problems worse by causing more weight gain, increasing your triglyceride and cholesterol production, and increasing your risk for degenerative diseases of aging.

The Importance of Knowing If Your Adrenal Glands Are Healthy or Burned Out

If your adrenal glands are burned out, it will take you longer to heal and you will need to make changes to your nutrition and lifestyle habits more slowly so that you can be successful during your transition. If you try to change everything at once, you may find yourself "falling apart" and suffering from incapacitating fatigue, headaches, depression, irritability, bloating and ankle swelling. Other problems to watch out for are more severe allergies and/or asthma, increased frequency of colds or flu, flare-up of skin disorders such as psoriasis and hives, and increased chemical sensitivities. (See chapter 4 for complete list of symptoms and problems.)

You may experience none, some or all of these symptoms and problems no matter how slowly you change your lifestyle habits and follow your program, but they can be tolerable and manageable if you make small rather than abrupt changes in your habits.

What About Fat-Weight Loss?

You need to heal your metabolism first to become insulin-sensitive and have healthy adrenal glands again—*before* you can lose all your fat weight. But remember that as you are healing you are also gaining muscle weight. Keep this in mind as you are going through your transition and be patient if it seems that it is taking too long to burn off excess storage fat. Keep these guidelines in mind:

- If you are insulin-sensitive, it means that you have the *potential* to gain fat weight quickly, but you can lose it quickly, too.
- If you are insulin-resistant, it means that you have probably already gained most of your fat weight and are having a hard time losing fat weight that you have already gained.
- If you have healthy adrenal glands, you can lose fat weight easily.

- If you have burned-out adrenal glands, it is easier for you to gain and harder for you to lose fat weight.

The following describes what will most likely happen to your fat weight when you begin to eat balanced meals, do your recommended exercise program consistently and follow the rest of the SPII recommendations.

- If you are insulin-sensitive and have healthy adrenal glands, *you should lose fat weight quickly.*
- If you are insulin-resistant and have healthy adrenal glands, *you should begin to lose fat weight slowly.*
- If you are insulin-sensitive and have burned-out adrenal glands, *you are most likely to gain fat weight before you begin to slowly lose fat weight.*
- If you are insulin-resistant and have burned-out adrenal glands, *you are more likely to gain more fat weight before you begin to slowly lose the fat weight you already have stored.*

Tips for Success

To ensure your success on this program, only make as many changes at one time as you can stick to because making too many changes at once usually means you will end up making none of them permanently. The good news is that any change you make will benefit you.

As you begin changing your habits, the most important place to start is with nutrition. Since you will be using food to regenerate, eating the right types of foods is essential for a successful transition process.

If you are under too much stress, it may be impossible for you to make *all* the necessary changes to your eating habits at first. If that is the case, stress management becomes a very important step for you.

If you find yourself having problems following the program, ask your physician to check for a glandular-based endocrine disorder. If you do not have a glandular-based endocrine disorder, you may need to self-medicate to feel good enough to continue the healing process.

Keep in mind that you are trying to become healthy—not just lose fat weight. If you try to lose fat weight before you become healthy, you will only damage your metabolism further. Be consistent, and your new lifestyle habits will get easier over time.

Now it's time to get started with your program. Let's move on to chapter 11 and Step One of the SPII program.

Eleven

Step One: Healthy Nutrition

lthough we all share the same basic physiology, we do not all share the same current metabolism. This is because your personal nutrition and lifestyle habits throughout your life have been different from those of your family and friends. However, the SPII program's nutrition principles are the same for everyone. You will still eat all the same real foods—the ones you can theoretically hunt, fish, grow and harvest—but your proportions of these foods will differ from other people's. It all depends on whether or not you are insulin-sensitive or insulin-resistant and have healthy or burned-out adrenal glands.

General Guidelines

If you begin eating real foods and balancing your food groups *and* you gain weight, you have a damaged metabolism. Resist the temptation to cut back on portions, skip meals or go on a fad diet to lose this weight. You will just dig yourself into a deeper metabolic "hole" if you do. You have to eat well to heal your metabolism. There is no other way.

Once you have healed your metabolism, you will burn off your fat weight without having to decrease the amount of food you eat by dieting.

When you begin changing your eating habits, keep in mind the principles listed below. If you follow these ten principles, you will be eating in a balanced, healthy way that will ensure you make it through your transition successfully.

One: Never skip a meal again.

Skipping meals causes hormonal chaos! When you skip or delay a meal, both adrenaline and cortisol levels increase. Any time these hormone levels increase because you are not eating, your body "eats" itself up. This may make the numbers on the scale go down, but you are not healing because your body is using up your functional and structural biochemicals along with your stored energy biochemicals (glycogen and fat).

Additionally, the next time you do eat, your insulin levels will rise even higher than they would have normally for the same amount of carbohydrates consumed. Your body then has two reasons to secrete insulin. The first is to counter your adrenaline and cortisol levels to keep your body from using itself up too quickly or too much, and the second is in response to the amount of carbohydrates in your meal to ensure excess sugar is taken up by your cells.

Two: Eat real, unprocessed foods as much as possible.

You use food to rebuild your functional, structural and energy proteins, fats and carbohydrates on a continuous basis. Foods that you use to rebuild your biochemicals are those that you can theoretically pick, gather, milk, fish or hunt. Therefore, it is important that you stay away from processed and damaged foods, as well as those filled with toxic chemicals.

I have designed the Schwarzbein Principle Square to help you visualize how your meals should consist of foods from the following four food groups: proteins, healthy fats, nonstarchy vegetables and real carbohydrates. You will also need to eat the right amount of protein and carbohydrates for your current metabolism type and activity level. Refer to your current metabolism type program. (See chapter 17, 18, 19 or 20.)

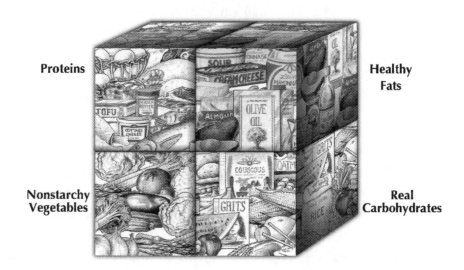

Proteins

Healthy Fats

Nonstarchy Vegetables

Real Carbohydrates

Figure 11-1. The Schwarzbein Square

Three: Eat balanced meals.

Eating balanced meals means consuming foods from the four food groups at every meal. It does not mean that you eat the same-sized portions of proteins, healthy fats, nonstarchy vegetables and real carbohydrates.

It is important to eat balanced meals for two reasons. First, since you are using food to rebuild with, you need to eat the foods that you are made from. Second, you need to keep your hormones balanced. Eating too many carbohydrates at one time raises your insulin levels too high; eating too much protein raises adrenaline and cortisol levels too high.

Ideally, you should eat smaller meals more frequently: three meals and two snacks a day. If that is not possible, make sure that you are eating at least three meals a day. Eating too much food at one time raises your insulin levels too high. Not eating enough food makes your adrenaline/cortisol levels rise too high.

In general, to identify a balanced meal, divide your plate into one-third slots and place the proteins, real carbohydrates and nonstarchy vegetables in each slot. Then add a healthy fat to each or some of the portions as well. For example, steak, corn on the cob and green salad comprise a protein, real carbohydrate and nonstarchy vegetable respectively. The steak already has fat in it. You can add butter as the healthy fat to the corn and olive oil, lemon and garlic as the dressing on your salad. This is a balanced meal.

Four: Choose a protein as the main nutrient in your meal.

You will be building your meal around this protein. You can choose meats, poultry, fish, eggs or tofu. Make sure that your protein choice is as fresh as possible and that it is not filled with chemicals, additives, preservatives or hormones. Buy organic food as much as possible.

Your body is made up mostly of proteins, so you will be using proteins to rebuild. However, eating too much protein or eating a protein alone triggers the release of adrenaline and cortisol; ironically this will cause you to use up your biochemicals instead of rebuild them. See Healthy Proteins section on page 231 in this chapter.

Five: Add some healthy fats to your meal.

The purpose of eating good fats is to rebuild your functional, structural and energy biochemicals.

The definition of a healthy fat has nothing to do with whether it is saturated or mono- or polyunsaturated, but everything to do with whether or not the fat is damaged.

Avoid all damaged fats. Some fats are damaged when the molecules of the fat are rearranged during the cooking or processing of the fat. This damaged fat is known as a trans-fat. You know a food product is more likely to have trans-fats in it if the package says "partially hydrogenated" or "hydrogenated."

Do not buy or eat products that contain these types of fats. In fact, this is a good time to go through your cupboards and refrigerator and throw away all foods that contain damaged fats. When you are looking for good fats, check the ingredients and look for saturated fats, or cold-pressed, pure-pressed, or expeller-pressed mono- or polyunsaturated oils.

Most margarine contains trans-fats, so begin eating butter or olive oil today. Refer to the Damaged Fats section on page 254 in this chapter.

Six: Add real carbohydrates to your meals.

A real carbohydrate is one that can be grown, picked or harvested. Avoid ingesting pesticides by buying organic fruits, whole grains, legumes and starchy vegetables as much as possible.

The amount of carbohydrates you eat should match your current metabolism and activity level. You can create hormonal imbalances if you do not eat enough carbohydrates or if you eat too many of them. Eating too few carbohydrates increases adrenaline/cortisol levels and causes your body to use up its biochemicals too quickly. Eating too many carbohydrates increases insulin levels and causes you to over-build and store fats.

Learn how to eat the correct amount of carbohydrates to balance your hormones. Refer to your current metabolism type program. (See chapters 17, 18, 19 or 20.)

Seven: Eat nonstarchy vegetables.

Nonstarchy vegetables add fiber, vitamins and minerals to your diet, as well as phytochemicals (plant chemicals). These healthy nutrients help your body rebuild tissues and regenerate more quickly.

Unfortunately, more and more vegetables contain fewer and fewer nutrients because of nutrient-depleted soil; therefore, I recommend that you supplement with a good pharmaceutical-grade multivitamin and mineral unless you can eat all organically grown foods, which you should do to avoid ingesting pesticides and other chemicals. See the supplementation discussion beginning on page 314 of this chapter.

Eight: Eat snacks.

It is better to eat smaller meals more frequently, so snacking is important. Each snack ideally should consist of all four food groups. At the minimum, include a protein and carbohydrate in every snack. See Snack Ideas section on page 308 of this chapter.

Nine: Eat solid food.

Drinking instead of eating your meals leads to hormone imbalances. Initially you will have a fast rise of insulin, and this will be followed by a fast rise of adrenaline and cortisol. This is exactly what you do not want to have happen. These fluctuating hormone levels can make you feel lousy and damage your metabolism. When you eat solid food, your body processes the meal more slowly, and you avoid these unwanted hormone fluctuations.

Ten: Make sure you drink enough water each day.

Your body is comprised of 50 to 60 percent water and it needs to be replenished. Drink at least eight glasses of water a day, more if you are exercising. Refer to "Why Drinking Enough Water Is Important" on page 281 in this chapter to understand the many benefits of water.

Healthy Proteins

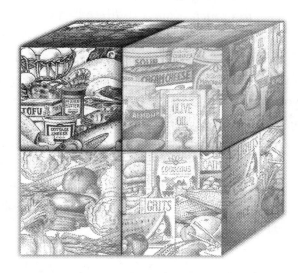

In my first book, *The Schwarzbein Principle*, I focused on the fact that eating too many man-made carbohydrates is the number-one reason for hormonal imbalances. I wrote that you should never eat a carbohydrate alone, and I explained why you should restrict how many carbohydrates you eat at one time.

I also explained that you do not need to restrict the amount of fat or protein you consume—based on the premise that your own body will tell you when it has had enough—as long as you are eating the correct amount of carbohydrates for your current metabolism and activity level. The amount of fat and protein you consume becomes naturally restricted over time because of feedback methods for their control. This premise still holds true if you have healthy adrenal glands and eat the correct amount of carbohydrates.

When people with healthy adrenal glands eat protein, their adrenaline and cortisol levels rise above normal, which signals to the body that they are satiated. If they continue to eat more protein at this time, they will end up feeling bloated and stuffed, or they may have a hard time sleeping that night. However, if you have burned-out adrenal glands, your feedback mechanisms may not be working because you are starting off with lower than normal adrenaline and cortisol levels, and when you eat too much protein your levels rise closer to normal. This actually makes you feel better in the short-term. However, eating too much protein is one of the causes of adrenal gland burnout, so you will not be able to recognize that you are actually harming instead of helping yourself.

Therefore, if your adrenal glands are burned out, you must initially monitor how much protein as well as how many carbohydrates you eat.

However, you still do not have to count, measure or restrict the amount of total fat you eat. Your body will regulate this for you as long as you are eating the correct amount of proteins and carbohydrates for your current metabolism and activity levels.

Guidelines for Consuming Proteins

How Much Protein to Eat

In general, you should eat a minimum of 1.0 to 1.25 grams of protein for every kilogram you weigh. To calculate your minimum range of protein intake, divide your weight in pounds by 2.2. This equals your weight in kilograms (kg). Then multiply your weight in kg first by 1.0 and then by 1.25. This will give you your minimum protein *range*. Next, divide each amount of protein in grams by 7 (there are 7 grams in 1 ounce of protein) to obtain the ounces of protein you should eat. Here are a few examples:

- A 100-pound person would weigh 100/2.2 or 45.5 kg, and should eat between 45.5 and 57 grams of protein a day—or about 7 to 8 ounces a day minimally.
- A 150-pound person would weigh 150/2.2 or 68 kg, and should eat between 68 and 85 grams of protein a day—or about 10 to 12 ounces a day minimally.

- A 200-pound person would weigh 200/2.2 or 91 kg, and should eat between 91 and 114 grams of protein a day—or about 13 to 16 ounces a day minimally.

Divide Your Proteins Throughout the Day

- If you eat five times a day, you must eat a *minimum* of 2 to 3 ounces of protein with each meal and 1 to 3 ounces of protein per snack.
- If you eat four times a day, you should eat a *minimum* of 2 to 4 ounces of protein with each meal and snack.
- If you eat three meals a day, you should eat a *minimum* of 3 to 5 ounces of protein with each meal.

What Types of Protein to Eat

- Try not to consume more than 7 to 10 servings a week of red meat if you are insulin-sensitive because you need a variety of protein sources. If you are insulin-resistant, keep your servings down to no more than three to five a week. You cannot eat as many servings because red meat contains hidden sugar in the form of glycogen. You can eat as many servings of white meats as you want, but strive for variety.
- Eat fish at least three times a week. The more the better. Eat more salmon, tuna and mackerel because they are high in omega-3 fatty acids. Omega-3 fatty acids, among their many health benefits, improve insulin sensitivity. If you are a vegetarian and do not eat fish, eat more walnuts and ground flaxseeds or flaxseed oil to obtain your omega-3 fatty acids.
- For variety, you can add organic soy products to your meal plans throughout the week.

General Guidelines

1) Never eat a protein by itself. Too much protein raises adrenaline/cortisol levels and will cause you to burn out your adrenal glands over time.

2) You are probably getting too much protein if you develop bad breath, get constipated, get stomachaches, cannot sleep well at night, get irritable, experience heart palpitations, sweat excessively, lose weight too quickly and/or you are getting arthritis-like stiffness, inflammation or pain after you start to eat this way.

3) First, check to be sure that you are eating balanced meals. If you are, you need to cut back on your protein portion size. Refer to guidelines 1 and 2, but never eat less than the recommended total minimal protein amount for the day. You may have to add another meal to get smaller amounts of protein at one time or take digestive enzymes and/or hydrochloric acid if you are having a hard time digesting proteins.

4) If your adrenal glands are burned out, you may not experience any of the above symptoms, so it is important for you to follow your protein guidelines.

The following box contains protein portion sizes to guide you in eating the right amount of protein and the following tables list good sources of proteins for you to choose from. If you are insulin-resistant be aware of hidden sugars and the higher saturated fat content of some of these protein choices. Make sure you read the fine print so that you eat the right foods for your current metabolism.

Protein Portions

Two-Ounce Portions

Two ounces of protein is approximately half the size of your palm and as thick as a deck of a cards. Examples of two-ounce protein portions include:

2 ounces beef, lamb, pork, chicken, turkey, fish
2 eggs
2 ounces canned tuna (⅓ can)
½ cup cottage cheese
2 ounces cheese
¾ cup tofu
½ cup tempeh
Nuts: ¼ cup soybeans, 2 ounces almonds, 3 ounces other nuts

Three-Ounce Portions

Three ounces of protein is approximately the size and thickness of a deck of cards. Examples of three-ounce protein portions include:

3 ounces beef, lamb, pork, chicken, turkey, fish
3 eggs
3 ounces canned tuna (½ can)
¾ cup cottage cheese
3 ounces cheese
1¼ cups tofu
¾ cup tempeh

Four-Ounce Portions

Four ounces of protein is approximately the size of your palm and as thick as a deck of cards. Examples of four-ounce protein portions include:

4 ounces beef, lamb, pork, chicken, turkey, fish
4 eggs
4 ounces tuna (⅔ can)
1 cup cottage cheese
4 ounces cheese (combine this with another protein; try to limit cheese to 2 ounces, unless you are a vegetarian)
1½ cups tofu
1 cup tempeh

Five-Ounce Portions

Five ounces of protein is approximately one and one-half the size of your palm and as thick as a deck of cards. Examples of 5-ounce protein portions include:

5 ounces beef, lamb, pork, chicken, turkey, fish

5 eggs

5 ounces tuna (⅝ can)

1¼ cups cottage cheese

5 ounces cheese (try to limit cheese to 2-ounce servings, unless you are a vegetarian)

2 cups tofu

1¼ cups tempeh

Eggs

You can eat eggs every day, as many as your body wants.

Meat and Poultry

Whenever possible buy hormone-free, antibiotic-free, range-fed meat and poultry.

Beef*	Pheasant	Squab
Chicken**	Pork (bacon	Turkey**
Duck*	and ham)*	Veal
Lamb*	Quail	

---

* Bacon and ham are cured with sugar. If you must eat bacon and ham, only do so occasionally and always make sure you are buying nitrate-free meats. Beef, duck and lamb contain glycogen, a hidden sugar. All contain saturated fats. Watch your portions if you are insulin-resistant. Avoid them if you are following the lower-saturated fat meal plans.

**Dark chicken and turkey meat have more saturated fat. Eat mostly white meat, especially if you are insulin-resistant or following the lower-saturated fat meal plans.

Additive- and Nitrate-Free Sausages

Do not eat packaged sausage or lunch meats because they contain nitrates that increase your risk for developing cancer. Many communities have at least one old-fashioned butcher shop that still makes homemade sausage. Ask your butcher if he or she makes them without nitrates and/or additives. Limit your sausage intake to three to four a week but do not eat any if you are on a lower-saturated fat plan.

Berliner	Chorizo	Liver sausage
Bockwurst	Duck sausage	Liverwurst
Bratwurst	Frankfurter	Polish sausage
Braunschweiger	Italian sausage	Pork sausage
(liverwurst)	Kielbasa	Pork and beef sausage
Brotwurst	Knackwurst	Turkey sausage
Chicken sausage	Liver cheese	

Paté

Chicken liver paté	Goose liver paté	Salmon paté
Duck liver paté	Rabbit liver paté	Shrimp paté

Unless you are insulin-sensitive and have healthy adrenal glands, you should limit eating paté to one to two times a week. However, do not eat paté if you are on a lower-saturated fat plan.

Cheese

Since most cheese is heat treated, which damages the fat contained in the cheese, all cheese should be used in moderation. In addition, aged cheeses are damaged fats. Whenever possible, choose white cheese over yellow. Most yellow cheeses are colored with artificial coloring.

The Best Cheese to Eat*

Cottage cheese**   Mozzarella (buffalo   Provolone
Feta   and regular)   Queso fresco
Fontina   Muenster   Ricotta, whole
Gjetost   Neufchâtel   or skim milk
Goat

Eat Only Occasionally

Bleu   Colby   Parmesan
Brick   Cream cheese   Port de salut
Brie   Edam   Romano
Camembert   Gouda   Roquefort
Caraway   Gruyère   Swiss
Cheddar   Limburger   Tilsit
Cheshire   Monterey Jack

Fish and Shellfish

All fish is an excellent source of protein. Eat more cold-water fish because of its omega-3 content. (See page 251 for a list of fish that contain omega-3.) Eat fresh wild fish instead of canned or smoked. Most smoked fish contain nitrates.

---

* You only need to eat low-fat cheeses if you are on a lower-saturated fat plan.
**Cottage cheese, while an excellent source of protein, also contains 6 grams of carbohydrate per cup. Count this as part of your carbohydrate consumption if you are insulin-resistant or have severely burned-out adrenal glands.

Protein Foods That Contain Carbohydrates

Nuts, Nut Butters and Seeds

Nuts, nut butters and seeds are good sources of both protein and fat. However, each serving below also contains six grams of carbohydrates. Count this as part of your carbohydrate consumption if you are insulin-resistant or have severely burned-out adrenal glands. Eat nuts raw or dry-roasted. All items are raw unless otherwise noted.

Food Item	Serving
Acorns	½ ounce
Almonds	1 ounce (23 nuts)
Almond butter	4 tablespoons
Almond paste	½ ounce
Amaranth seed	⅓ ounce
Brazil nuts (butternuts)	1½ ounces
Cashews	¾ ounce
Cashew butter	1½ tablespoons
Chinese chestnuts	½ ounce
Coconut cream*	¼ cup
Coconut liquid from coconut*	¾ cup
Coconut meat*	½ cup, shredded
Coconut milk*	½ cup
Cottonseed kernels (roasted)	1 ounce
European chestnuts	½ ounce
Filberts or hazelnuts	1½ ounces
Ginkgo nuts	½ ounce
Hickory nuts	1 ounce
Japanese chestnuts	¾ ounce
Lotus seeds	1½ ounces
Macadamia nuts**	1½ ounces
Peanuts	1 ounce
Peanut butter	2 tablespoons
Pecans	1 ounce (15 halves)

*Do not eat if you are following the lower-saturated fat meal plan.
**Eat only half of a handful if you are following the lower-saturated fat meal plan.

Protein Foods That Contain Carbohydrates (cont'd)

Pine nuts	1 ounce
Pistachio nuts	1 ounce (47 kernels)
Pumpkin and squash kernels	1 ounce (hulled)
Pumpkin and squash seeds	½ ounce (42 seeds)
Safflower kernels (dried)	½ ounce
Sesame butter (tahini)	1½ tablespoons
Sesame seed kernels (dried)	1 ounce
Sunflower seed butter	1½ tablespoons
Sunflower seed kernels (dried)	¼ cup
Walnuts	2 ounces
Watermelon seed kernels	⅜ cup

Soy Products

Soy products contain both protein and carbohydrates. Count the carbohydrate content of them if you are insulin-resistant. Each of the following selections contains fifteen grams of carbohydrate.

Food Item	Serving
Miso (diluted)	¼ cup
Natto	½ cup
Soy milk*	1 cup
Soy protein	1½ ounces
Tempeh	½ cup
Tofu	1 cup

---

*Always count soy milk as a carbohydrate and do not drink it if you are insulin-resistant.

Healthy Fats

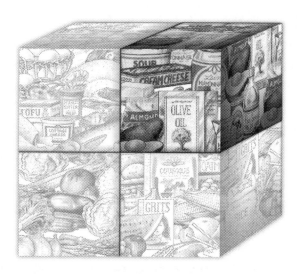

Do not be afraid to eat real foods that contain healthy fats, including cholesterol. Not all fats are harmful; in fact, healthy fats, including cholesterol, are essential for optimum health. Eating healthy fats will keep you happier and healthier longer by allowing your body to maintain hormone balance and slowing down accelerated aging. Although in theory you do not have to count or measure your fat intake, strive for moderation. You should not overeat fats, just like you should not overeat carbohydrates or proteins. This is not a high-fat or low-fat eating plan.

Here are some reasons that eating healthy fats is essential to maintaining optimum health:

- Eating healthy fats, including cholesterol, is essential to maintaining a healthy metabolism because you use these nondamaged fats for energy and to rebuild your functional and structural fats.

- Healthy fats are your body's only source for essential fatty acids, which are necessary for good health.

- Healthy fats in your diet keep you satiated and satisfied and thus help prevent overeating.

- Healthy fats are required for a healthy immune system, for the absorption of fat-soluble vitamins, as an energy source, and to slow down the absorption of carbohydrates and proteins in your meal.

Fatty Acids

There are three types of healthy fatty acids—saturated, monounsaturated and polyunsaturated. All fatty acids are made of carbon molecules that are chemically bonded together. Carbon needs to be chemically bonded to four other molecules. In a chain, carbon bonds to two other carbons leaving two empty sides.

When these sides are completely filled with hydrogen molecules the fatty acid is saturated.

Saturated Fatty Acid Molecule

When two carbon molecules that are next to each other are each missing a hydrogen molecule, the carbon molecules will attach twice to the carbon next to it. This is a double bond, and when there is only one double bond in the fatty acid, it is a monounsaturated fat.

Monounsaturated Fatty Acid Molecule

```
    H       H       H       H       H       H       H       H
    |       |       |       |       |       |       |       |
 —  C   —   C   =   C   —   C   —   C   —   C   —   C   —   C   —
    |       |       |       |       |       |       |       |
    H                       H       H       H       H       H
```

Polyunsaturated fats have more than one double bond.

Polyunsaturated Fatty Acid Molecule

```
    H       H       H       H       H       H       H       H
    |       |       |       |       |       |       |       |
 —  C   —   C   =   C   —   C   —   C   —   C   =   C   —   C   —
    |       |       |       |       |               |
    H                       H       H                       H
```

When you deprive your body of dietary fats, you end up depleted of two essential polyunsaturated fatty acids called alpha linolenic acid (ALA) and linoleic acid (LA). Without these essential fatty acids, your body will not function properly. (Also see Essential Fatty Acids on page 247 in this chapter.)

This does not mean that it is okay for you to overeat fats. However, unlike proteins and carbohydrates, you do not have to worry about monitoring your total fat intake.

When you eat fat, your body secretes the hormone cholecystokinin (CCK). CCK goes to your brain and announces that food has arrived. CCK also makes your gallbladder contract, releasing bile to help you absorb fats. If CCK is overproduced, you will become nauseous. If you ignore this feeling and keep eating more fat, you will either become more nauseated or vomit. This is how your body regulates your total fat intake for you. Other symptoms of too much fat in your diet are abdominal pain or cramping, loose bowel movements and stools that float in the toilet.

It is important to monitor the amount of the different types of fatty acids you consume. Make sure to eat foods from all three fatty acids types: saturated, monounsaturated and polyunsaturated.

Saturated Fats

In theory, saturated fats are not bad for you. They are used as a form of energy, are important in brain function and are needed to build cell membranes.

However, if you have a badly damaged metabolism and cannot burn saturated fats for energy or use them to rebuild biochemicals, they can keep your blood-sugar levels higher. The higher blood-sugar levels will cause higher insulin levels, which in turn leads to increased cholesterol and triglyceride production, higher blood pressure, further weight gain or the inability to lose weight, and increased inflammation of your joints and bones. Over time, diabetes, blood-pressure levels, fat-weight problems, plaque buildup in your arteries and arthritis may get worse.

If you already have any of these conditions, you may need to be on a lower-saturated fat plan until your metabolism heals. (Refer to the Special Dietary Recommendations starting on page 319 in this chapter.)

This does not mean you are going on a low-fat diet. You will need to eat plenty of monounsaturated and healthy polyunsaturated oils instead of saturated fats. You will also need to make sure that your ratio of omega-3 to omega-6 fatty acid intake is at least 1-to-3.

Foods High in Saturated Fat—Avoid or Eat Sparingly on a Lower-Saturated Fat Plan

The following is a list of foods to avoid completely or eat in small quantities on a low saturated fat plan.

Dairy and Related Products

- Cream—Mostly avoid, but you may use a teaspoon in your morning decaffeinated coffee or a small amount of unsweetened whipped heavy cream on berries (low glycemic index fruits).
- Milk—Avoid all milk. You should not be drinking milk anyway—unless you have diabetes and are having a low blood-sugar reaction. Then you can drink whole milk to treat your hypoglycemia.
- Sour cream/Cream cheese—You should always eat very small amounts of sour cream or cream cheese anyway. But avoid it completely for the time being.
- Whole-milk cheeses (cheddar, Swiss, jack, muenster)—Avoid all whole-milk cheeses at this time, but you may use part-skim-type cheeses such as low-fat cottage cheese, part-skim mozzarella, buffalo mozzarella and part-skim ricotta.
- Whole-milk yogurt—Avoid all low-fat and nonfat yogurts. Low-fat or nonfat milk yogurts are filled with extra sugar and chemicals. When you are exercising consistently, you can begin eating small amounts of organic whole-fat plain yogurt.

Meat, Poultry and Fish

- Bacon—Avoid eating bacon at this time, even if it is nitrate free.
- Chicken, turkey and chicken or turkey skin—Avoid eating chicken and turkey skin and eat more white meat than dark meat chicken and turkey.

Meat, Poultry and Fish (cont'd)

- Duck—Avoid eating duck at this time.
- Ground meats—avoid all ground meats except ground sirloin and low-fat ground turkey meat.
- Meats—Highly marbled or prime grades of beef, lamb or pork should always be avoided, but you may eat lean cuts of pork now. Later on you may reintroduce lean cuts of beef and lamb.
- Ribs—Avoid all at this time.
- Sausage—Avoid all at this time.

Breads and Grains

- Avoid all baked goods made with milk or animal fat—read labels.

Fruits and Nuts

- Coconut—Avoid completely at this time.
- Macadamia nuts—Eat only small amounts in any one day (half of a handful).

Fats and Oils

- Butter—Cut down on butter at this time and use more olive oil.
- Coconut oils—Avoid completely at this time.
- Cream sauces—Avoid completely at this time.
- Lard—Avoid completely at this time.
- Palm or palm kernel oils—Avoid completely at this time.

Essential Fatty Acids

Essential fatty acids (EFAs) are a special group of polyunsaturated oils that cannot be made by the body and must be obtained from foods or supplements. There are only two EFAs: alpha linolenic acid (ALA) and linoleic acid (LA).

Essential fatty acids and their conversion into prostaglandins are involved in a number of vital functions in the body. These include:

- Transport and metabolism of cholesterol and triglycerides

- Normal brain development and function

- Cell membrane structure

- Production of prostaglandins that regulate blood clotting, blood pressure, inflammation, immune function, blood-sugar levels, fertility, reproduction and pain

- Replenishment of skin oils to speed healing and decrease drying and wrinkling

Omega-3 and Omega-6 Fatty Acids

There are two major families of essential fats: omega-3 and omega-6 fatty acids. ALA heads up the omega-3 family and LA the omega-6 family. These two fatty acids are then converted to the different prostaglandins.

ALA requires conversion to docosahexaenoic acid (DHA) and eicosapentaenoic acid (EPA) to produce the beneficial prostaglandins.

LA is converted to gamma linolenic acid or GLA, which then can make prostaglandins that inhibit inflammation, lower blood pressure, inhibit blood clotting, lower blood-sugar levels and decrease the symptoms of premenstrual tension.

However, some of the GLA has to go on to produce arachidonic acid that promotes inflammation, increases blood pressure, causes blood clotting and raises blood-sugar levels.

Research indicates that it is the ratio of omega-3 to omega-6 fatty acids that is most important. It is important to maintain a balance between the omega-3 and omega-6 fatty acids to maintain a balance between inflammatory and anti-inflammatory responses, higher and lower blood pressure, increased and decreased blood clotting, and many other functions in the body. For example, if you get injured, you need to be able to clot your blood or you will bleed to death. It is only when the ability to clot is excessive that you end up with an increased risk of ischemic strokes and heart attacks.

The standard American diet (SAD) is very unbalanced with too many damaged omega-6 fatty acids and inadequate amounts of omega-3 fatty acids. Therefore, the production of the various prostaglandins in the body is imbalanced, and we make too many blood clotting, blood-pressure raising and inflammatory prostaglandins.

In addition to this imbalance, other factors inhibit the conversion of essential fatty acids into the different prostaglandins. These include:

- Alcohol consumption

- Aging

- High insulin levels

- High sugar intake

- Hydrogenated fats and trans-fats in the diet

- Hormonal responses to stress

- Inadequate nutrients, including deficiencies of vitamin C, vitamin B_6, zinc and magnesium

- Viral infections

Foods Containing Omega-3 Fats

The omega-3 fats are found especially in fatty fish, wild game, breast milk and omega-3 eggs. (Although all eggs contain some omega-3 fatty acids, these eggs are produced from chickens that are fed flaxseeds.) All these foods contain preformed DHA and EPA, which are directly converted into healthy prostaglandins.

The omega-3 fats in vegetarian sources such as flaxseeds and walnuts contain ALA, which requires conversion to DHA and EPA to produce the beneficial prostaglandins. The flaxseeds must be ground to absorb the fats; flaxseed oil is also available. Most people can adequately convert ALA to DHA and EPA; however, people with diabetes, high blood-pressure disease (hypertension) and respiratory (lung) conditions may not efficiently convert the vegetarian sources, so the preformed DHA and EPA food sources or supplements are recommended.

Recommended Daily Intake of Omega-3 and Omega-6 Fats

Although there is no recommended dietary allowance (RDA) for omega fats, it is recommended that we consume between 1 and 3 grams of omega-3 fats per day. By following the SPII program, you will consume adequate but not excessive amounts of omega-6 fatty acids. Eat more of the omega-3 sources listed on page 251 in this chapter.

Some people may need GLA—found in black currant, borage and evening primrose oils—to balance their prostaglandins. The most common reasons for needing to supplement with GLA is the body's inability to produce it because of excessive alcohol consumption, stress, high sugar intake and high insulin levels.

Balancing Omega-3 and Omega-6 Fatty Acids

A good ratio of omega-3 to omega-6 fats to strive for is a 1-to-3 ratio. This means you need to eat at least 1 gram of omega-3 fatty acid for every 3 grams of omega-6 fatty acids you eat. If you eat too many omega-3 fatty acids, you can end up with excessive thinning of your blood, leading to easy bruising and increased risk of gastrointestinal bleeding or a hemorrhagic stroke. Too much omega-6 or too little omega-3 in your diet can cause increased inflammation, joint and muscle aches, and high blood pressure, as well as increased insulin resistance. Refer to the charts on the next two pages for sources and content of omega-3 and omega-6 fatty acids. You will notice that there are more foods that contain omega-6 fatty acids than there are those that contain omega-3 fatty acids. You may need to supplement with ground flaxseeds or take an omega-3 supplement to meet your daily omega-3 fatty acid requirement.

Food Sources of Omega-3 Fatty Acids

Food	Serving Size	Omega-3 Content (gms)
FISH		
Fatty fish: wild salmon, sardines mackerel, bluefin or albacore tuna bluefish	3½ ounces	1.0–2.5
Medium fat fish: trout, rockfish, oysters, mussels	3½ ounces	0.5–0.8
Low-fat fish: halibut, crab, cod, flounder, scallops, lobster, clams, swordfish, sole, orange roughy, shrimp	3½ ounces	0.1–0.4
MEAT		
Lamb	3½ ounces	0.5
Meat, poultry	3½ ounces	0.2
Dairy products	1 ounce cheese	0.1
OILS		
Flax oil	1 tablespoon	6.6
Flax meal	1 tablespoon	1.6
Canola oil	1 tablespoon	1.6
NUTS AND SEEDS		
Walnuts	2 tablespoons	1.0
Chia seeds	2 tablespoons	1.1
LEGUMES AND TOFU		
Soybeans, cooked	1 cup	1.1
Tofu, firm	½ cup	0.7
VEGETABLES		
Purslane	3½ ounces	0.4
Broccoli, kale, leafy greens	½ cup	0.1
Peas	½ cup	0.1

Food Sources of Omega-6 Fatty Acids

Food	Serving Size	Omega-6 Content (gms)
PLANT FOODS		
FATS AND OILS		
Safflower oil	1 tablespoon	10.0
Sunflower oil	1 tablespoon	9.0
Corn oil	1 tablespoon	8.0
Soybean oil	1 tablespoon	7.0
Peanut oil	1 tablespoon	4.5
Canola oil	1 tablespoon	2.5
Olive oil	1 tablespoon	1.2
Mayonnaise	1 tablespoon	5.0
NUTS AND SEEDS		
Seeds (sesame, pumpkin, sunflower)	¼ cup	9.0
Nuts (peanuts, walnuts, Brazil and pine nuts)	1 ounce	4.0
Nuts (almonds, cashews, pecans, hazelnuts)	1 ounce	2.0
LEGUMES/WHOLE GRAINS		
Tofu, firm	½ cup	5.4
Soybeans (cooked from dry)	½ cup	3.6
Tofu, medium	½ cup	3.5
Soy milk	1 cup	1.6
Legumes	½ cup	0.2
Wheat germ	2 tablespoons	1.0
Grains (wheat, rice, oats, etc.)	½ cup cooked	0.5
VEGETABLES AND FRUITS		
Avocado	1 whole	3.5
Vegetables and fruits	½ cup or 1 medium fruit	0.05
ANIMAL FOODS		
MEAT, POULTRY AND FISH		
Poultry (light and dark meat)	3½ ounces	2.0
Pork (lean)	3½ ounces	0.7
Beef (lean)	3½ ounces	0.3
Fish (high-fat varieties)	3½ ounces	0.2
Fish (low-fat varieties)	3½ ounces	0.1

Recommended Oils and Fats

Use mostly monounsaturated oils and some saturated fats; use only pure-pressed, cold-pressed or expeller-pressed polyunsaturated oils.

Monounsaturated	Polyunsaturated	Saturated
Almond oil	Corn oil	Most other vegetable oils
Apricot kernel oil	Cottonseed oil	Butter*
Avocado oil	Essential fatty acids	Cheese
Canola oil	(borage, flaxseed, primrose)	Chicken fat
Hazelnut oil	Herring oil	Coconut oil
Mustard oil	Menhaden (fish) oil	Cream**
Oat oil	Safflower oil	Duck fat
Olive oil	Salmon oil	Eggs*
Peanut oil	Sardine oil	Ghee (clarified butter)
Rice oil	Sesame oil	Meats
Most nuts	Soybean oil	Nutmeg oil
Most other nut	Sunflower oil	Sheanut oil
oils	Wheat germ oil	Turkey fat

*Contains some polyunsaturated fatty acids—use caution when cooking.
**Buy only heavy whipping cream without any added chemicals.

Best Oils to Use

- Extra-virgin olive oil
- Peanut oil
- Cold-, pure- or expeller-pressed vegetable oils (do not cook with these oils)
- Essential fatty acids—primrose, flaxseed, salmon, borage (do not cook with these oils)
- Mayonnaise that is made from canola or other cold-, pure- or expeller-pressed oil and contains no partially hydrogenated or hydrogenated oils

Damaged Fats

It is important to avoid ingesting damaged fats—trans-fats, oxidized, hydrogenated and fake fats—because they disrupt normal cellular function, which increases your risk for degenerative diseases of aging.

Healthy polyunsaturated fatty acids become damaged when their molecular structure is altered and they become trans-fats. Hydrogenation is one process that damages polyunsaturated fatty acids. Cholesterol and other fats are damaged by oxidation. All fake fats are considered damaged because they do not occur in nature.

Saturated fats cannot be damaged because they have a very stable molecular structure; therefore, high temperatures will not cause a rearrangement in their molecular structure. You can theoretically damage monounsaturated fats because they contain one double bond and are vulnerable at that site for molecular damage. But this only happens with *very* high temperatures, so you do not need to be concerned about damaging them.

Damaged Polyunsaturated Fats

It is very easy to damage polyunsaturated fats. Polyunsaturated fats have more than one double bond, making them very susceptible to molecular damage.

Foods that are cooked with polyunsaturated fats that are heat-processed from their natural state into oils are damaged and are not good for you. For example, corn oil in the corn is not damaged. It is found in its natural state inside the corn. However, during the refining process that is used to get corn oil out of the corn and into a bottle, high temperatures are required that damage the polyunsaturated corn oil by rearranging its molecules. This is a trans-fat and is very harmful because the body cannot use it for function, structure or energy.

```
                    Cis Configuration—Healthy

                         H       H
         |               |       |         |         |        Hydrogen
      —  C  —  C     =   C    —  C    —    C     —    molecules are
         |               |                 |         |        on same side
```

Trans-Fats

Trans-fats clog up tissues and disrupt normal biochemical reactions, killing off your cells. You would compound the problem if you were to use the corn oil for cooking because you would create more trans-fats.

The same holds true for foods cooked with pure-pressed polyunsaturated oils. Although the polyunsaturated oil begins as a healthy cis-fat, heat damages this type of oil by creating trans-fats.

Hydrogenation is a process where liquid polyunsaturated oils are turned into solid fats with the addition of hydrogen molecules. During this process the risk of creating trans-fats from the healthy cis-fats is high.

```
                   Trans Configuration—Damaged

                        H
         |              |                    |         |        Hydrogen
                                                                molecules are
      —  C  —   C    =  C    —   C    —      C     —    on opposite
         |              |                    |         |        side
                        H
```

Oxidized Fats

Oxidized fats are another type of damaged fats. Oxidation of fats occurs when fats are exposed to oxygen in the air. This damage can occur with or without heat.

Oxidation that occurs without cooking is apparent when butter turns dark yellow or oils turn brown. These are rancid fats. Rancid fats are not good for you because they are "free radicals," and free radicals damage your tissues.

To avoid oxidizing all fatty acids and cholesterol, keep them away from sunlight and air. In other words, keep them in airtight opaque containers or in the refrigerator.

Another way to oxidize cholesterol is during cooking. To avoid damaging cholesterol, do not burn your food, and cook fatty meats at low, even temperatures.

Fake Fats

Fake fats are damaged fats, too. Your body cannot absorb fake fats. Fake fats, like Olestra, were invented so that people on low- or nonfat diets could enjoy the texture and flavor of fats without cholesterol and added calories. The problem with this is that by avoiding real fats you become essential fatty acid-deprived, your insulin levels go too high and you burn out your adrenal glands because cholesterol is used to make adrenal gland hormones. Fake fats also interfere with your body's ability to absorb the fat-soluble vitamins A, D, E and K. There is nothing to gain and everything to lose by eating them.

The Do's and Don'ts of Fats

Here are some simple do's and don't do's for fat intake.

The Do's

- Eat healthy, not damaged fats.
- Eat fresh fats and keep fats refrigerated.
- Keep monounsaturated and polyunsaturated oils in opaque, airtight containers.
- Read labels to avoid buying fats with added chemicals.
- Cook fatty meats at low, even temperatures to avoid damaging fats.
- Cook your eggs at low, even temperatures. (Egg yolks have essential fatty acids and other polyunsaturated fats that can be damaged at high heat.)

The Don'ts

- Do not cook with polyunsaturated oils.
- Do not cook with butter at high temperatures. Butter contains polyunsaturated oils and can be damaged with high heat. You can use saturated or monounsaturated fats to cook with because they are more resistant to damage from high temperatures.
- Do not use most low-fat or nonfat products as the fat is usually replaced with sugars and/or artificial chemicals.
- Do not eat a fat by itself.
- Do not eat too many or too few fats because this will damage your metabolism.

The next few pages contain charts of foods that you should try to avoid for the most part unless specified. Read the fine print for exceptions.

Fats, Foods, Oils and Sugars to Avoid

Avoid Fats That Contain Damaged Fats, Chemicals and/or Sugar

Bottled salad dressings
Buttermilk
Cream substitutes
Cream containing chemicals
Deep-fat-fried foods
Half-and-half
High-fat meats that have been
  cooked at high temperatures
Hydrogenated oils
Imitation mayonnaise
Imitation sour cream

Lard/shortening
Margarine
Nondairy creamers
Palm oil
Pressurized whipped cream
  and dessert toppings
Processed foods and fast
  foods using hydrogenated oils
Rancid fats
Sandwich spreads

Other Unhealthy Items to Avoid

Do Not Eat Highly Processed Meat and Sausages

Barbecue loaf
Beer salami
Beerwurst
Beerwurst salami
Bologna
Corned beef loaf

Honey loaf
Honey-roll sausage
Lebanon bologna
Luxury loaf
Mother's loaf
Pastrami

Peppered loaf
Pepperoni
Picnic loaf
Pork headcheese
Salami
Vienna sausage

Do Not Eat Man-Made or Refined Grain Products*

Bagels
Banana bread
Biscuits
Bread sticks**

Bread stuffing
Chinese noodles
Cold cereal
Corn cakes

Cornbread
Cornbread stuffing
Cream of rice
Cream of wheat

*You may eat these foods in moderation as long as you are insulin-sensitive and they are made from whole
  grains and are not highly processed and filled with chemicals, sugar and damaged fats. Avoid these foods if
  you are insulin-resistant or have severely burned-out adrenal glands.
**You will probably not be able to find these foods without sugar and/or damaged fats.

Do Not Eat Man-Made or Refined Grain Products* (cont'd)

Croissants	Muffins	Scones
Croutons	Navajo bread**	Sourdough bread
Crumpets	Noodles	Spaghetti
Dinner rolls	Pancakes	Waffles
Egg bread	Pasta	White English
Flour tortilla	Phyllo dough	muffins**
French bread	Pie crust	White hamburger
Ice cream cone**	Pizza dough	and hot-dog buns**
Irish soda bread	Popovers**	White rice
Italian bread	Puff pastry	Wonton wrappers
Macaroni		

*You may eat these foods in moderation but you may only have them if you are insulin-sensitive if they do not contain damaged fats. If you are insulin-sensitive, you may eat these foods in moderation if they are made from whole grains and are not highly processed and filled with chemicals, sugar and damaged fats.
**You will probably not be able to find these foods without sugar and/or damaged fats.

Do Not Eat Sugar and Desserts

Banana chips	Fruit butters*	Processed yogurt
Brown sugar	Fruit leathers	(low-fat, nonfat
Cakes*	Gelatin desserts	or flavored yogurt)
Candy	Granola and other	Pudding
Caramel or other	snack bars*	Sherbet*
flavored popcorn	Honey**	Strudel
Cheesecake*	Ice cream*	Sweet rolls
Cocoa	Jams, jellies, pre-	Syrups (fudge,
Coffeecake	serves, marmalade*	corn, high-fructose
Cookies	Milk shakes	corn, malt, maple,
Dessert toppings	Molasses	sorghum, butter-
Doughnuts	Pastries*	scotch or caramel)
Eclairs	Pie*	Toaster pastries
Frosting	Protein bars (with	White sugar
Frozen desserts	man-made chemicals)	

*Do not eat sugar and desserts if you are insulin-resistant. However, if you are insulin-sensitive with healthy adrenal glands, you may have small amounts of these desserts as long as they are made from whole ingredients, including whole fats, and they do not contain a lot of added sugar. For example, a homemade pie made with a whole-grain crust and fresh fruit is a better choice than a frozen apple pie made with white flour and syrupy apple compote.
**Honey is the best sugar to eat but only in small quantities.

Do Not Eat Processed Snack Foods

Beef jerky	Pizza**	Taro chips*
Pork skins	Popcorn*	Tortilla chips*
Corn chips*	Potato chips*	Trail mix packaged
Corn nuts	Pretzels	with chocolate chips
Meat-based sticks	Sesame sticks	and other sweets

_____

*Only eat baked chips and those without damaged fats. Eat air-popped popcorn, or use canola oil to pop corn.

**You can eat sauceless whole-grain thin-crust pizza or thin-crust pizza made with sugarless sauce as long as you are insulin-sensitive.

Do Not Eat Processed Foods

Canned foods	Fast foods	Packaged foods
Dried soups	Mixes	

Do Not Eat Condiments
(They Contain Sugar and Chemical Additives)

Barbecue sauces	Ketchup	Relishes
Fish sauces	Meat extender	Sweet pickles
Gravies	Meat tenderizer	Worcestershire
Hoisin sauce	Oyster sauce	

Carbohydrates

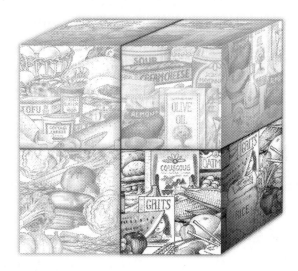

Carbohydrates are foods such as breads, grains, cereals, fruits, fruit juices, starchy vegetables, legumes, sugary foods, some milk products and alcohol.

Your body uses carbohydrates mostly for energy; therefore, the amount of carbohydrates that you eat should match your current metabolism and activity level.

If you eat too many carbohydrates or eat them by themselves, your insulin levels will rise too high. If you eat too few carbohydrates, your adrenaline/cortisol levels will rise too high. The amount of carbohydrates you should eat will depend on your current metabolism type. Refer to your current metabolism type program (chapter 17, 18, 19 or 20) to determine your starting carbohydrate amount.

Carbohydrate Guidelines

- Eat real carbohydrates as much as possible—man-made carbohydrates usually contain a lot of refined sugars and other chemicals. Read labels carefully. A real carbohydrate is one that can be grown, picked or harvested.

- Eat carbohydrates to match your current metabolism and activity level. (See your personal program in chapter 17, 18, 19 or 20.)

- Never eat a carbohydrate by itself. Eating carbohydrates alone causes a release of high amounts of insulin followed by a high release of adrenaline/cortisol if you are insulin-sensitive with healthy adrenal glands. If you are insulin-resistant, eating carbohydrates alone makes your insulin levels stay high or go even higher. If your adrenal glands are burned out, eating carbohydrates alone will never heal them.

- Avoid pesticides by buying organic fruits, whole grains, legumes and starchy vegetables as much as possible.

- Eating too few or too many carbohydrates is equally damaging.

Starchy Vegetables

All items are cooked unless otherwise noted. Each of the following serving sizes contains approximately fifteen grams of carbohydrate.

Food Item	Serving
Acorn squash	½ cup
Artichokes	1 artichoke
Beets	1 cup
Burdock root (raw)	½ root
Butternut squash	⅔ cup
Carrots	1 cup
Corn	½ cup
Green peas	½ cup
Jerusalem artichokes	½ cup
Leeks	1 cup
Lima beans	½ cup

Lotus root	½ cup
Okra	1 cup
Parsnip	⅔ cup
Potato (baked)	½ medium
Pumpkin	1 cup
Rutabaga (raw)	¼ large
Sweet potato or yam	½ medium
Turnip	½ cup

Legumes

All items are cooked unless otherwise noted. Each of the following serving sizes contains approximately fifteen grams of carbohydrate.

Food Item	Serving
Adzuki beans	¼ cup
Black beans	⅓ cup
Broadbeans (fava beans)	½ cup
Chickpeas (garbanzo, Bengal)	⅓ cup
Cowpeas (black-eyed peas)	½ cup
Cranberry (Roman) beans	⅓ cup
French beans	⅓ cup
Great Northern beans	⅓ cup
Garbanzo beans	⅓ cup
Hyacinth beans	⅓ cup
Hominy	½ cup
Kidney beans	⅓ cup
Lentils	⅓ cup
Lupins	1 cup
Moth beans	⅓ cup
Mung beans	⅓ cup
Mungo beans (dry)	½ cup
Navy beans	⅓ cup

Legumes (cont'd)

Pigeon peas	⅓ cup
Pink beans	⅓ cup
Pinto beans	⅓ cup
Split peas	⅓ cup
White beans	⅓ cup
Yellow beans	⅓ cup

Grains

Always buy grains in their natural state and avoid eating processed grains. Never eat grains that are "flavored" or that have additives such as imitation bacon bits.

Each of the following serving sizes contains approximately fifteen grams of carbohydrate.

Food Item (cooked unless noted)	Serving
Barley	⅓ cup
Brown rice	⅓ cup
Buckwheat (whole-grain)	⅓ cup
Buckwheat groats (kasha)	⅓ cup
Bulgur (tabouli)	⅓ cup
Corn bran (crude)	¼ cup
Corn grits, white or yellow	½ cup
Couscous farina	⅓ cup
Millet	⅓ cup
Oats	⅔ cup
Polenta	⅓ cup
Popcorn (air-popped)	2½ cups
Quinoa	⅓ cup
Rye	¼ cup

Semolina (whole-grain, dry)	2 tablespoons
Triticale (dry)	2½ tablespoons
Wheat (whole-grain, dry)	1½ tablespoons
Wheat bran (crude, dry)	½ cup
Wheat germ (crude, dry)	⅓ cup
Wild rice	½ cup

Whole-Grain Flour and Meals

Each of the following serving sizes contains approximately fifteen grams of carbohydrate. All items are dry.

Food Item	Serving
Almond meal	½ cup
Amaranth flour	2 tablespoons
Arrowroot flour	2 tablespoons
Brown rice flour	2 tablespoons
Buckwheat flour (whole-grain)	3½ tablespoons
Corn flour (whole-grain)	2½ tablespoons
Cornmeal	2 tablespoons
Cottonseed flour	1½ ounces
Oat bran flour	⅔ cup
Peanut flour	⅔ cup
Pecan flour	¾ cup
Potato flour	1½ tablespoons
Rye flour	3 tablespoons
Semolina flour (whole-grain)	2 tablespoons
Sesame flour	2½ tablespoons
Soy flour	½ cup
Sunflower seed flour	¾ cup
Semolina (whole-grain)	¼ cup
Sesame flour	1½ ounces
Triticale flour	2½ tablespoons
Whole-wheat flour	3 tablespoons

Yogurt

Each of the following serving sizes contains approximately fifteen grams of carbohydrate.

Food Item	Serving
Plain whole milk yogurt	1 cup
Plain whole milk, goat	1 cup
Plain whole milk, Indian buffalo	1 cup
Plain whole milk, sheep	1 cup
Soy	1 cup

Man-Made Carbohydrate Options

The goal is to eliminate all man-made carbohydrates. However, if you do eat them, some man-made carbohydrates are better than others. Each of these man-made carbohydrate selections contains fifteen grams of carbohydrates. *Remember, you should eat real carbohydrates whenever possible. Fresh-baked bread is preferable because it contains no additives.*

Please read labels and avoid all man-made carbohydrates that have partially hydrogenated and/or hydrogenated fats.

Bread

Food Item	Serving
Bread crumbs (whole wheat)	1½ tablespoons
Corn tortilla	1 medium tortilla
Cracked-wheat bread	1 slice
Cracker meal	1½ tablespoons
Low-carbohydrate bread*	2 slices

Any bread that contains 7½ grams of carbohydrates or less.

Oat bran bread	1 slice
Oatmeal bread	1 slice
Pumpernickel bread	1 regular slice
Rice bran bread	1 slice
Rye bread	1 large slice
Wheat bran bread	1 slice
Wheat germ bread	1 slice
Wheatberry	1 slice
Whole-grain hamburger/hot-dog bun	½ bun
Whole-grain raisin bread	1 slice
Whole-wheat English muffins	½ muffin
Whole-grain dinner roll	1 roll
Whole-grain pita	1 small pita
Whole-grain, 7-grain bread	1 slice

Crackers

Most crackers contain many additives, including hydrogenated fats. Look for crackers that are low-carbohydrate, whole-grain and do not contain hydrogenated fats. Each selection below contains fifteen grams of carbohydrate.

Food Item	Serving
Rice cakes	2 cakes
Rice crackers	4 crackers
Rye crispbread	2 crackers
Rye wafers (Wasa)	2 crackers
Rusk toast	1½ ounces
Wheat crackers (Ak-Mak)	4 crackers
Wheat Euphrates	5 crackers
Wheat melba toast	3 toasts
Whole-wheat matzo	½ (6"x 4")

Fruits

Fruits are high in simple sugar. However, they also contain vitamins, minerals and fiber, so they are much healthier than candy and desserts.

If you are addicted to sugary foods because your adrenal glands are burned out, switching from candy, sodas and desserts to fruit is a good start in tapering off sugary foods.

If you are *insulin-sensitive and have healthy adrenal glands*, fruits raise both insulin and adrenaline/cortisol levels.

If you are *insulin-resistant*, fruit will keep your insulin levels higher and therefore must be counted as carbohydrates.

If you have *burned-out adrenal glands*, fruit will "push" your adrenal glands to squeeze out more adrenaline and cortisol.

If you have *burned-out adrenal glands,* and you are using fruit when you have uncontrollable sugar cravings, do not count the fruit as a carbohydrate. You need to add in complex carbohydrates above your fruit intake in order to heal your adrenal glands. Refer to either the **"Insulin-Sensitive with Burned-Out Adrenal Glands Program"** on page 431 or the **"Insulin-Resistant with Burned-Out Adrenal Glands Program"** on page 449 for the best way to use fruit to self-medicate.

The Fruit Servings lists on the next two pages divide the different fruits by their glycemic index (GI)—lowest, intermediate, highest. If you need to heal your metabolism, the best fruit choices are the ones with the lowest GI. If you already have a good metabolism—i.e., you are insulin-sensitive and have healthy adrenal glands—you only need to count the fruits with the intermediate or high GI as carbohydrates. Consider the low-GI fruits in the same way you would nonstarchy vegetables as long as you are eating less than three portion sizes a day (45 grams).

The Glycemic Index

The glycemic index of food is a measure of how fast insulin levels rise in response to a given food entering the portal vein at any given moment. The faster and higher the amounts of sugar that enter the portal vein, the higher the levels of insulin—and the higher the GI of that food. In general, I ask people to ignore the GI of individual foods because combining the complex carbohydrate with proteins, healthy fats and nonstarchy vegetables can change the GI. However, I do want you to consider the GI of fruit because of its simple sugar content.

Fruit Servings by Glycemic Index (GI)

Each portion size is equal to fifteen grams of carbohydrates.

Lowest GI

These fruits are appropriate for everyone except those with diabetes whose blood sugar rises after eating them.

Blackberries	¾ cup
Blueberries	½ cup
Boysenberries	¾ cup
Grapefruit	½ medium or ½ cup
Raspberries	1 cup
Strawberries	1¼ cups

Intermediate GI

You may eat these if you are insulin-sensitive.

Apple	1 small
Applesauce (unsweetened)	½ cup
Apricots	2 medium
Apricot halves	4 halves
Cantaloupe	1¼ cups

Fruit Servings by Glycemic Index (GI) (cont'd)

Cherries	12 cherries
Honeydew	⅛ medium
Kiwi	1 large
Mango	½ small
Nectarine	1 small
Orange	1 small
Papaya	1 cup
Peach	1 medium
Pear	½ large
Pineapple (raw)	¾ cup
Plums	2 medium

Highest GI

You may eat these if you are insulin-sensitive and your adrenal glands are healthy.

Banana	½ small
Dates	2 medium
Figs	2 medium
Grapes	15 small
Prunes	3 medium
Raisins	2 tablespoons
Watermelon	1¼ cups

Fruit

Each of the following serving sizes contains approximately fifteen grams of carbohydrate. All fruits are raw, except when noted.

Food Item	Serving
Acerola (West Indian cherry)	15 fruits
Apple	1 small

Apples (dried)	3 rings
Applesauce (unsweetened)	½ cup
Apricots	2 medium
Apricots (dried)	7 halves
Avocados (California)	1 avocado
Avocados (Florida)	½ avocado
Bananas	½ small
Bananas (dehydrated)	1 tablespoon
Blackberries	¾ cup
Blueberries	½ cup
Boysenberries	¾ cup
Breadfruit	⅛ small
Carambola (starfruit)	1½ cups (sliced)
Cherimoya (custard apple)	2 ounces
Cherries	12 cherries
Crabapples	½ cup (sliced)
Cranberries (unsweetened)	1 cup, whole
Currants (European, fresh)	1 cup
Currants (red or white)	1 cup
Currants (Zante, dried)	2 tablespoons
Dates	2 medium
Elderberries	½ cup
Figs	2 medium
Figs (dried)	1 medium
Gooseberries	1 cup
Grapefruit	½ medium or ½ cup
Grapes (American)	15 grapes
Grapes (European)	7 grapes
Groundcherries (cape-gooseberries)	1 cup
Guavas (common)	1½ fruits
Guavas (strawberry)	15 guavas
Jackfruit	2 ounces
Java-plum (Jambolan)	¾ cup

Fruit (cont'd)

Jujube	¼ cup
Jujube (dried)	1 tablespoon
Kiwi fruit (Chinese gooseberries)	1 large
Kumquats	5 kumquats
Lemons	3 medium
Limes	2 medium
Litchis	7 fruits
Litchis (dried)	2 tablespoons
Loganberries	¾ cup
Longans	31 fruits
Longans (dried)	2 tablespoons
Loquats	5 large
Mammey-apple	1 medium
Mangos	½ small
Melons (cantaloupe)	1¼ cups (cubes)
Melons (casaba)	1½ cups (cubes)
Melons (honeydew)	⅛ medium
Mulberries	1 cup
Nectarines	1 small
Oranges	1 small
Papayas	1 cup
Passion fruit (granadilla)	3 fruits
Peaches	1 medium
Peaches (dried)	2 halves
Pears	½ large
Pears (dried)	1 half
Persimmons (Japanese)	½ medium
Persimmons (Japanese, dried)	½ medium
Persimmons (native)	2 medium
Pineapple	¾ cup
Plantains (cooked)	⅓ cup
Plums	2 medium

Pomegranates (Chinese apple)	½ fruit
Pomelo	¾ cup
Prickly pears	1½ medium
Prunes	3 medium
Quinces	1 medium
Raisins (dark/golden seedless)	2 tablespoons
Raspberries	1 cup
Rhubarb	7 stalks
Rose-apples	2 medium
Sapotes (marmalade plum)	½ medium
Soursop (guanabana)	½ cup
Strawberries	1¼ cups
Sugar-apples (sweetsop)	½ fruit
Sun-dried tomatoes	⅙ ounce
Tamarinds	15 fruits
Tangerines	2 small
Tomatoes (green and red)	1 medium
Tomatillos	1 large
Watermelon	1¼ cups

Eat fruits in their natural state. Do not eat fruit cocktail or fruits canned in syrup. Eat organic, "spray-free" fruits.

The following are a few juices that are good for you. Each selection contains the GI equivalent of fifteen grams of carbohydrates.

Note: Do not drink these if you are insulin-resistant.

Food Item	Serving
Carrot	3 fluid ounces
Vegetable	6 fluid ounces
Tomato	6 fluid ounces

Nonstarchy Vegetables

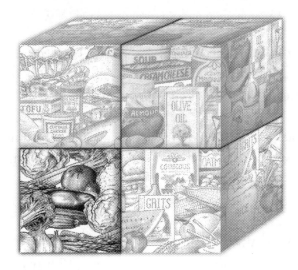

Nonstarchy vegetables are a source of fiber, vitamins and minerals. The fiber slows the digestion and absorption of your carbohydrates, proteins and fats. This helps balance your hormones and at the same time allows only a small amount of food to enter your bloodstream at any given moment. This is important because your body is able to process food better in smaller quantities.

Fiber also helps add bulk to your bowel movements and is what your good colon bacteria use as food to thrive. This helps keep your colon healthy and happy.

The vitamins and minerals found in nonstarchy vegetables are used as coenzymes, which are chemicals that speed up biochemical reactions. This helps you regenerate more efficiently.

Nonstarchy Vegetables Guidelines

- Eat at least five servings of nonstarchy vegetables a day and include at least one serving with each meal, including breakfast.

- Eat organically grown vegetables as much as possible to avoid pesticides.

- Vary your choices as different vegetables contain different anti-oxidants and phytochemicals that help keep you healthy.

- You may eat frozen vegetables as long as there are no added preservatives or sugars. Watch out for hidden salt in frozen vegetables if you are insulin-resistant or have burned-out adrenal glands, and/or you have water-retention problems such as ankle swelling and bloating.

- Consider any vegetable that contains five grams or less of carbohydrates per half-cup serving to be a nonstarchy vegetable.

- Carrots and tomatoes are considered both starchy and non-starchy vegetables. When you eat them raw, consider them non-starchy. When you cook them, consider them starchy. (Cooking breaks down their fiber content.)

Nonstarchy Vegetables

Amaranth leaves
Arrowhead
Arugula
Asparagus
Balsam-pear
Bamboo shoots
Bean sprouts
Beet greens
Bell peppers
  (red, green, yellow)
Borage
Broadbeans
Broccoli
Brussels sprouts
Butterbur (fuki)
Cabbage
Cardoon
Carrots (raw)
Cassava
Cauliflower
Celeriac
Celery
Celtuce
Chayote fruit
Chicory (witloof)
Chicory greens
Chives
Chrysanthemum
  (garland)
Collard greens
Coriander

Cowpeas (leafy tips)
Cucumber
Dandelion greens
Dock
Eggplant
Endive
Eppaw
Fennel
Gardencress
Garlic
Ginger root
Gourd
Green beans
Hearts of palm
Horseradish-tree,
  leafy tips/pods
Jicama (raw)
Jalapeño peppers
Jew's ear (pepeao)
Jute potherb
Kale
Kohlrabi
Lamb's quarter
Lettuce
Mushrooms
Mustard greens
Nopales
Onions
Parsley
Peppers (sweet green,
  red and yellow)

Pokeberry shoots
Pumpkin flowers/
  leaves
Purslane
Radishes
Radicchio
Salsify
Scallop squash
Sesbania flower
Snap beans
Snow peas
Shallots
Spinach
Spaghetti squash
Summer squash
  (crookneck,
  scallop,
  straight neck,
  zucchini)
Sweet potato leaves
Swiss chard
Taro (leaves or
  shoots)
Tomatoes (raw)
Tree fern
Turnip greens
Watercress
Waxgourd (Chinese
  preserving melon)
Yardlong bean

Herbs and Spices

Spices and herbs do not contain sugar or increase insulin secretion. Use them freely.

Healthy Condiments

Balsamic and other vinegars   Natural mustard

Garlic cloves   Olives

Homemade sauces   Peanut sauce (made without sugar)

Low-sodium tamari soy sauce   Salsa (made without sugar)

Beverages

It is important to drink enough fluids throughout the day. Drink at least eight glasses of water per day, more if you are exercising. Also, drink more water initially if you are still consuming beverages with caffeine, sugar or alcohol, as these chemicals deplete water from your body.

What to Drink

Water

This is the best choice. Your body is comprised of 50 to 60 percent water that needs to be replenished daily. For variety and to spice up your water, add a lemon, lime or orange slice for flavor. Or drink the bottled water that has the essence of fruit already instilled.

Sparkling waters

You may drink them in place of still water if they contain less than 50 milligrams of sodium.

Caffeine-free herbal teas

You can count these as part of your water intake as long as they are not diuretic teas.

Decaffeinated coffee

If you need to drink coffee, drink water-processed decaffeinated coffee with organic whole cream. Both milk and half-and-half contain milk sugar (lactose). You may have a small amount of milk in your coffee if you are insulin-sensitive and have healthy adrenal glands. Do not use half-and-half because it is filled with other chemicals.

Vegetable juices

You can have wheat grass, spinach and/or celery juice, or any other juice you can come up with that is made from nonstarchy vegetables.

Carrot and tomato juices

You can have carrot or tomato juice as long as you are not insulin-resistant, but you must count them as a carbohydrate. If you are insulin-resistant, do not drink carrot or tomato juice because they contain too many carbohydrates for your current metabolism.

Real fruit juices

You can have real fruit juices one to three times a week as long as you are insulin-sensitive, have healthy adrenal glands and exercise consistently. However, it is better to eat the fruit rather than drink it because the fiber in the fruit lowers the amount of sugar entering your body. However, if you feel like drinking something other than water, real fruit juices can be an alternative, but you must dilute them—four parts juice to one part water. Do not drink more than two glasses of diluted juice daily.

Fruit smoothies

You can have fruit smoothies one to three times a week as long as you are insulin-sensitive, have healthy adrenal glands and exercise consistently but you must add in protein powder or another protein source. Remember to count these as carbohydrates if they are made with intermediate- or high-GI fruits—even if you add in protein powder or other protein sources. (See Fruit Servings by GI on page 269 in this chapter.) Do not drink smoothies in place of a meal; do not add in frozen yogurt, sherbet, sorbet or ice cream; and do not drink more than eight ounces in one day.

What to Avoid

Milk

It is best to avoid drinking milk because it contains a great deal of hidden sugar in the form of lactose. But if you are insulin-sensitive and have healthy adrenal glands, you may drink milk in moderation (one to two glasses a day). If you must have it, use organic whole milk because the fats in it will help slow the absorption of the sugar in the milk. This will keep your insulin levels more balanced. If you cannot tolerate the taste of whole milk, try diluting it with water.

Do not drink milk if you are insulin-resistant unless you are having a low blood-sugar reaction. If you have Type I or Type II diabetes and are on diabetic drugs that can cause hypoglycemia (low blood sugar), milk is something you can drink to help bring your blood sugar up quickly during a hypoglycemic episode. However, the most important treatment of hypoglycemia is to determine what caused it and prevent it from happening in the future.

What Not to Drink

Alcohol

Avoid alcohol, but if you must drink it, drink red wine and keep it to a half of a glass or three to four ounces per day. Only drink alcohol if you are insulin-sensitive and have healthy adrenal glands. Do not save up the equivalent of your daily drink to have it all at once during one night. In other words, you should not drink three and a half glasses of wine once a week.

Drinking one beer a day or a half a glass of white wine is equivalent to a half of a glass of red wine in terms of alcohol content, but studies are not showing the same benefits to drinking beer and white wine that they are attributing to drinking small amounts of red wine.

If you are insulin-resistant, you should not have any alcohol. Alcohol makes you more insulin-resistant. If you have burned-out adrenal glands, you are probably using alcohol to self-medicate and this can cause further burnout.

You can stop drinking alcohol cold turkey as long as you have healthy adrenal glands. Taper off alcohol if you have burned-out adrenal glands. (Refer to your personal program—chapter 17, 18, 19 or 20—to help you taper off alcohol.)

High-fructose beverages

Avoid all beverages with high-fructose corn syrup. Fructose, a sugar found in fruits and vegetables, is more damaging to cells than white sugar when it is ingested in high amounts. Fructose is found naturally in low amounts in fruits and some vegetables, but in very high amounts in high-fructose corn syrup. Read the labels and stay away from high-fructose corn syrup products.

Artificially sweetened beverages

Avoid all beverages with artificial sweeteners. Aspartame, saccharine, sucralose and other artificial sugars all damage the cells of your body. Keep these toxic chemicals out of your system because they will age you faster.

Caffeinated beverages

Avoid all beverages with caffeine. If you are insulin-resistant, caffeine makes insulin resistance worse. You should stop drinking caffeine cold turkey if you do not have burned-out adrenal glands. If your adrenal glands are burned out, you will need to taper off caffeine or you may experience a "crash." You may need to use caffeine to self-medicate, so you should taper off caffeine last.

Prepackaged vegetable juices

Do not drink prepackaged vegetable juices in cans because they usually contain too much salt.

Why Drinking Enough Water Is Important

Here are a few points to help you understand why drinking enough water is important.

- Most people are chronically dehydrated.
- Some people mistake thirst for hunger.
- Being dehydrated affects your ability to burn fats efficiently.
- Drinking a glass of water at night can help eliminate false midnight hunger pangs.
- Lack of water can cause fatigue.
- Drinking enough water may help decrease joint and back pain.
- Even being slightly dehydrated can affect your thinking processes.
- Drinking enough water can help decrease the risk of colon and breast cancers.

Visit *www.drinkbetterwater.com* online for a listing of good water sources.

Food Bars and Meal-Replacement Shakes

I have been asked countless times why I do not recommend food bars, protein shakes or other types of liquid shakes as meal replacements. The answers are simple:

- They are not real food.
- They do not contain healthy ingredients.
- They are not a balanced meal; they either have too many carbohydrates or too many proteins.
- They usually are filled with refined or artificial sugars.
- They usually contain too much salt.
- They are poor sources of protein.
- They contain damaged fats and other toxic chemicals.
- They go through your digestive system and enter your bloodstream too quickly, causing unwanted hormonal fluctuations.

However, if you can find food bars* that do not contain chemicals and are made from healthy foods, you may eat them as a snack as long as you balance them with the food groups that are missing.

————————

*Please share your findings with me at www.SchwarzbeinPrinciple.com.

Tear out and use the charts below and on the following pages as a quick reference to healthy meal planning. To achieve balance, eat a variety of foods.

Healthy Meal Planning

General Guidelines

- Do not skip meals. Three meals with two snacks a day are ideal.
- Each meal should contain a protein, a healthy fat, a nonstarchy vegetable and a real carbohydrate. Each snack should consist ideally of all four food groups. At the minimum, include a protein and a carbohydrate in every snack.
- Never eat a carbohydrate alone; never eat a protein alone; never eat a fat alone.
- Drink at least eight glasses of water a day, more if you are exercising.
- Always avoid processed foods, sodas and sweets.
- Avoid eating damaged fats.
- Eat solid food, not liquid meal substitutes.

Proteins

- Eat only fresh meats. Avoid processed meats.
- Use only nitrate-free meats.
- Whenever possible use hormone-free, antibiotic-free, range-fed meats and poultry.
- Never eat a protein alone!

Good Proteins

Beef*	Nuts*
Cheese (mozzarella, feta, ricotta, goat, muenster)	Pork
	Salmon
Chicken	Scallops
Chicken (dark meat)*	Shrimp
Cottage cheese, 4% whole*	Tempeh*
Crab	Tofu*
Duck*	Tuna
Eggs	Turkey
Hamburger*	Turkey (dark meat)*
Lamb*	Veal

_____

*These contain glycogen, a hidden sugar. Watch your portions if you are insulin-resistant.

Write your starting personal protein count per meal here. (You can determine your ounces from the Guidelines for Consuming Proteins section on page 232 in this chapter: _____ounces x _____meals.

Healthy Oils and Fats

- Use mostly monounsaturated fats and some saturated fats; use only pure-pressed, cold-pressed or expeller-pressed polyunsaturated fats.
- Eat fresh fats and keep fats refrigerated.
- Read the labels and do not buy any fats with added chemicals.
- Do not use polyunsaturated oils for cooking as heat damages these fats.
- Do not use margarine, partially hydrogenated oils or hydrogenated oils—read labels!
- Do not use low-fat or nonfat products because the fat is usually replaced with sugars.
- Do not use spray vegetable oils.

Healthy Oils

Monounsaturated	Saturated	Polyunsaturated (do not heat)
Canola oil	Butter*	Corn oil
Sesame oil	Cream (heavy whipping)**	Cottonseed oil
Grapeseed oil	Ghee (clarified butter)	Sunflower oil
Soybean oil		
Olive oil		
Peanut oil		

*Also contains polyunsaturated oils.
**Buy only heavy whipping cream without any added chemicals.

Foods with Healthy Fats

Avocado*	Nuts*
Eggs	Nut butters*
Flaxseeds (ground)	Olives
Mayonnaise (from pure-pressed vegetable oils)	Salad dressing (no sugar added)
	Seeds*

*These contain glycogen, a hidden sugar. Watch your portions if you are insulin-resistant.

Carbohydrates

- Both real and man-made carbohydrates raise insulin levels in the blood; insulin is a fat-storing hormone.
- Carbohydrate intake should be monitored closely.
- Never eat a carbohydrate alone!
- Eat carbohydrates in proportion to your current metabolism and activity level.
- Eat real carbohydrates whenever possible; eat man-made carbohydrates as rarely as possible.
- Avoid pesticides by buying organic fruits, grains, legumes and vegetables as much as possible.

Write your starting personal carbohydrate count per meal here. (You can determine your grams from your Personal Program for Your Current Metabolism in chapter 17, 18, 19 or 20: _____grams x _____meals.)

Please remember that your starting carbohydrate count should change as your metabolism improves.

Changes over time: _____grams x_____meals
                       _____grams x_____meals
                       _____grams x_____meals

Real Carbohydrates

Each selection contains fifteen grams of carbohydrates.

Starchy Vegetables	**Legumes**	**Grains**
1 large artichoke	1 cup cooked tomato	⅓ cup barley
1 cup carrots (cooked)	⅓ cup black beans	⅓ cup brown rice
½ cup corn	⅓ cup chickpeas	⅓ cup bulgur
½ cup lima beans	½ cup black-eyed peas	⅓ cup couscous
½ cup green peas	⅓ cup kidney beans	⅔ cup oatmeal
½ medium potato	⅓ cup lentils	⅓ cup quinoa
½ medium sweet potato	⅓ cup pinto beans	2½ cups popcorn (air
or yam	⅓ cup split peas	kettle-popped)

Yogurt

1 cup plain, whole-milk yogurt

1 cup soy yogurt

Fruit (also see separate list)

Lowest GI: berries, grapefruit

Intermediate GI: apples, oranges, melon

Highest GI: grapes, bananas

Man-Made Carbohydrates

These are some of the man-made carbohydrates that are not as bad for you. Choose brands without damaged fats and/or other additives and chemicals.

Each selection contains fifteen grams of carbohydrates.

1 medium corn tortilla   Whole-grain crackers*

Whole-grain bread*   1 small whole-grain pita

Whole-grain cereal*

*Read the label; serving size varies

Nonstarchy Vegetables

- Eat at every meal and snack, including breakfast.
- Eat fresh and organic as much as possible.
- It is important to eat at least five servings of nonstarchy vegetables a day.

Healthy Nonstarchy Vegetables

Asparagus	Cucumber	Peppers—all colors
Bean sprouts	Eggplant	Snap peas
Broccoli	Green beans	Spinach
Cabbage	Leeks	Sprouts
Carrots (raw only)	Lettuce	Tomatoes (raw only)
Celery	Mushrooms	
Cauliflower	Onions	

Beverages

- Drink at least eight glasses of water per day; more if you are exercising. Flavor with lemon, lime or orange slices.
- Sparkling waters. You may drink them in place of still water if they contain less than fifty milligrams of sodium.
- Drink herbal tea or fresh vegetable juice (not canned because of excess salt).
- Decaffeinated coffee. If you need to drink coffee, drink water-processed decaffeinated coffee with whole cream. Both milk and half-and-half contain sugar. You may have milk if you are insulin-sensitive with healthy adrenal glands. Do not use half-and-half because it is filled with other chemicals. If you have burned-out adrenal glands, you may have to continue caffeinated tea or coffee for a while. Caffeinated green tea is better than black tea, which is better than coffee.
- You can have carrot and tomato juice as long as you are not insulin-resistant.
- You can have real fruit juices as long as you dilute them, you exercise consistently and you are not insulin-resistant or do not have burned-out adrenal glands. The same goes for fruit smoothies.
- Avoid all products with artificial sweeteners, high-fructose corn syrup and caffeine. Taper off caffeine if your adrenal glands are burned out or use caffeine to get you through your transition.
- Avoid milk, but if you must have it use organic whole milk. Never drink milk if you are insulin-resistant unless you are having a real hypoglycemic episode (low blood-sugar reaction). If you have Type I diabetes, you may drink milk to treat a hypoglycemic episode.
- Avoid alcohol. If you are insulin-resistant or have burned-out adrenal glands you must not drink alcohol. Taper off alcohol if your adrenal glands are burned out, and stop cold turkey if they are not. If you are insulin-sensitive with healthy adrenal glands and feel that you must drink, limit your intake to a half a glass of red wine or one beer a night. Do not drink your week's worth of alcohol in one night!

Fruit Servings

Each portion size is equal to fifteen grams of carbohydrates.

Lowest GI

These fruits are appropriate for everyone except those with diabetes whose blood sugar rises after eating them.

Blackberries	¾ cup
Blueberries	½ cup
Boysenberries	¾ cup
Grapefruit	½ medium or ½ cup
Raspberries	1 cup
Strawberries	1¼ cups

Intermediate GI

You may eat these only if you are insulin-sensitive.

Apple	1 small
Applesauce (unsweetened)	½ cup
Apricots	2 medium
Apricot halves	4 halves
Cantaloupe	1¼ cups
Honeydew	⅛ medium
Kiwi	1 large
Mango	½ small
Nectarine	1 small
Orange	1 small
Papaya	1 cup
Peach	1 medium
Pear	½ large
Pineapple (raw)	¾ cup
Plums	2 medium

Highest GI (fruit that contains the most sugar)

You may eat these only if you are insulin-sensitive and have healthy adrenal glands.

Banana	½ small
Cherries	12 cherries
Dates	2 medium
Figs	2 medium
Grapes	5 small
Prunes	3 medium
Raisins	2 tablespoons
Watermelon	1¼ cups

Foods High in Saturated Fat—Avoid or Eat Sparingly on a Lower-Saturated Fat Plan

The following is a list of foods to avoid completely or eat in small quantities on a low saturated fat plan.

Dairy and Related Products
- Cream (one teaspoon in morning decaffeinated coffee is okay or a small amount whipped on low GI fruits)
✓ • Milk
✓ • Sour cream/Cream cheese
✓ • Whole-milk cheeses (cheddar, Swiss, jack, muenster)
✓ • Whole-milk yogurt

Meat, Poultry and Fish
✓ • Bacon
- Chicken, turkey and chicken or turkey skin (white meat is okay)
✓ • Duck
- Ground meats (ground sirloin is okay)
✓ • Meats (lean cuts of pork are okay now; later you may add lean cuts of beef and lamb)
✓ • Ribs
✓ • Sausage

Breads and Grains
- Avoid all baked goods made with milk or animal fat—read labels.

Fruits and Nuts
✓ • Coconut
- Macadamia nuts (½ handful is okay)

Fats and Oils
- Butter (use more olive oil for now)
✓ • Coconut oils
✓ • Cream sauces
✓ • Lard
✓ • Palm or palm kernel oils

✓ *Avoid these foods completely until you are exercising consistently and your metabolism is improving.*

Menu Plans

Here are a variety of sample menu plans to get you started in creating your own balanced meals. These menu plans will help you understand how to combine foods from the four food groups of healthy proteins, healthy fats, nonstarchy vegetables and real carbohydrates.

Feel free to mix and match entrée items. For example, you can use a fish dish from one day with the side dishes from another day. For each specific carbohydrate count there are regular, low-saturated fat and vegetarian menu plans. Use the plan that you need to follow. If you do not know which plan you should follow, refer to your personal program (chapter 17, 18, 19 or 20).

Only the carbohydrates or foods that contain carbohydrates have been quantified in each meal plan. The low-saturated fat menu plans already are lower in saturated fats so there is nothing for you to calculate or quantify.

However, if you have burned-out adrenal glands, you *will* have to calculate your protein requirements using the "Guidelines for Consuming Proteins" chart on page 232 earlier in this chapter together with the "Protein Portions" suggestions that follow it. (You can also calculate your protein portion if you have healthy adrenal glands.) As an example: if you weigh 150 pounds, you need to eat a minimum of 10 to 12 ounces of protein a day. This should be spread out proportionately throughout the day. For example you should eat 2 to 3 ounces of protein per each meal and snack. You can get your minimum protein requirement at breakfast by eating 3 ounces of protein as 2 scrambled eggs (2 ounces protein) and one-quarter cup of cottage cheese (1 ounce protein) or 3 scrambled eggs or three-quarters of a cup cottage cheese. The balance of your meals and snacks should contain 7 to 9 ounces of protein, spread out proportionately.

Please note that snack items have not been included, so you will need to refer to the different snack ideas that follow this section to fill in your daily menu plans.

Some of the menu plans contain recipes from my two cookbooks, *The Schwarzbein Principle Cookbook* and *The Schwarzbein Principle Vegetarian Cookbook*. You do not have to use these exact recipes, but they are very delicious! Have fun eating!

General Information About Menu Plans

When bread is indicated use Ezekial, Vogel or Alvarado. When crackers are indicated use Ak-Mak, Lavosh, Wasa or Ryvita.

When raw vegetables are indicated you may use carrots, celery, jicama, tomatoes, onions, cucumber, broccoli, cauliflower and/or peppers.

Mixed greens may include a variety of lettuce, spinach, onions, tomatoes, grated carrots, cucumber, celery and/or peppers.

Meats such as turkey, sausage and bacon should be nitrate-free. So should tofu substitutes. All meats should be lean, and if you are following the lower saturated fat meal plans, skinless too.

Nut butters should be organic and sugar free. Eat low-fat or part-skim-milk cheeses if you are following the lower-saturated fat meal plan.

If you are diabetic, substitute low GI fruits wherever intermediate or high GI fruits appear in the meal plans or snack ideas. If you are insulin-resistant but not diabetic, intermediate fruits are acceptable, but subsitute the high GI fruits with low or intermediate GI fruits.

Note: If you are a diabetic, raw carrots and tomatoes may cause blood-sugar levels to increase.

15-Gram Regular Sample Menu Plan #1

Each meal contains approximately 15 grams of carbohydrates per meal.

MEALS	MONDAY	TUESDAY	WEDNESDAY	THURSDAY	FRIDAY	SATURDAY	SUNDAY
Breakfast	Scrambled eggs with goat cheese and spinach. 1¼ cups strawberries.	¾ cup oatmeal. Grilled nitrate-free chicken sausage with peppers.	Sliced turkey on 1 slice Ezekial toast with ricotta cheese, sliced onion and tomato.	Scrambled eggs, nitrate-free turkey sausage and ½ cup roasted potatoes with onions and peppers.	Melted mozzarella cheese and spinach in 1 corn tortilla. Grape tomatoes.	Mexican scrambled eggs with peppers, onion and lean ground lean beef. ½ cup beans. Salsa.	Vegetable frittata (SPVC** recipe). ½ cup roasted potatoes.
Lunch	Chicken salad with cold-pressed oil mayonnaise on mixed greens with ½ sliced apple and ½ avocado. Raw carrots.	Tomato stuffed with tuna salad mixed with cold-pressed oil mayonnaise, onion, celery and olives. 4 Ak-Mak crackers.	Quiche (crustless; SPC* recipe). 1 cup berries. Mixed-greens salad with vinaigrette dressing.	Salmon on mixed greens. ½ cup red potatoes. Raw veggies.	Homemade taco salad (no shell) with lean ground beef, mixed greens, onions, ½ cup beans, salsa and olives.	Chicken stir-fry with veggies in olive oil. ½ cup brown rice.	Lean hamburger patty. ½ cup corn. Tomato, feta cheese and green onion salad with vinaigrette dressing.
Dinner	Lean steak. ½ cup oven-roasted red potatoes with rosemary. Broccoli. Mixed-greens salad with vinaigrette dressing.	Grilled salmon. ½ sweet potato. Sautéed spinach. Mixed-greens salad with vinaigrette dressing.	Pecan chicken (SPC* recipe). ½ cup bulgur. Green beans. Tomato and onion salad with vinaigrette dressing.	Beef stroganoff (SPC* recipe) on ½ cup wild rice. Asparagus. Hearts of romaine salad and feta cheese with vinaigrette dressing.	Grilled halibut. ½ cup butternut squash. Sautéed green beans. Mixed-greens salad with vinaigrette dressing.	Mint pesto chicken kabob with vegetables. (SPC* recipe) ½ cup couscous. Butterleaf lettuce salad and goat cheese with vinaigrette dressing.	Grilled lamb chops. ½ cup roasted potatoes. Grilled zucchini. Mixed-greens salad with vinaigrette dressing.

*SPC Schwarzbein Principle Cookbook
**SPVC Schwarzbein Principle Vegetarian Cookbook

Note: 15-gram carbohydrate meal plans require two 7½- to 15-gram carbohydrate snacks (see snack section that follows). It is important to eat smaller meals more frequently throughout the day to heal your metabolism.

15-Gram Regular Sample Menu Plan #2
Each meal contains approximately 15 grams of carbohydrates per meal.

MEALS	MONDAY	TUESDAY	WEDNESDAY	THURSDAY	FRIDAY	SATURDAY	SUNDAY
Breakfast	Scrambled eggs with peppers and onions. 1 slice whole-grain bread with butter.	⅔ cup oatmeal with heavy organic cream. Nitrate-free turkey sausage with onions and peppers.	½ cup cottage cheese. 2 celery sticks with 1 tablespoon almond butter. 3 Ak-Mak crackers.	1 tablespoon organic, sugar-free peanut butter on ½ apple. ½ cup cottage cheese. 2 celery sticks.	Deviled eggs. Sliced tomatoes. 1 apple.	Open-faced lean turkey sandwich on 1 slice whole-grain bread with goat cheese, tomato and onion.	Goat cheese and spinach omelet. ½ cup potatoes.
Lunch	Chicken salad with goat cheese, ½ sliced pear salad, ¼ cup pecans and onions. Vinaigrette dressing.	Leftover lean steak on arugula salad with tomato, peppers and ⅔ cup corn. Vinaigrette dressing.	Shrimp salad with tomato, cucumber, ¼ avocado and ½ cup papaya. Vinaigrette dressing.	Greek salad with chicken, onions, cucumbers, 1 small orange and feta cheese. Vinaigrette dressing.	Chicken fajitas with onions, peppers (*SPC** recipe) and ⅓ cup black beans. Mixed-greens salad with vinaigrette dressing.	Lean chicken breast. Red cabbage, ½ orange and ¼ cup walnut salad with goat cheese. Vinaigrette dressing.	Mozzarella cheese and vegetable quesadilla on 1 corn tortilla. Tomato salad with vinaigrette dressing.
Dinner	Lean steak. Broccoli and cauliflower mix. ½ baked potato. Mixed-greens salad with vinaigrette dressing.	Salmon steak on bed of ⅓ cup lentils. Asparagus spears. Mixed-greens salad with vinaigrette dressing.	Lamb chops. ⅓ cup tabbouleh. Grilled zucchini. Mixed-greens salad with vinaigrette dressing.	Roast lean turkey. ½ sweet potato with butter. Green beans with slivered almonds. Mixed-greens salad with vinaigrette dressing.	Trout with mushrooms. ½ cup corn. Asparagus. Mixed-greens salad with vinaigrette dressing.	Tofu stir-fry with sesame seeds, cabbage and onions. ⅓ cup brown rice. Mixed-greens salad with vinaigrette dressing.	Mint pesto chicken kabob with peppers, onions and mushrooms. ⅓ cup brown rice. Mixed-greens salad with vinaigrette dressing.

Note: 15-gram carbohydrate meals require two 7½- to 15-gram carbohydrate snacks (see snack section that follows). It is important to eat smaller meals more frequently throughout the day to heal your metabolism.

**SPC Schwarzbein Principle Cookbook*
***SPVC Schwarzbein Principle Vegetarian Cookbook*

15-Gram Low-Saturated Fat Menu Plan
Each meal contains approximately 15 grams of carbohydrates per meal.

MEALS	MONDAY	TUESDAY	WEDNESDAY	THURSDAY	FRIDAY	SATURDAY	SUNDAY
Breakfast	⅔ cup oatmeal with 2 tablespoons almonds and 1 tablespoon flaxseeds. 2 hard-boiled eggs. Raw veggies.	Scrambled tofu with onions and mushrooms. ½ cup red potatoes.	4 ounces plain whole yogurt, ¼ cup low-fat cottage cheese and ½ cup strawberries—mixed. 2 sticks celery with organic almond butter.	Mediterranean omelet with 2 tablespoons feta cheese, tomatoes and onions. ¾ cup melon.	Scrambled egg with spinach and onions. 1 slice whole-grain toast with organic almond butter.	Lean turkey breast on 1 slice whole-grain bread with sliced tomatoes.	Salmon (leftover) on 2 Lavosh crackers with low-fat ricotta cheese, sliced onion and tomato.
Lunch	½ tuna sandwich with tomato and lettuce on whole-grain bread. Mix tuna with cold-pressed oil mayonnaise, onions and celery. Spinach salad with vinaigrette dressing.	Shrimp salad with tomato, cucumber, ¼ avocado and ½ cup papaya.	Grilled skinless chicken salad with tomato, peppers and ½ cup corn. Vinaigrette dressing.	Taco salad (no shell) with lean ground turkey, onions, lettuce, tomato, ⅓ cup beans and salsa.	Stir-fry tofu with vegetables. ⅓ cup brown rice. Mixed-greens salad with vinaigrette dressing.	Skinless, lean chicken breast. Red cabbage, ½ orange and ¼ cup walnut salad with 2 tablespoons goat cheese. Vinaigrette dressing.	Lean turkey patty. ½ cup corn. Broccoli. Mixed-greens salad with vinaigrette dressing.
Dinner	Baked chicken (skinless) breast. Broccoli and cauliflower mix. ⅓ cup couscous. Mixed-greens salad with vinaigrette dressing.	Salmon steak on bed of ⅓ cup lentils. Asparagus spears. Mixed-greens salad with vinaigrette dressing.	Roasted skinless turkey breast. ½ yam. Sautéed spinach. Mixed-greens salad with vinaigrette dressing.	Halibut. ½ cup roasted red potatoes. Zucchini. Mixed-greens salad with vinaigrette dressing.	Mint pesto chicken kabob with peppers, onions and mushrooms. (*SPC** recipe) 1 roasted medium red potato. Mixed-greens salad with vinaigrette dressing.	Broiled salmon. ⅓ cup white beans. Roasted vegetables in olive oil. Mixed-greens salad with vinaigrette dressing.	Trout with mushrooms. ½ acorn squash. Asparagus spears. Mixed-greens salad with vinaigrette dressing.

Note: 15-gram carbohydrate meal plans require two 7½- to 15-gram carbohydrate snacks (see snack section that follows). It is important to eat smaller meals more frequently throughout the day to heal your metabolism. This is not a low-fat plan. Make sure to include healthy fats (olive oil, nuts, avocado and olives) with each meal.

**SPC Schwarzbein Principle Cookbook*
***SPVC Schwarzbein Principle Vegetarian Cookbook*

15-Gram Vegetarian Sample Menu Plan *Each meal contains approximately 15 grams of carbohydrates per meal.*							
MEALS	**MONDAY**	**TUESDAY**	**WEDNESDAY**	**THURSDAY**	**FRIDAY**	**SATURDAY**	**SUNDAY**
Breakfast	Melted mozzarella cheese on 1 slice whole-grain toast. Cherry tomatoes.	Scrambled eggs with onions, peppers and ¼ avocado on 1 corn tortilla.	⅔ cup oatmeal with ¼ cup soy protein or scrambled eggs. Carrot sticks.	4 ounces whole plain yogurt, ¼ cup cottage cheese and ½ cup strawberries—mixed. 2 celery sticks.	Tofu scramble with ½ cup tomatoes and onions. 4 Ak-Mak crackers.	2 tablespoons organic almond butter on 1 slice whole-grain toast. Carrot sticks.	Goat cheese and spinach omelet. ½ cup potatoes in olive oil.
Lunch	Tofu egg salad with cold-pressed oil mayonnaise. 2 Ak-Mak crackers. Raw veggies. ½ small apple.	½ cup cottage cheese. ¼ cup lentils, sliced tomatoes and green onions with vinaigrette dressing.	Tofu burger with lettuce, onion and tomato on ½ slice whole-grain bread. Mixed-greens salad with vinaigrette dressing.	Crustless quiche with vegetables. (*SPVC*** recipe) 1 small pear. Mixed-greens salad with vinaigrette dressing.	1 cup vegetarian chili using ⅓ cup beans and tofu. Endive and tomato salad with vinaigrette dressing.	1 tempeh taco on 1 corn tortilla with salsa. Mixed-greens salad with vinaigrette dressing.	Cheese and vegetable quesadilla on 1 corn tortilla. Tomato and cucumber salad with vinaigrette dressing.
Dinner	Ricotta-stuffed bell peppers with ⅓ cup brown rice. Hearts of romaine salad with vinaigrette dressing.	Tofu stir-fry. ⅓ cup bulgur with butter. Grilled vegetables. Mixed-greens salad with vinaigrette dressing.	Baked chili relleños. ⅓ cup black beans. Mixed-greens salad with vinaigrette dressing.	1 enchilada with corn tortilla stuffed with ricotta and tofu. Zucchini. Mixed-greens salad with vinaigrette dressing.	Nitrate-free tofu sausage with ⅓ cup polenta. Broccoli. Mixed-greens salad with vinaigrette dressing.	Nitrate-free tofu salad with tomato, lettuce and ½ cup artichoke hearts. Mixed-greens salad with vinaigrette dressing.	Vegetarian patty. ½ cup acorn squash. Green beans with slivered almonds. Mixed-greens salad with vinaigrette dressing.

Note: 15-gram carbohydrate meal plans require two 7½- to 15-gram carbohydrate snacks (see snack section that follows). It is important to eat smaller meals more frequently throughout the day to heal your metabolism.

**SPC Schwarzbein Principle Cookbook*
***SPVC Schwarzbein Principle Vegetarian Cookbook*

20-Gram Regular Sample Menu Plan #1

Each meal contains approximately 20 grams of carbohydrates per meal.

MEALS	MONDAY	TUESDAY	WEDNESDAY	THURSDAY	FRIDAY	SATURDAY	SUNDAY
Breakfast	Scrambled eggs with mushrooms. 2 cups strawberries.	1 cup oatmeal with butter. Grilled chicken breast. Tomatoes.	Poached eggs. ¾ cup roasted potatoes with peppers and onions.	Melted mozzarella cheese and spinach in 2 small corn tortillas with tomatoes	2 tablespoons organic almond butter on 1 small apple. Carrot sticks. Muenster cheese.	Mexican scrambled eggs with peppers, onion and lean ground beef. ⅓ cup beans. Salsa.	Vegetable Frittata ¾ cup roasted potato. Asparagus.
Lunch	Tuna salad with cold-pressed canola mayonnaise on mixed greens with ½ sliced apple and ¼ avocado. Raw carrots. 2 Ak-Mak crackers.	Roast lean turkey. Carrot-ginger soup. 3 Ak-Mak crackers.	Shredded lean beef. ½ cup black beans. Mixed-greens salad with vinaigrette dressing.	Salmon on mixed greens with snap peas, ½ cup red potatoes and ¼ avocado. Vinaigrette dressing.	Chicken on mixed greens with ⅓ cup black beans, onions, tomatoes and ¼ avocado. Vinaigrette dressing.	Chicken stir-fry with veggies. (*SPC** recipe) ⅓ cup brown rice. ¼ avocado. Mixed-greens salad with vinaigrette dressing.	Lean-meat hamburger patty. ½ cup corn. Tomato, feta cheese and green onion salad with ¼ cup green peas. Vinaigrette dressing.
Dinner	Lean steak. ¾ cup oven-roasted red potatoes with rosemary. Broccoli. Mixed-greens salad with vinaigrette dressing.	Grilled salmon. ⅔ sweet potato. Sautéed spinach. Mixed-greens salad with vinaigrette dressing.	Pecan chicken. (*SPC** recipe) ½ cup bulgur. Green beans. Tomato and onion salad with ¼ avocado. Vinaigrette dressing.	Beef stroganoff (*SPC** recipe) on ⅔ cup wild rice. Asparagus. Hearts of romaine salad with feta cheese. Vinaigrette dressing.	Grilled halibut. 1 cup butternut squash. Sautéed green beans. Mixed-greens salad with vinaigrette dressing.	Mint pesto chicken kabob with vegetables. (*SPC** recipe) ½ cup couscous. Butterleaf lettuce salad with goat cheese. Vinaigrette dressing.	Grilled lamb chops. ¾ cup roasted potatoes. Grilled zucchini. Mixed-greens salad with vinaigrette dressing.

Note: 20-gram carbohydrate meal plans require two 15- to 20-gram carbohydrate snacks (see snack section that follows). It is important to eat smaller meals more frequently throughout the day to heal your metabolism.

**SPC Schwarzbein Principle Cookbook*
***SPVC Schwarzbein Principle Vegetarian Cookbook*

20-Gram Regular Sample Menu Plan #2

Each meal contains approximately 20 grams of carbohydrates per meal.

MEALS	MONDAY	TUESDAY	WEDNESDAY	THURSDAY	FRIDAY	SATURDAY	SUNDAY
Breakfast	Scrambled eggs on 2 corn tortillas with mozzarella cheese and tomato slices or salsa.	2 tablespoons almond butter on 3 Ak-Mak crackers. ½ cup cottage cheese. Raw veggies.	Scrambled eggs with green and red peppers and grated mozzarella cheese. ¾ cup oatmeal with heavy cream, if desired.	½ cup cottage cheese with ½ cup strawberries and ½ small apple Raw veggies.	Spinach omelet with red peppers and goat cheese. ¾ cup sautéed potatoes.	Poached eggs. Nitrate-free turkey sausage. Sliced tomatoes. 1½ slices whole-grain toast.	Greek omelet with olives, tomato, onion and feta cheese. ¾ cup honeydew melon.
Lunch	Open-faced lean roast beef sandwich on 1 slice whole-grain bread with lettuce, tomato, onions and cold-pressed canola mayonnaise. Raw veggies. ½ cup strawberries.	Cold salmon on mixed-greens salad with vinaigrette dressing. Raw veggies. ¾ cup cold red potatoes. ¼ avocado.	Mint pesto chicken kabob with veggies. (*SPC** recipe) ½ cup couscous. Mixed-greens salad with vinaigrette dressing.	Grilled tofu on ½ cup tabbouleh with peppers, tomatoes and broccoli.	Tuna salad with cold-pressed mayonnaise on mixed greens with roasted peppers, tomatoes and onions. 4 Ak-Mak crackers. ½ orange.	Lean turkey burger with fontina cheese on 2 slices whole-grain bread with lettuce, tomato, mustard and cold-pressed mayonnaise. Mixed-greens salad with vinaigrette dressing.	Seafood salad on bed of lettuce and mixed raw vegetables garnished with ½ cup fresh pineapple. Vinaigrette dressing. 3 Ak-Mak crackers.
Dinner	Broiled halibut. Asparagus. ¾ cup red potatoes with butter. Mixed-greens salad with vinaigrette dressing.	Lean pork chop. ¾ cup peas with mushrooms. Tomato and red onion salad with vinaigrette dressing.	1 veggie burger (no bun) with melted muenster cheese and ¼ avocado. ⅓ cup brown rice. Mixed-greens salad with vinaigrette dressing.	Roast chicken. Cauliflower. Small baked potato with butter and chives. Mixed-greens salad with vinaigrette dressing.	Beef fajitas with bell peppers and onions on 2 corn tortillas. (*SPC** recipe) Mixed-greens salad with vinaigrette dressing.	Grilled salmon. ½ cup couscous. Brussels sprouts. Mixed-greens salad with vinaigrette dressing.	Chicken kabob with peppers, onion and mushrooms. ½ cup brown rice. Mixed-greens salad with vinaigrette dressing.

Note: 20-gram carbohydrate meal plans require two 15- to 20-gram carbohydrate snacks (see snack section that follows). It is important to eat smaller meals more frequently throughout the day to heal your metabolism.

**SPC Schwarzbein Principle Cookbook*
***SPVC Schwarzbein Principle Vegetarian Cookbook*

20-Gram Lower-Saturated Fat Sample Menu Plan

Each meal contains approximately 20 grams of carbohydrates per meal.

MEALS	MONDAY	TUESDAY	WEDNESDAY	THURSDAY	FRIDAY	SATURDAY	SUNDAY
Breakfast	⅔ cup oatmeal with 2 tablespoons almonds and 1 tablespoon flaxseeds. 2 hard-boiled eggs. Raw veggies. ½ cup berries.	Scrambled tofu with onions and mushrooms. ¾ cup red potatoes.	Part-skim mozzarella cheese on 2 small corn tortillas. Raw veggies.	Mediterranean omelet with tomatoes and onions. 1 slice whole-grain bread. ½ cup strawberries.	Scrambled egg with spinach and onions. 1 slice whole-grain toast. 2 tablespoons organic almond butter.	White-meat turkey on 1 slice whole-grain toast with sliced tomatoes, ¼ avocado and lettuce.	Salmon (leftover) on 3 Lavosh crackers with part-skim ricotta cheese and sliced onion and tomato.
Lunch	½ tuna sandwich mixed with cold-pressed oil mayonnaise, onions, celery, ½ apple, tomato and lettuce. Spinach salad with vinaigrette dressing. Carrot sticks.	Quesadilla made with 2 small corn tortillas, part-skim mozzarella cheese, spinach and tomatoes. Mixed-greens salad with vinaigrette dressing.	Grilled skinless, white-meat chicken salad with ½ cup quinoa and raw carrots.	Taco salad (no shell) with lean ground turkey, onions, lettuce, tomato, ½ cup beans and salsa.	Crustless quiche (SPC* recipe) with spinach and onions. 1 medium peach. Mixed-greens salad with vinaigrette dressing.	Broiled salmon on mixed greens with ¾ cup red potatoes and asparagus. Vinaigrette dressing.	Lean turkey patty. ½ cup corn. Broccoli. Mixed-greens salad with balsamic vinegar.
Dinner	Skinless, white-meat baked chicken. ½ cup lentils. Broccoli with lemon. Mixed-greens salad with vinaigrette dressing.	Halibut. ½ cup couscous. Zucchini squash. Mixed-greens salad with vinaigrette dressing.	Chicken taco on 1 small corn tortilla with ½ cup beans and salsa. Mixed-greens salad with vinaigrette dressing.	Roasted white-meat, skinless turkey. ½ cup yam. Sautéed spinach. Mixed-greens salad with vinaigrette dressing.	Salmon. ½ cup bulgur. Roasted vegetables. Mixed-greens salad with vinaigrette dressing.	Lean pork chops. ½ cup roasted red potatoes. Green beans. Mixed-greens salad with vinaigrette dressing.	Stir-fry skinless, white-meat chicken with vegetables. ½ cup brown rice. Mixed-greens salad with vinaigrette dressing.

*SPC Schwarzbein Principle Cookbook
**SPVC Schwarzbein Principle Vegetarian Cookbook

Note: 20-gram carbohydrate meal plans require two 15- to 20-gram carbohydrate snacks (see snack section that follows). It is important to eat smaller meals more frequently throughout the day to heal your metabolism. This is not a low-fat plan. Make sure to include healthy fats (olive oil, nuts, avocado and olives) with each meal.

20-Gram Vegetarian Sample Menu Plan
Each meal contains approximately 20 grams of carbohydrates per meal.

MEALS	MONDAY	TUESDAY	WEDNESDAY	THURSDAY	FRIDAY	SATURDAY	SUNDAY
Breakfast	Melted mozzarella cheese on 1 slice whole-grain toast. Cherry tomatoes. ½ cup strawberries.	Scrambled eggs with onions and peppers on 2 small corn tortillas.	⅔ cup oatmeal with ¼ cup soy protein or scrambled eggs. Carrot sticks. ⅓ cup berries.	4 ounces whole plain yogurt with ½ cup cottage cheese and 1 cup berries—mixed. 2 celery sticks.	Tofu scramble with ½ cup tomatoes, ¼ cup corn, onions and ¼ cup potatoes.	2 tablespoons organic almond butter on 1 piece whole-grain toast. 1 hard-boiled egg. Carrot sticks.	Goat cheese and spinach omelet. ½ slice whole-grain toast. ⅓ cup potatoes.
Lunch	Tofu egg salad. 3 Ak-Mak crackers. Raw veggies. ½ small apple.	½ cup cottage cheese. ⅓ cup lentils. Sliced tomatoes and onions.	Tofu burger with lettuce, onion and tomato on 1 slice whole-grain bread. Mixed-greens salad with vinaigrette dressing.	¼ cup couscous with feta cheese, tomatoes and 2 tablespoons pine nuts. ½ cup cottage cheese. ½ cup fresh pineapple.	1 cup vegetarian chili using ½ cup beans and tofu. Endive and tomato salad with vinaigrette dressing.	2 tempeh tacos on 2 small corn tortillas. Salsa. Mixed-greens salad with vinaigrette dressing.	Cheese and vegetable quesadilla on 2 small corn tortillas. Tomato and cucumber salad with oil-and-vinegar dressing.
Dinner	Ricotta-stuffed bell peppers (*SPVC*** recipe). ⅓ cup brown rice. Hearts of romaine salad with vinaigrette dressing.	Tofu stir-fry. ⅔ sweet potato with butter. Grilled vegetables. Mixed-greens salad with vinaigrette dressing.	Baked chili relleños (*SPVC*** recipe). ½ cup black beans. Mixed-greens salad with vinaigrette dressing.	1 enchilada with 1 corn tortilla stuffed with ricotta and ⅓ cup cottage cheese. Zucchini. Mixed-greens salad with vinaigrette dressing.	Tofu nitrate-free sausage with ½ cup polenta. Broccoli. ¼ avocado. Mixed-greens salad with vinaigrette dressing.	Tofu salad with tomato, ¼ avocado, lettuce and ½ cup artichoke hearts. 2 Ak-Mak crackers. Mixed-greens salad with vinaigrette dressing.	Vegetarian patty. 1 cup acorn squash. Green beans with slivered almonds. Mixed-greens salad with vinaigrette dressing.

Note: 20-gram carbohydrate meal plans require two 15- to 20-gram carbohydrate snacks (see snack section that follows). It is important to eat smaller meals more frequently throughout the day to heal your metabolism.

**SPC Schwarzbein Principle Cookbook*
***SPVC Schwarzbein Principle Vegetarian Cookbook*

25-Gram Regular Sample Menu Plan

Each meal contains approximately 25 grams of carbohydrates per meal.

MEALS	MONDAY	TUESDAY	WEDNESDAY	THURSDAY	FRIDAY	SATURDAY	SUNDAY
Breakfast	Scrambled eggs with goat cheese and spinach. ½ cup potato. ¼ cup strawberries.	1¼ cups oatmeal. Grilled chicken nitrate-free sausage with peppers.	Turkey on 1 slice whole-grain bread with ricotta cheese, sliced onion and tomato. ⅔ cup melon.	Poached eggs. Nitrate-free turkey sausage. Sliced tomatoes. 1 slice whole-grain toast. ⅓ cup blueberries.	Scrambled eggs with mushrooms. 1 slice whole-grain toast. ½ apple.	Mexican scrambled eggs with peppers, onions and lean ground beef. ⅓ cup beans. Salsa. 1 corn tortilla.	Vegetable egg frittata. ¾ cup roasted potatoes. Sliced tomatoes.
Lunch	Grilled chicken on mixed greens with ¼ avocado, ¼ cup pecans and 1 orange. Raw vegetables.	Chicken stir-fry with broccoli, onions and cabbage on ¾ cup brown rice.	Quiche (crustless; *SPC** recipe). ½ cup boysenberries and ½ small sliced banana. Mixed-greens salad with vinaigrette dressing.	Salmon on mixed greens with feta cheese, ⅔ cup sliced red potatoes and ⅓ avocado. Raw veggies.	Taco salad with lean ground beef, lettuce, tomato, ¼ avocado, ½ cup beans and salsa.	Tomato stuffed with tuna salad mixed with pure-pressed canola mayonnaise. 4 Ak-Mak crackers. ½ apple.	¾ cup cottage cheese. 3 Ak-Mak crackers. ½ cup fresh pineapple. Tomato, feta cheese and green onion salad with vinaigrette dressing.
Dinner	Lean steak. 1 medium baked potato. Broccoli. Mixed-greens salad with vinaigrette dressing.	Grilled salmon. ½ cup red potatoes. ⅓ cup corn. Sautéed spinach. Mixed-greens salad with vinaigrette dressing.	Pecan chicken (*SPC** recipe). ½ cup couscous. Green beans. Tomato, onion and ¼ avocado salad with vinaigrette dressing.	Beef stroganoff (*SPC** recipe) on ¾ cup wild rice. Asparagus. Hearts of romaine salad with vinaigrette dressing.	Grilled swordfish. ½ cup butternut squash. Sautéed green beans. ⅔ cup melon. Mixed-greens salad with vinaigrette dressing.	Mint pesto chicken kabob with peppers, onions and mushrooms. (*SPC** recipe) ⅔ cup yam with butter. Hearts of romaine and feta cheese salad with vinaigrette dressing.	Grilled lamb chops. ¾ cup brown rice. Grilled zucchini. Mixed-greens salad with vinaigrette dressing.

**SPC Schwarzbein Principle Cookbook*
***SPVC Schwarzbein Principle Vegetarian Cookbook*

Note: 25-gram carbohydrate meal plans require two 15- to 25-gram carbohydrate snacks or one 25-gram carbohydrate snack (see snack section that follows). It is important to eat smaller meals more frequently throughout the day to heal your metabolism.

25-Gram Low-Saturated Fat Sample Menu Plan
Each meal contains approximately 25 grams of carbohydrates per meal.

MEALS	MONDAY	TUESDAY	WEDNESDAY	THURSDAY	FRIDAY	SATURDAY	SUNDAY
Breakfast	Scrambled eggs and spinach. ½ cup potatoes. ½ cup strawberries.	1¼ cup oatmeal. Egg, over easy. Fresh red peppers.	White-meat turkey breast on 1 slice whole-grain toast with part-skim ricotta cheese, sliced onion and tomato. ⅔ cup melon.	Poached eggs. 1 slice whole-grain toast. Sliced tomatoes. ⅓ cup blueberries.	Scrambled eggs with mushrooms. 1 slice whole-grain toast. 1 small tangerine.	Mexican scrambled eggs with peppers, onions, ground sirloin, ½ cup corn and salsa. 1 corn tortilla.	Vegetable egg frittata. ¾ cup roasted potatoes. Sliced tomatoes.
Lunch	Skinless white-meat grilled chicken on mixed greens with ¼ avocado, ¼ cup pecans and 1 orange. Raw veggies.	Taco salad with lean ground sirloin, lettuce, tomato, ¼ avocado, ½ cup beans and salsa.	Tomato stuffed with tuna salad mixed with cold-pressed canola mayonnaise. 3 Ak-Mak crackers. 1 apple.	Salmon on mixed greens with ½ cup sliced red potatoes and ½ avocado. Raw veggies.	Quiche (crustless; *SPC** recipe). ½ cup berries and ½ small sliced banana. Mixed-greens salad with vinaigrette dressing.	White-meat chicken stir-fry with broccoli, onions and cabbage on ½ cup brown rice.	¾ cup low-fat cottage cheese. 3 Ak-Mak crackers. ½ cup fresh pineapple. Tomato and green onion salad with vinaigrette dressing.
Dinner	Halibut steak. 1 medium baked potato. Broccoli. Mixed-greens salad garnished with ¼ cup pecans. Vinaigrette dressing.	Grilled salmon. ½ cup white beans. Sautéed spinach. ⅓ cup boysenberries. Mixed-greens salad with vinaigrette dressing.	Pecan chicken (*SPC** recipe). ½ cup couscous. Green beans. Tomato, onion and ⅓ avocado salad with vinaigrette dressing.	Roasted skinless turkey breast. ½ cup wild rice. Asparagus. ½ cup strawberries. Hearts of romaine salad with vinaigrette dressing.	Grilled swordfish. ½ cup butternut squash. Sautéed green beans. Mixed-greens salad with ½ cup artichoke hearts. Vinaigrette dressing.	Mint pesto chicken kabob (white meat) with peppers, onions and mushrooms. (*SPC** recipe) ⅔ cup yam. Hearts of romaine salad with vinaigrette dressing.	Grilled lean pork chops. ½ cup brown rice. Grilled zucchini. Mixed-greens salad with vinaigrette dressing.

**SPC Schwarzbein Principle Cookbook*
***SPVC Schwarzbein Principle Vegetarian Cookbook*

Note: 25-gram carbohydrate meal plans require two 15- to 25-gram carbohydrate snacks or one 25-gram carbohydrate snack (see snack section that follows). It is important to eat smaller meals more frequently throughout the day to heal your metabolism. This is not a low-fat plan. Make sure to include healthy fats (olive oil, nuts, avocado and olives) with each meal.

25-Gram Vegetarian Sample Menu Plan

Each meal contains approximately 25 grams of carbohydrates per meal.

MEALS	MONDAY	TUESDAY	WEDNESDAY	THURSDAY	FRIDAY	SATURDAY	SUNDAY
Breakfast	Eggs with goat cheese and spinach. ½ cup potato. ¼ cup strawberries.	1 cup oatmeal with butter. Grilled tofu nitrate-free sausage with peppers.	Tempeh. 1 slice whole-grain bread. Ricotta cheese, sliced onion and tomato. ⅔ cup melon.	Tofu scramble. (*SPVC*** recipe) 1 slice whole-grain toast. ¼ cup potatoes. Sliced tomatoes.	2 tablespoons organic almond butter on 1 slice whole-grain toast. 1 hard-boiled egg. 1 small tangerine.	Mexican scrambled eggs with peppers, onions, ⅓ cup beans and salsa. 1 corn tortilla.	Vegetable egg frittata. (*SPVC*** recipe) ½ cup roasted potatoes. ⅓ cup blueberries.
Lunch	Grilled tofu on mixed greens with ½ avocado, ¼ cup pecans and 1 orange. Raw veggies.	Tomato stuffed with tofu egg salad mixed with pure-pressed canola mayonnaise. 3 Ak-Mak crackers. 1 apple.	¾ cup cottage cheese with ½ cup pineapple and 1 cup strawberries. Mixed-greens salad with vinaigrette dressing.	Tofu on mixed greens with feta cheese and ⅔ cup sliced red potatoes with vinaigrette dressing. Raw veggies.	Taco salad with tempeh, lettuce, tomato, ¼ avocado, ½ cup beans and salsa.	Tofu stir-fry with broccoli, onions and cabbage on ½ cup brown rice.	¾ cup cottage cheese. 2 Ak-Mak crackers. ½ cup fresh pineapple. Tomato, feta cheese and green onion salad with vinaigrette dressing.
Dinner	Ricotta-stuffed bell peppers (*SPVC*** recipe). ⅔ cup oven-roasted red potatoes. Broccoli. Mixed-greens salad with vinaigrette dressing.	Tofu sausage with ½ cup couscous. Sautéed spinach. Mixed-greens salad with ¼ cup corn. Vinaigrette dressing.	Tempeh. ½ cup brown rice. Green beans. Tomato, onion and ¼ avocado salad with vinaigrette dressing.	Tofu stroganoff on ½ cup wild rice. (*SPVC*** recipe) Asparagus. Hearts of romaine salad with ¼ avocado. Vinaigrette dressing.	Vegetarian patty. ½ cup butternut squash. Sautéed green beans. Mixed-greens salad with ½ cup artichoke hearts. Vinaigrette dressing.	Asian mint pesto tofu kabob with peppers, onions and mushrooms. (*SPVC** recipe) ⅔ cup yam with butter. Hearts of romaine and feta cheese salad with vinaigrette dressing.	Baked chili rellenos with ½ cup black beans. (*SPVC*** recipe) Mixed-greens salad with vinaigrette dressing.

Note: 25-gram carbohydrate meal plans require two 15- to 25-gram carbohydrate snacks or one 25-gram carbohydrate snack (see snack section that follows). It is important to eat smaller meals more frequently throughout the day to heal your metabolism.

**SPC Schwarzbein Principle Cookbook*

***SPVC Schwarzbein Principle Vegetarian Cookbook*

30-Gram Regular Sample Menu Plan #1

Each meal contains approximately 30 grams of carbohydrates per meal.

MEALS	MONDAY	TUESDAY	WEDNESDAY	THURSDAY	FRIDAY	SATURDAY	SUNDAY
Breakfast	Scrambled eggs. 1 corn tortilla with mozzarella cheese, tomato slices or salsa. 1 small orange.	1 tablespoon organic, sugar-free peanut butter. 5 Ak-Mak crackers. ½ cup cottage cheese. Raw veggies.	Scrambled eggs with green and red peppers and grated mozzarella cheese. 1 cup oatmeal with heavy cream, if desired.	½ cup cottage cheese with 1 cup strawberries and ½ small banana. Raw veggies.	Spinach omelet with goat cheese and red peppers. ½ cup sautéed potatoes. 1 slice whole-grain toast.	Poached eggs. Nitrate-free turkey sausage. Sliced tomatoes. 1 slice whole-grain toast. ½ cup blueberries.	Greek omelet with olives, tomato, onions and feta cheese. ½ cup honeydew melon. 1 slice whole-grain toast.
Lunch	Lean roast beef sandwich on whole-grain bread with lettuce, tomato, onions and pure-pressed canola mayonnaise. Raw veggies.	Cold salmon on mixed greens and raw veggies with vinaigrette dressing. ¾ cup cold red potatoes. ½ avocado.	Turkey and avocado sandwich on whole-grain bread with lettuce, tomato, mustard and pure-pressed canola mayonnaise. Mixed-greens salad with vinaigrette dressing.	Grilled tofu or chicken on ⅔ cup tabbouleh with peppers, tomatoes and broccoli.	Tuna salad with pure-pressed mayonnaise on mixed greens, roasted peppers, tomatoes and onions. 4 Ak-Mak crackers. 1 orange.	Lean turkey burger with muenster cheese on 2 slices whole-grain bread with lettuce, tomato, mustard and pure-pressed mayonnaise. Small mixed-greens salad with vinaigrette dressing.	Seafood salad on bed of lettuce and mixed raw vegetables garnished with ¾ cup fresh pineapple. 4 Ak-Mak crackers.
Dinner	Broiled halibut. Asparagus. ½ cup red potatoes. ½ cup cooked carrots with butter. Mixed-greens salad with vinaigrette dressing.	Lean pork chop. 1 cup peas with mushrooms. Tomato and red onion salad with vinaigrette dressing.	Lean steak. 1 medium baked potato with butter and chives. Broccoli. Mixed greens and ¼ avocado salad with vinaigrette dressing.	Roast chicken. Cauliflower. ⅔ cup brown rice. Mixed-greens salad with vinaigrette dressing.	Beef fajitas, bell peppers and onions. (*SPC* recipe) 2 corn tortillas. Mixed-greens salad with vinaigrette dressing.	Grilled salmon. ⅔ cup couscous. Brussels sprouts. Mixed-greens salad with vinaigrette dressing.	Mint pesto chicken kabob with peppers, onion and mushrooms. (*SPC** recipe) ⅔ cup brown rice. Mixed-greens salad with vinaigrette dressing.

Note: If you are insulin-sensitive and have healthy adrenal glands or burned-out adrenal glands, 30-gram meal plans require two 7½- to 20-gram snacks. However, if you are insulin-resistant, you may eat 30 grams of carbohydrate without snacking, though this is not ideal. It is important to eat smaller meals more frequently throughout the day to heal your metabolism faster.

*SPC Schwarzbein Principle Cookbook
**SPVC Schwarzbein Principle Vegetarian Cookbook

30-Gram Regular Sample Menu Plan #2
Each meal contains approximately 30 grams of carbohydrates per meal.

MEALS	MONDAY	TUESDAY	WEDNESDAY	THURSDAY	FRIDAY	SATURDAY	SUNDAY
Breakfast	Scrambled eggs with goat cheese and spinach. ½ cup potatoes. ¾ cup strawberries.	1⅓ cups oatmeal. Nitrate-free grilled chicken sausage with peppers in olive oil.	Turkey on 1 slice whole-grain bread with ricotta cheese, sliced onion, tomato and ¼ avocado. 1 small orange.	Poached eggs. Nitrate-free turkey sausage. 1 slice whole-grain toast with butter. ½ cup potatoes. Sliced tomatoes.	String cheese. 1 tangerine. ½ banana. Handful of almonds. Grape tomatoes.	Mexican scrambled eggs with peppers, onion and lean ground beef cooked in butter. ⅓ cup beans. Salsa. 1 corn tortilla.	Basic frittata. (*SPVC*** recipe) ½ cup roasted potatoes with olive oil. 1 cup melon.
Lunch	Grilled chicken on mixed greens with ½ avocado, ¼ cup pecans and 1 orange. Raw veggies.	Quiche (crustless; *SPC** recipe). ¾ cup berries and ½ sliced banana.	Tomato stuffed with tuna salad mixed with cold-pressed canola mayonnaise. 4 Ak-Mak crackers. 1 apple.	Salmon on mixed greens with feta cheese and 1 cup sliced red potatoes with vinaigrette dressing. Raw veggies.	Taco salad with lean ground beef, lettuce, tomato, ½ avocado, ½ cup beans and salsa.	Chicken stir-fry with broccoli, onions and cabbage in olive oil. 1 cup brown rice.	Cottage cheese. 4 Ak-Mak crackers. ¾ cup fresh pineapple. Tomato, feta cheese and green onion salad with vinaigrette dressing.
Dinner	Lean steak. 1 cup oven-roasted red potatoes. Broccoli. Mixed-greens salad with vinaigrette dressing.	Grilled salmon. ⅔ cup couscous. Sautéed spinach. Mixed-greens salad with vinaigrette dressing.	Pork loin. ⅔ cup couscous. Green beans. Tomato and onion salad with vinaigrette dressing.	Beef stroganoff (*SPC** recipe) on ⅔ cup wild rice. Asparagus. Hearts of romaine salad with vinaigrette dressing.	Grilled swordfish. 1 cup butternut squash. Sautéed green beans. Mixed-greens salad with vinaigrette dressing.	Mint pesto chicken kabob with peppers, onions and mushrooms. (*SPC** recipe) 1 yam with butter. Hearts of romaine and feta cheese salad with vinaigrette dressing.	Grilled lamb chops. 1 sweet potato with butter. Grilled zucchini. Mixed-greens salad with vinaigrette dressing.

Note: If you are insulin-sensitive and have healthy adrenal glands or burned-out adrenal glands, 30-gram meal plans require two 7½- to 20-gram snacks. However, if you are insulin-resistant, you may eat 30 grams of carbohydrate without snacking, though this is not ideal. It is important to eat smaller meals more frequently throughout the day to heal your metabolism faster.

**SPC Schwarzbein Principle Cookbook*
***SPVC Schwarzbein Principle Vegetarian Cookbook*

30-Gram Low-Saturated Fat Sample Menu Plan

Each meal contains approximately 30 grams of carbohydrates per meal.

MEALS	MONDAY	TUESDAY	WEDNESDAY	THURSDAY	FRIDAY	SATURDAY	SUNDAY
Breakfast	1½ cups oatmeal with 1 tablespoon flaxseeds and 2 tablespoons almonds. 2 hard-boiled eggs. Raw veggies.	Scrambled tofu with onions and mushrooms. 1 cup red potatoes.	8 ounces whole plain yogurt, ¼ cup low-fat cottage cheese and 1 cup strawberries—mixed. 2 celery sticks with almond butter.	Mediterranean omelet with 2 tablespoons feta cheese, tomatoes and onions. 1 slice whole-grain toast. ¼ cup melon.	Scrambled eggs with spinach and onions. 1 slice whole-grain toast with almond butter. 1 orange.	Skinless turkey breast on 2 slices whole-grain toast with sliced tomatoes and lettuce.	Salmon (leftover) on 4 Lavosh crackers with part-skim ricotta cheese, sliced onion and tomato.
Lunch	Tuna sandwich on 2 slices whole-grain bread with tomato and lettuce. Mix tuna with pure-pressed oil mayonnaise, onions, celery. Spinach salad/w vinaigrette dressing. Carrot sticks.	Quesadilla (2 corn tortillas, skim-milk mozzarella cheese, spinach and tomatoes). Mixed-greens salad with vinaigrette dressing.	Grilled breast of skinless chicken and mixed-greens salad with vinaigrette dressing. ⅔ cup quinoa. Raw carrots.	Taco salad (no shell) with lean ground turkey, onions, lettuce, tomato, ½ cup beans and salsa. ⅓ avocado.	Veggie burger (no bun). ½ avocado. Raw vegetable salad with vinaigrette dressing. 1 medium apple.	Broiled salmon on mixed greens with ½ cup red potatoes and asparagus with vinaigrette dressing.	Lean turkey patty. ½ cup corn. ½ cup roasted beets. Broccoli. Mixed-greens salad with vinaigrette dressing.
Dinner	Baked skinless chicken breast. ⅔ cup lentils. Broccoli with lemon. Mixed-greens salad with vinaigrette dressing.	Halibut. ½ cup couscous. Zucchini squash. Mixed-greens salad with vinaigrette dressing.	Lean steak. Grilled vegetables in olive oil. 1 small baked potato with salsa. Mixed-greens salad with vinaigrette dressing.	Roasted skinless breast of turkey. 1 small yam. Spinach sautéed in olive oil. Mixed-greens salad with vinaigrette dressing.	Lean pork chops. 1 cup roasted red potatoes with rosemary and olive oil. Green beans. Mixed-greens salad with vinaigrette dressing.	Broiled salmon. ⅔ cup white beans. Roasted vegetables in olive oil. Mixed-greens salad with vinaigrette dressing.	Stir-fry chicken breast with vegetables. ⅓ cup brown rice. Mixed-greens salad with vinaigrette dressing.

Note: If you are insulin-sensitive and have healthy adrenal glands or burned-out adrenal glands, 30-gram meal plans require two 7½- to 20-gram snacks. However, if you are insulin-resistant, you may eat 30 grams of carbohydrate without snacking, though this is not ideal. It is important to eat smaller meals more frequently throughout the day to heal your metabolism faster. This is not a low-fat plan. Make sure to include healthy fats (olive, oil, nuts, avocado and olives) with each meal.

*SPC Schwarzbein Principle Cookbook
**SPVC Schwarzbein Principle Vegetarian Cookbook

30-Gram Vegetarian Sample Menu Plan
Each meal contains approximately 30 grams of carbohydrates per meal.

MEALS	MONDAY	TUESDAY	WEDNESDAY	THURSDAY	FRIDAY	SATURDAY	SUNDAY
Breakfast	Melted mozzarella cheese on 2 slices whole-grain toast. Cherry tomatoes.	Scrambled eggs with onions and peppers. ⅓ cup pinto beans. 1 corn tortilla.	⅔ cup oatmeal with ¼ cup soy protein or scrambled eggs. 1 cup cantaloupe. Carrot sticks.	6 ounces whole plain yogurt, ½ cup cottage cheese and 1 cup strawberries—mixed. 2 celery sticks.	Tofu scramble (*SPVC*** recipe) with ½ cup tomatoes, ¼ cup corn and onions. ½ cup potatoes.	2 tablespoons organic almond butter or 1 tablespoon organic, sugar-free peanut butter on 1 slice whole-grain toast. 1 apple.	Goat cheese and spinach omelet. ½ cup potatoes. 1 slice whole-grain toast.
Lunch	Tofu egg salad with pure-pressed oil mayonnaise. (*SPVC*** recipe) 4 Ak-Mak crackers. Raw veggies. 1 small apple.	½ cup cottage cheese. ½ cup lentils. Sliced tomatoes and onions.	Tofu burger with lettuce, onions and tomato on 2 slices whole-grain bread. Mixed-greens salad with vinaigrette dressing.	½ cup couscous with feta cheese and tomatoes. ½ cup cottage cheese with ½ cup fresh pineapple garnished with slivered almonds.	1¼ cups vegetarian chili using ½ cup beans and tofu. Endive and tomato salad with vinaigrette dressing.	Tempeh tacos (*SPVC*** recipe) Mixed-greens salad with vinaigrette dressing.	Cheese and vegetable quesadilla on 2 6-inch corn tortillas. Tomato and cucumber salad with oil-and-vinegar dressing.
Dinner	Ricotta-stuffed bell peppers with 1 cup brown rice. (*SPVC*** recipe) Hearts of romaine salad with vinaigrette dressing.	Tofu stir-fry. 1 sweet potato with butter. Grilled vegetables. Mixed-greens salad with vinaigrette dressing.	Baked chili rellenos (*SPVC*** recipe). ⅓ cup black beans. ⅓ cup brown rice. Mixed-greens salad with vinaigrette dressing.	Tofu enchilados suizas. (*SPVC*** recipe) Zucchini. Mixed-greens salad with vinaigrette dressing.	Tofu nitrate-free sausage with ½ cup polenta. Broccoli. Mixed-greens salad with vinaigrette dressing.	Tofu salad with tomato, ½ avocado, lettuce and ½ cup artichoke hearts. 3 Ak-Mak crackers. Mixed-greens salad with vinaigrette dressing.	Vegetarian patty. 1 cup acorn squash. Green beans with slivered almonds. Mixed-greens salad with vinaigrette dressing.

**SPC Schwarzbein Principle Cookbook*
***SPVC Schwarzbein Principle Vegetarian Cookbook*

Note: If you are insulin-sensitive and have healthy adrenal glands or burned-out adrenal glands, 30-gram meal plans require two 7½- to 20-gram snacks. However, if you are insulin-resistant, you may eat 30 grams of carbohydrate without snacking, though this is not ideal. It is important to eat smaller meals more frequently throughout the day to heal your metabolism faster.

45-Gram Regular Sample Menu Plan

Each meal contains approximately 45 grams of carbohydrates per meal.

MEALS	MONDAY	TUESDAY	WEDNESDAY	THURSDAY	FRIDAY	SATURDAY	SUNDAY
Breakfast	Scrambled eggs with onions and peppers. 1½ cups oatmeal. 1 orange.	Poached eggs. Sliced tomatoes. 1 slice whole-grain toast. 2 kiwis.	Turkey on 2 slices whole-grain bread with ricotta cheese, sliced onion and tomato. 1 apple.	2 hard-boiled eggs. 2 table-spoons almond butter on 1 slice whole-grain toast. ½ grapefruit. Cherry tomatoes.	Breakfast sandwich made with scrambled eggs, bacon, muenster cheese and sliced tomato on 2 slices whole-grain toast. 1 cup raspberries.	Vegetable quiche (crustless; SPC* recipe). 1½ cups pineapple. ½ cup blueberries.	Eggs over easy. Grilled nitrate-free chicken sausage with peppers and onions. 1 cup roasted potatoes. 1 slice whole-grain toast.
Lunch	Grilled chicken on mixed greens with ⅓ cup corn and ⅓ cup black beans. Raw veggies with vinaigrette dressing. 1 apple.	1 cup cottage cheese salad with raw, chopped vegetables and 2 tablespoons sunflower seeds. 5 Ak-Mak crackers. 1 large apple.	Salmon on mixed greens and 1 cup sliced red potatoes with vinaigrette dressing. 1 pear.	Chicken stir-fry with veggies and olive oil. 1 cup brown rice. ½ cup corn.	2 chicken tacos on 2 corn tortillas with lettuce, tomato, ⅓ cup beans and ¼ avocado.	Lean beef patty on 1 slice whole-grain toast with lettuce, tomato and ½ avocado. 1 cup strawberries.	Chicken Caesar salad (no croutons) with ½ avocado. 6 Ak-Mak crackers. 1 peach.
Dinner	Roast lean pork loin. ⅔ cup couscous. Asparagus. Mixed-greens salad with tomatoes and cucumber with olive oil dressing.	Grilled lean lamb chops. Green beans. 1 sweet potato with butter. 1 cup berries. Mixed-greens salad with vinaigrette dressing.	Beef stroganoff (SPC* recipe). ⅔ cup brown rice. Sautéed spinach. 1 cup cooked carrots. Mixed-greens salad with vinaigrette dressing.	Mint pesto grilled chicken kabob with peppers, onions and mushrooms. (SPC* recipe) 1 cup couscous. Mixed-greens salad with vinaigrette dressing.	Grilled swordfish. 1 medium corn on the cob. 1 cup red potatoes. Sautéed spinach. Mixed-greens salad with vinaigrette dressing.	Grilled salmon. ⅔ cup polenta. ½ cup mango salsa. Asparagus. Mixed-greens salad with vinaigrette dressing.	Lean New York strip steak. 1 large baked potato with butter and chives. Broccoli. 1 cup melon. Mixed-greens salad with vinaigrette.

*SPC Schwarzbein Principle Cookbook
**SPVC Schwarzbein Principle Vegetarian Cookbook

Note: If you are insulin-sensitive and have healthy adrenal glands, you may eat only three meals a day, but keep in mind that eating smaller meals more frequently is better for you. If you are extremely active, add in at least two snacks with at least 20 grams of carbohydrates per snack.

45-Gram Vegetarian Sample Menu Plan

Each meal contains approximately 45 grams of carbohydrates per meal.

MEALS	MONDAY	TUESDAY	WEDNESDAY	THURSDAY	FRIDAY	SATURDAY	SUNDAY
Breakfast	Scrambled eggs with onions and peppers. 1½ cups oatmeal. 1 orange.	Poached eggs. Sliced tomatoes. 1 slice whole-grain toast. 2 kiwis.	Tofu mushroom and spinach scramble. 1 cup red potatoes. 1 cup strawberries.	2 hard-boiled eggs. Cherry tomatoes. 2 tablespoons almond butter on 1 slice whole-grain toast. 1 apple.	Breakfast sandwich made with scrambled eggs, muenster cheese and sliced tomato. 2 slices whole-grain toast. 1 cup raspberries.	Vegetable quiche crustless; (SPVC** recipe). 1½ cups pineapple. ½ cup blueberries.	Eggs over easy. 1 cup roasted potatoes with peppers and onions. ½ grapefruit.
Lunch	Grilled tofu on mixed greens with ⅓ cup corn and ⅓ cup black beans. Raw veggies with vinaigrette dressing. 1 apple.	1 cup cottage cheese salad with chopped raw vegetables and 2 tablespoons flaxseeds. 5 Ak-Mak crackers. 1 large apple.	Grilled tofu on mixed greens with 1 cup sliced red potatoes with vinaigrette dressing. 1 pear.	Tomato stuffed with tofu egg salad mixed with cold-pressed mayonnaise. 6 Ak-Mak crackers. ½ avocado. ½ mango.	2 tofu tacos on 2 soft corn tortillas with lettuce, tomato, ½ cup beans and ¼ avocado.	Vegetarian patty (limit to 5-gram carbohydrate content) on 2 slices whole-grain toast with lettuce, tomato and ½ avocado. 1 cup strawberries.	1 cup cottage cheese with 1 cup mixed berries, ½ sliced banana and ¼ cup walnuts. Mixed-greens salad with vinaigrette dressing.
Dinner	Mint tofu pesto kabob. (SPVC** recipe) ⅔ cup couscous. Asparagus. Mixed greens, tomato and cucumber salad with olive oil dressing. Mixed-greens salad with vinaigrette dressing.	Ricotta-stuffed bell peppers. (SPVC** recipe) 1 sweet potato with butter. 1 cup berries. Mixed-greens salad with vinaigrette dressing.	Tempeh stroganoff (SPC* recipe). ⅔ cup brown rice. Spinach sautéed in olive oil. 1 cup cooked carrots. Mixed-greens salad with vinaigrette dressing.	Grilled tofu kabob with peppers, onions and mushrooms. 1 cup couscous. Mixed-greens salad with vinaigrette dressing.	Quesadilla made with 2 corn tortillas with mixed vegetables and mozzarella cheese. 1 corn on the cob. Sliced tomatoes. Mixed-greens salad with vinaigrette dressing.	Grilled tofu sausage. 2/3 cup polenta. 1/2 cup mango salsa. Asparagus. Mixed-greens salad with vinaigrette dressing.	Tofu loaf. 1 large baked potato with butter and chives. Broccoli. Cucumber salad with sour-cream-and-vinegar dressing. 1 cup cantaloupe. Mixed-greens salad with vinaigrette dressing.

*SPC Schwarzbein Principle Cookbook
**SPVC Schwarzbein Principle Vegetarian Cookbook

Note: If you are insulin-sensitive and have healthy adrenal glands, you may eat only three meals a day, but keep in mind that eating smaller meals more frequently is better for you. If you are extremely active, add in at least two snacks with at least 20 grams of carbohydrates per snack.

Snacks

Along with eating balanced meals, eat balanced snacks as well. A few suggestions for snacks appear below. To make your snacks balanced, add some nonstarchy vegetables such as celery, carrots, tomatoes, cucumbers, peppers, broccoli and cauliflower.

You can mix and match any carbohydrate with any protein combination. All the foods that contain carbohydrates are italicized. There are four snack lists—one that contains 7.5 carbohydrate grams, one that contains 15 carbohydrate grams, one that contains 20 carbohydrate grams and one that contains 25 carbohydrate grams. Substitute low glycemic fruits if you are insulin-resistant or have burned-out adrenal glands. Be creative, but keep your snacks healthy.

Carbohydrate Snacks

7.5-Gram Carbohydrate Snacks
Each snack contains approximately 7.5 grams of carbohydrates.
- ✓ ¼ cup *sunflower seeds*
- ✓ 1½ tablespoons *cashews*
- ✓ ⅓ cup *almonds* with string cheese
- ✓ 3 tablespoons organic, sugar-free *peanut butter* on celery sticks
- ✓ 3 tablespoons *hummus* with raw carrots, bell pepper, celery sticks
- ✓ 1½ tablespoons organic *cashew butter* on celery sticks
- ✓ 2 low-carbohydrate, *whole-grain crackers* (e.g., Ak-Mak) with mozzarella cheese
- ✓✓ ½ cup *cottage cheese* with raw carrot sticks
  ½ small *apple** with string cheese or goat cheese
  1 small *fig** with Swiss cheese
- ✓✓ ½ cup *strawberries* with ¼ cup *cottage cheese*
- ✓ 2 tablespoons *almond butter* on celery sticks
  ½ *pear** with string cheese or goat cheese

---
*If you are insulin-resistant, substitute the following fruits: ¼ cup blueberries, ½ cup other berries or ¼ grapefruit.
✓ You may eat on a low-saturated fat meal plan.
✓✓ You may eat on a low-saturated fat meal plan if you substitute low-fat or part-skim cheese.

7.5-Gram Carbohydrate Snacks
✓ 1 *Lavosh cracker* with tuna salad
✓ 1 tablespoon organic, sugar-free *peanut butter* with ⅓ small *apple**
   2 low-carbohydrate, *whole-grain crackers* with herring and sour cream
✓ ½ serving *tofu* "egg salad" with raw carrot sticks
✓ ¼ cup *walnuts* with ½ cup *strawberries*
   ½ cup *blueberries* with unsweetened whipping cream and Camembert cheese
✓ 2 *Ak-Mak crackers* with egg salad
✓ ⅓ cup *edamame* beans (shelled)

15-Gram Carbohydrate Snacks
Each snack contains approximately 15 grams of carbohydrates.
✓✓ ½ cup *blueberries* with mozzarella cheese
✓ ½ small *banana** and 1 tablespoon organic, sugar-free *peanut butter*
   4 dried *apricot halves* spread with goat cheese
✓ 1 small *kiwi** and ¼ cup *walnuts*
✓ 1 small *apple** and 1 tablespoon organic, sugar-free *peanut butter*
✓✓ 12 *cherries** with mozzarella cheese
✓ 1 tablespoon *raisins** and ½ cup *pumpkin seeds*
✓✓ ¼ cup *unsweetened applesauce** and ¼ cup *cottage cheese*
   ½ cup *whole-milk yogurt* and ½ cup *strawberries*
✓ ½ *mango** and marinated organic tofu
✓ 1¼ cups *strawberries* and mozzarella cheese
✓✓ 1 corn *tortilla*, tomatoes and queso fresco cheese

---

*If you are insulin-resistant, substitute the following fruits: ¼ cup blueberries, ½ cup other berries or ¼ grapefruit.
✓ You may eat on the low-saturated fat meal plan.
✓✓ You may eat on the low-saturated fat meal plan if you substitute low-fat or part-skim cheese.

Carbohydrate Snacks (cont'd)

15-Gram Carbohydrate Snacks

    ✓   4 *Ak-Mak crackers* and egg salad

    ✓✓   ¾ cup fresh *pineapple** and ricotta cheese

    ✓   1 slice 15-gram *whole-grain bread* with chicken salad

        4 *whole-grain crackers* (e.g., Ak-Mak), cucumber and goat cheese

    ✓   ½ medium *pear** and ¼ cup *pecans*

    ✓   ¼ cup *hummus* on 2 *Lavosh crackers*; raw vegetables

    ✓   ⅔ cup *edamame* beans (shelled)

20-Gram Carbohydrate Snacks

Each of the following snacks contains approximately 20 grams of carbohydrates.

        20 *grapes** and Swiss cheese

    ✓   ½ small *banana** and 2 tablespoons organic, sugar-free *almond butter*

        5 dried *apricot halves** spread with goat cheese

    ✓   1 medium *kiwi** and ¼ cup *walnuts*

    ✓   1 small *apple** and 2 tablespoons organic sugar-free *peanut butter*

    ✓✓   ⅓ small baked *potato* and ½ cup *cottage cheese*

    ✓✓   12 *cherries** with mozzarella cheese

    ✓✓   ½ cup *unsweetened applesauce** and ¼ cup *cottage cheese*

        ¾ cup *whole-milk yogurt* and ¾ cup *strawberries*

    ✓✓   2 corn *tortillas*, tomatoes and queso fresco cheese

    ✓✓   ½ *mango** and ½ cup *cottage cheese*

    ✓   4 *Finn crisp crackers* and egg salad

    ✓✓   1 cup fresh *pineapple** and ricotta cheese

    ✓   1 slice 15-gram *whole-grain bread* with ¼ *avocado* and chicken salad

        6 *whole-grain crackers* (e.g., Ak-Mak), cucumber and goat cheese

---

*If you are insulin-resistant, substitute the following fruits: ¼ cup blueberries, ½ cup other berries or ¼ grapefruit.

✓ You may eat on the low-saturated fat meal plan.

✓✓ You may eat on the low-saturated fat meal plan if you substitute low-fat or part-skim cheese.

20-Gram Carbohydrate Snacks
✓ ½ medium *pear** and ½ cup *pecans*
✓ ⅓ cup *hummus* on 2 *Lavosh crackers*; raw vegetables
✓ ⅔ cup *edamame* beans (shelled)

25-Gram Carbohydrate Snacks
Each of the following snacks contains approximately 25 grams of carbohydrates.

    20 *grapes** and Swiss cheese
✓ ½ medium *banana** and 2 tablespoons organic *almond butter*
    7 dried *apricot halves** spread with goat cheese
✓ 2 small *kiwis** and ¼ cup *walnuts*
✓ 1 medium *apple** and 2 tablespoons organic, sugar-free *peanut butter*
✓✓ ½ small baked *potato* and ½ cup *cottage cheese*
✓✓ 15 *cherries** with mozzarella cheese
✓✓ ¾ cup *unsweetened applesauce** and ½ cup *cottage cheese*
    1 cup *whole-milk yogurt* and ¾ cup *strawberries*
✓✓ 2 corn *tortillas,* tomatoes, ¼ *avocado* and queso fresco cheese
✓✓ ¾ *mango** and ½ cup *cottage cheese*
✓ 6 *Ak-Mak crackers* and egg salad
✓✓ 1¼ cups fresh *pineapple* and ricotta cheese
✓ 1 slice 15-gram *whole-grain bread** with ¼ *avocado* and chicken salad and ½ small *apple**
    7 *whole-grain crackers* (e.g., Ak-Mak), cucumber and goat cheese
✓ 1 small *pear** and ¼ cup *pecans*
✓ ⅓ cup *hummus* on 3 *Lavosh crackers*; raw vegetables
✓ 1¼ cups *edamame* beans (shelled)

*If you are insulin-resistant, substitute the following fruits: ¼ cup blueberries, ½ cup other berries or ¼ grapefruit.
✓ You may eat on the low-saturated fat meal plan.
✓✓ You may eat on the low-saturated fat meal plan if you substitute low-fat or part-skim cheese.

Two-Gram Sodium Diet

The two-gram sodium diet is highly recommended for those who have a medical reason to restrict their salt intake such as congestive heart failure, kidney failure and salt-sensitive high blood pressure. Consult with your physician regarding your personal salt restriction needs.

The two-gram salt restriction *can* also be used by those of you who are having a difficult time with your transition. If you are insulin-resistant *or* have burned-out adrenal glands, you may find yourself retaining fluids as you improve your eating habits. By restricting your salt intake for a few months, you can alleviate your bloating and ankle swelling.

If you find yourself craving salt or feeling light-headed, you may have overdone your restriction. Be very cautious of salt restriction if you are on any medications that cause salt or other electrolyte wasting. If you do not know if your medications do this, ask your physician or pharmacist.

Foods Allowed on Two-Gram Sodium Diet

Bread Three or fewer servings of allowed bread or crackers. One slice of bread should not exceed 150 mg of sodium.

Cereals Whole-grain cooked cereals prepared without salt.

Cheese Eat only the low-sodium allowed cheeses.

Fats Nondamaged vegetable-oil-based unsalted salad dressings. Unsalted butter to be used as desired. Nuts without salt.

Fruits Eat fruits according to carbohydrate allowance.

Grains, legumes, starchy vegetables (cooked without salt) Potatoes, rice, legumes, barley, quinoa and oats, according to carbohydrate allowance.

Meat (cooked without salt) Beef, lamb, fresh pork, veal, chicken or unsalted fish. Low-sodium canned tuna or salmon. Eggs. Tofu.

Foods Allowed on Two-Gram Sodium Diet

Soups* Unsalted broth; homemade unsalted soups made from cream, vegetables or meats.

Vegetables Any fresh or frozen vegetable without sauces or additives.

Yogurt (plain) Limited to eight ounces per day.

———

*Be aware of hidden sugars in vegetable soups if you are insulin-resistant.

Foods to Avoid on Two-Gram Sodium Diet*

Bread Salted crackers, cheese crackers, cheese breads or any other bread that contains more than 150 mg of sodium per slice.

Cereals Quick-cooking cereals.

Cheese All other cheeses that are not allowed.

Fats Commercial dressings containing salt. Salted butter, nuts or nut butters. Olives.

Fruits None to avoid.

Grains, legumes, starchy vegetables None to avoid unless cooked with salt.

Meat Salted or prepared meats such as bacon, ham, dried beef, salt pork, sausage, frankfurters, luncheon meats, corned beef, canned meats, poultry or fish prepared with salt. Also avoid shellfish and frozen meat entrees.

Soups Regular broth, bouillon, bouillon cubes, canned soups, and dried or dehydrated soups.

Vegetables Sauerkraut or any vegetable processed in brine. Canned vegetables, frozen vegetables, and vegetable juices that contain salt greater than 150 mg per serving.

———

*You should already be avoiding some of these foods because they are processed and/or man-made foods.

Supplementation with Vitamins, Antioxidants and Minerals

Your minimum vitamin regimen should include the following pharmaceutical-grade supplements: a well-balanced multivitamin and mineral, extra calcium and magnesium, a stress B-complex, and omega-3 fatty acids.

Pharmaceutical-Grade vs. Nonpharmaceutical Supplements

Many people want to know why I only recommend pharmaceutical-grade supplements instead of most nonpharmaceutical ones. Here is my answer:

- The nonpharmaceutical supplements are not regulated; therefore, what the label says they contain is not always what is bioavailable. There are a few exceptions to this, but it is very difficult to know which brands do provide what they say on their labels.
- The companies that manufacture these nonpharmaceutical supplements look for the cheapest ingredients, and these ingredients are not always the most biologically available—that is, you cannot easily absorb them from your intestine into your bloodstream.
- There is always a risk of heavy metal contamination in the nonpharmaceutical brands.
- Many companies load their nonpharmaceutical products with cheap fillers.

Note: Do not think you are getting a good deal because a vitamin is inexpensive. Usually if the supplement you are taking is very inexpensive, it is made with the very cheapest ingredients.

To read about my pharmaceutical vitamin line, visit my Web site at *www.SchwarzbeinPrinciple.com.*

There are many different supplements for many different symptoms, problems and diseases. I have listed only some of them that I have found to be helpful for insulin sensitivity, adrenal gland function, symptoms related to too much insulin or too little adrenaline, tapering off tobacco and tapering off alcohol. I have not, however, listed the recommended doses for the different supplements because these are constantly changing as new research emerges.

Instead, I have listed a few different nutrition books at the end of this section that can help you formulate a healthy supplement regimen for yourself. Or you can work with one of my healthcare providers through my Web site or office to formulate your personal regimen.

Supplements

Supplements That Help Improve Insulin Sensitivity and/or Carbohydrate Cravings

- **Alpha lipoic acid** Decreases carbohydrate cravings, helps control blood-sugar levels, and prevents and treats peripheral nerve damage.
- **Carnitine** Decreases carbohydrate cravings and mobilizes fat.
- **Chromium** Decreases carbohydrate cravings and improves insulin sensitivity.
- **CoEnzyme Q-10** Stabilizes blood-sugar levels and improves circulation.
- **Conjugated linolenic acid (CLA)** Improves insulin sensitivity; helps you burn off midsection fat.
- **Gamma linolenic acid (GLA)** Decreases carbohydrate cravings, improves the utilization of energy and helps you feel more satiated.
- **Garlic** Decreases and stabilizes blood-sugar levels and improves immunity.
- **Glutamine** Decreases carbohydrate cravings.
- **L-glutamine** Decreases sugar cravings.

Supplements (cont'd)

- **L-taurine** Decreases carbohydrate cravings and aids in the release of insulin.
- **Omega-3 fatty acids** Improve insulin sensitivity.
- **Stress B-complex** Improves the metabolism of sugar and helps decrease carbohydrate cravings. (The B vitamins work best together.)
- **Vanadium** Helps insulin action at the cellular level.
- **Zinc** Helps prevent zinc deficiency often seen with diabetes.

Supplements That Help Adrenal Gland Function

- **CoEnzyme-A** Reduces stress and supports proper functioning of the adrenal glands.
- **CoEnzyme Q-10** Carries oxygen to all the glands, including the adrenal glands.
- **Extra pantothenic acid (B_5)** The adrenal glands do not function properly without pantothenic acid.
- **L-tyrosine** Relieves stress put on the adrenal glands, becomes adrenaline and aids in the functioning of the adrenal glands. **Caution:** Do not use if you are taking an MAO-inhibitor antidepressant drug.
- **Nicotinamide Adenine Dinucleotide (NADH)** NADH is a form of B_3 (niacin) that is essential for the production of neurotransmitters and cellular energy.
- **Vitamin C with bioflavonoids** Vital for proper functioning of the adrenal glands.

Supplements That Relieve Adrenaline Withdrawal Symptoms

The following supplements can help relieve adrenaline withdrawal symptoms such as irritability, anxiety, depression, carbohydrate cravings, increased susceptibility to infections, digestion problems, PMS, and salt and water retention.

- **Betaine HCL** For protein digestion.
- **Digestive enzymes** For protein, fat and carbohydrate digestion.
- **Caprilyc acid, acidophilus** and **fructooligosaccharides (FOS)** For help recolonizing your intestines with healthy bacteria.
- **Garlic** For help with immune function.
- **GLA, DHA** and **EPA** For brain function, mood stability and carbohydrate cravings.
- **L-glutamine** For help with carbohydrate cravings.
- **L-taurine** As a diuretic along with vitamin B_6 for salt and water retention.
- **L-Tryptophan***, **5-HTP***, **SAM-e*** and **St. John's Wort*** For depression, irritability, PMS and carbohydrate cravings.
- **Phosphytidal serine, acetyl-carnitine and GABA** For irritability and anxiety
- **Quercetin** and **MSM** For help with allergies.

Cautions:

L-Tryptophan and 5-HTP—Do not use if you take antidepressants.

SAM-e—Do not use if you have bipolar disorder.

St. John's Wort—Do not use if you take antidepressants.

Tapering Off Tobacco

A good vitamin protocol can help you get off tobacco products *and* protect you from their harmful effects.

Tobacco causes many harmful effects in your body, including increased risk of heart attacks, strokes, impotence in men, earlier menopause in women, Type II diabetes and several different types of cancers. If you are currently smoking, do yourself, your family and friends a favor, and start to quit now. Refer to steps 1 and 3 of the SPII program to learn how to eat well and taper off tobacco products, and try the following supplements as well:

- Vitamins C, E, A and a good sublingual B-complex* help block the effects of smoking and decrease your need for tobacco by helping you deal with stress.
- CoEnzyme Q-10, CoEnzyme A and alpha lipoic acid also help block the damaging effects of smoking.
- Zinc helps boost your immune system.
- Calcium, magnesium and GABA help calm you down.
- Flaxseed or fish oils help your body maintain even energy levels and calms your nerves.

Tapering Off Alcohol

A good vitamin protocol can help you get off alcohol products *and* protect you from their harmful effects.

Alcohol, like tobacco, causes nutrient depletion, especially zinc and magnesium. It also increases the production of free radicals in your body, damages your liver and brain, and may increase the risk of breast cancer. Try the following to help you either completely stop or taper way down on your alcohol consumption:

- A good sublingual B-complex* helps correct nutrient deficiencies, reduce alcohol cravings and supports your adrenal glands.
- Alpha lipoic acid helps protect the liver and pancreas from alcohol damage.
- Calcium and magnesium help calm you down and remedy magnesium deficiency.
- Extra vitamin C helps the immune system fight off the toxic effects of alcohol and is vital for adrenal gland function.
- GABA, inositol and niacinamide help calm your body and prevent anxiety and stress.
- Glutathione, N-Acetylcysteine and L-Methionine help protect the liver and reduce alcohol cravings.
- Zinc helps boost your immune system and remedies zinc deficiency.

———————

Check out my Web site at www.SchwarzbeinPrinciple.com *for a good sublingual (under the tongue) sugar-free B-complex.*

Good Reading for Good Nutrition

Following is a list of recommended books to help you choose your supplement regimen:

- *Prescription for Nutritional Healing, 3rd Edition.* James F. Balch, M.D. Avery, 2000.
- *The Life Extension Foundation's Disease Prevention and Treatment, 3rd edition,* The Life Extension Foundation, 2000.
- *PDR for Nutritional Supplements.* Medical Economic, Inc., 2001.
- *Drug-Induced Nutrient Depletion Handbook, 2nd Edition.* Ross Pelton, R.P.H., Ph.D., CCN. Lexi-Comp, Inc., and Natural Health Resources, Inc., 2001.

Special Dietary Recommendations

The SPII program involves making changes to five different areas of your lifestyle. It is not just a program for changing your eating habits. You also need to learn to manage your stress, taper off toxic chemicals, follow a cross-training exercise program and take hormone replacement therapy if you need to. Food is very healing, but in order to follow the basic SPII food recommendations, you need to follow the rest of the program, too.

It is easier to make changes to all these areas at one time if your metabolism is not already badly damaged. However, if you have already damaged your metabolism and have a degenerative disease of aging, you will need to modify the SPII nutrition program slightly.

Lowering Saturated-Fat Intake

The most common change made to the SPII eating program is lowering saturated-fat intake. This is usually needed if you already have a degenerative disease of aging, you are not following an exercise routine, you cannot follow your recommended carbohydrate count immediately because of a carbohydrate or sugar addiction, or you are under tremendous amounts of stress. Refer to the saturated fat section starting on page 244 in this chapter to learn about what foods you need to avoid or eat sparingly.

In this program, saturated fats and carbohydrates—not just large quantities of carbohydrates—are used as energy. However, if you do not use the saturated fats as energy because you are not exercising, they will keep your blood sugar levels higher and cause your insulin levels to be high as well. This is the opposite of what you are trying to accomplish, so until you add in your exercise routine, lower your carbohydrate intake and/or manage your stress better you will need to lower your saturated-fat intake.

The extent to which you need to lower your saturated-fat intake depends on your response to the eating program. You may only have to cut back on red meat and dairy products, or you may have to avoid all the foods listed in the Saturated Fats section on page 245 in this chapter. Monitor your cholesterol/triglyceride levels, blood-sugar readings, blood-pressure readings and your fat-weight changes to determine how much saturated fat you should consume.

This does not mean you are going on a low-fat diet. You will need to eat plenty of monounsaturated and healthy polyunsaturated oils in place of saturated fat in order to remain healthy. Make sure your ratio of omega-3 to omega-6 fatty acid intake is at least 1 to 3. You may have to supplement with ground flaxseeds, flaxseed oil or fish oil to get enough omega-3 fatty acids in your diet. See Essential Fatty Acids section on page 247–253 in this chapter.

Other Special Conditions and Dietary Recommendations

The following recommendations are for those of you who already have a degenerative disease of aging and cannot follow the SPII program in its entirety. You may find that your problems initially get worse instead of better. Your insulin levels have to go higher than your adrenaline levels in order for you to heal, and this may make your condition worse. Following the recommendations ahead will help you stay in your transition. Follow your current metabolism-type program (see chapter 17, 18, 19 or 20) and incorporate the following recommendations.

Cholesterol abnormalities

If you are insulin-resistant or have burned-out adrenal glands, you may notice your cholesterol levels rising after you start your transition. This is a normal response to insulin levels rising higher than adrenaline levels during the healing phase. If you do not already have plaque in your arteries, or a history of heart bypass surgery, there is no reason to be alarmed by this *initial* change. A short-term rise in these levels will not harm you. As your metabolism heals and your hormone levels normalize, these numbers will come back down.

However, if you have known artery disease, are not exercising or are worried about these numbers, follow the low-saturated fat meal plans. Although saturated fats in theory are not bad for you, they will keep your blood-sugar levels higher and cause your insulin levels to be high as well if you cannot use them as energy. When your insulin levels remain high, you produce more triglycerides and cholesterol in your liver. These produced fats are the ones that cause the highest risk for heart disease.

Also, you should not drink any alcohol, milk, juice or fruit smoothies, nor should you smoke or use any tobacco products with this condition. Caffeine also raises cholesterol levels, but you may need to continue your caffeinated beverages if your adrenal glands are burned out to help get you through your transition.

Have your homocysteine level checked, and if it is high, take extra folate, vitamin B_6 and vitamin B_{12} to help lower your level.

If you are on a statin cholesterol-lowering medication, take extra CoEnzyme Q-10.

Dementia

If you are a caretaker of a person who has dementia, please help that person follow these recommendations.

If the dementia is due to hardening of the arteries and you cannot exercise at all or do not exercise consistently, follow the lower-saturated fat meal plans. Although saturated fats in theory are not bad for you, they will keep your blood-sugar levels higher and cause your insulin levels to be high as well if you cannot use them as energy. When insulin levels remain high, you produce more triglycerides and cholesterol in your liver. These produced fats are the ones that cause the highest risk for plaque in your arteries.

Also, you should not drink any alcohol, milk, juice or fruit smoothies, nor should you smoke or use any tobacco products with this condition. Caffeine also raises insulin levels but you may need to continue your caffeinated beverages if your adrenal glands are burned out to help get you through your transition.

Have your homocysteine level checked, and if it is high, take extra folate, vitamin B_6 and vitamin B_{12} to help lower your level.

Depression
No change is needed, but consider eating more of the foods that contain tryptophan. See list in chapter 6.

Early menopause
No change is needed.

High blood-pressure disease
If you have salt-sensitive blood pressure, you should follow the salt-restrictive diet until your metabolism heals. High insulin and/or high cortisol and/or low adrenaline are causes for salt-sensitive high blood pressure. Also, you should not drink any alcohol, milk, juice or fruit smoothies, nor should you smoke or use any tobacco products with this condition. Caffeine also raises blood pressure, but you may need to continue your caffeinated beverages if your adrenal glands are burned out to help get you through your transition.

However, if you are having a hard time controlling your blood pressure, and/or you are not exercising consistently, follow the low-saturated fat meal plans. Although saturated fats in theory are not bad for you, they will keep your blood-sugar levels higher and cause your insulin levels to be high as well if you cannot use them as energy. When insulin levels remain high, your blood pressure can also increase.

Morbid obesity

If you are insulin-resistant or have burned-out adrenal glands and do not or cannot exercise consistently *and* you carry fifty or more pounds of excess fat weight, try your regular program first. If you find yourself gaining weight very rapidly, switch to the low-saturated fat meal plans. Although saturated fats in theory are not bad for you, they will keep your blood-sugar levels higher and cause your insulin levels to be high as well if you cannot use them as energy. Also, you should not drink any alcohol, milk, juice or fruit smoothies, nor should you smoke or use any tobacco products with this condition. Caffeine also causes weight gain, but you may need to continue your caffeinated beverages if your adrenal glands are burned out to help get you through your transition.

Osteoarthritis

If you are insulin-resistant or have burned-out adrenal glands, do not exercise consistently and have osteoarthritis, you may notice your pain getting worse as you begin your transition. Try stopping all the nightshade vegetables (eggplant, potatoes, tomatoes, and green, yellow and red peppers) and decreasing your salt and saturated-fat intake to help with your pain. Although saturated fats in theory are not bad for you, they will cause your insulin levels to be high if you cannot use them as energy.

Also, you should not drink any alcohol, milk, juice or fruit smoothies, nor should you smoke or use any tobacco products with this condition. Caffeine also makes arthritis worse, but you may need to continue your caffeinated beverages if your adrenal glands are burned out to help get you through your transition.

Osteoporosis

If you have severe osteoporosis, make sure you are not eating too many proteins or too few proteins and/or carbohydrates. Eating too many proteins or too few carbohydrates increases the secretion of adrenaline/cortisol, causing bone breakdown. If you eat too few proteins you will not have the material to make new bones.

Also, you should not drink any alcohol or smoke or use any tobacco products with this condition. Caffeine also causes bone loss, but you may need to continue your caffeinated beverages if your adrenal glands are burned out to help get you through your transition.

Plaque in your heart arteries

If you have hardening of your arteries and are insulin-resistant *or* have burned-out adrenal glands and you do not or cannot exercise consistently, you need to keep your saturated-fat intake lower until you heal your metabolism again. Although saturated fats in theory are not bad for you, they will keep your blood-sugar levels higher and cause your insulin levels to be high as well if you cannot use them as energy. When insulin levels remain high, you produce more triglycerides and cholesterol in your liver. These produced fats are the ones that cause the highest risk for heart disease.

Also, you should not drink any alcohol, milk, juice or fruit smoothies, nor should you smoke or use any tobacco products with this condition. Caffeine also increases blood pressure and therefore your risk for heart attacks, but you may need to continue your caffeinated beverages if your adrenal glands are burned out until they have healed.

Have your homocysteine level checked, and if it is high, take extra folate and vitamins B_6 and B_{12} to help lower your level.

If you are on a statin cholesterol-lowering medication, take extra CoEnzyme Q-10.

Some forms of cancer

Discuss your dietary restrictions with your oncologist and if you do not have any restrictions, follow the regular meal plans. Because the treatment for most cancers not only destroys cancer cells but healthy cells as well, you are usually starting out with a badly damaged metabolism.

If you have lost weight during your therapy, it will all come back plus more. Do not be discouraged—this is the only way your body knows how to heal from the loss of lean body tissue—by rebuilding both lean body tissue and fat stores. With time your metabolism will heal, and you will be able to burn off your excess fat weight. You must make sure you are eating enough, as well as eating a variety of, different vegetables because they contain many antioxidants.

You could also go on the lower-saturated fat meal plans to minimize the amount of fat weight you will gain as you heal.

Also, you should not drink any alcohol or smoke or use any tobacco products with this condition.

Stroke

If you have suffered a stroke due to hardening of the arteries and cannot or do not exercise consistently, follow the low-saturated-fat meal plans. Although saturated fats in theory are not bad for you, they will keep your blood-sugar levels higher and cause your insulin levels to be high as well if you cannot use them as energy. When insulin levels remain high, you produce more triglycerides and cholesterol in your liver. These produced fats are the ones that cause the highest risk for plaque in your arteries.

Also, you should not drink any alcohol, milk, juice or fruit smoothies, nor should you smoke or use any tobacco products with this condition. Caffeine also raises blood pressure and therefore increases the risk of stroke, but you may need to continue your caffeinated beverages if your adrenal glands are burned out.

Have your homocysteine level checked, and if it is high, take extra folate, vitamin B_6 and vitamin B_{12} to help lower your level.

Type II diabetes

If you have Type II diabetes, follow the lower carbohydrate meal plans and make modifications as needed for whatever other problems you have, such as cholesterol abnormalities, plaque in your arteries, morbid obesity and/or high blood pressure.

Good Nutrition Leads to Good Health

Good nutrition, including supplementation with vitamins, antioxidants, minerals, and essential amino and fatty acids, is essential to healing or maintaining your metabolism.

Once you have made the necessary changes to your eating habits, you are well on your way to balancing out your hormones to obtain optimum health. However, this is only one step of five in the SPII program. It is time to master the rest.

Twelve

Step Two: Managing Stress and Getting Enough Sleep

Managing Stress

M anaging your stress is an important step to ensuring a successful transition.

Stress causes your body to use up its biochemicals—but this is not always bad. Your body needs to use them up so that you can accomplish your daily activities. Therefore, you do not want to eliminate all stress from your life. You do, however, need to learn how to manage your stress better to keep your body from using up biochemicals faster than it can rebuild them. Otherwise, you will damage your metabolism, which leads to accelerated metabolic aging, degenerative diseases and earlier death.

The Stress Hormones—Adrenaline and Cortisol

There are two types of stresses—immediate life-threatening stresses and chronic non-life-threatening stresses. In the twenty-first century, the types of stress you encounter are usually not the immediate life-threatening kinds of stress, but artificial, non-life-threatening ones, such as chronic job stress or being busy all day with self-imposed tasks. Your body, however, reacts to these two types of stress in the same way—by secreting adrenaline and cortisol, the body's two major stress hormones. If the stress is acute and life-threatening, these two hormones can save your life. However, if the stress is non-life-threatening and chronic, these same hormones can shorten your life by causing your body to use up its biochemicals faster.

Therefore, one of the most important steps in antiaging is learning how to counterbalance the continuous high secretion of stress hormones. If stress hormone levels have risen because of your personal stress, you need to learn how to bring them back down through stress management techniques. More importantly, you need to eliminate the stress that caused them to be high in the first place.

Daily Psychological Stresses

In this section, stress is defined as the psychological stresses that you encounter on a day-to-day basis, not as the stress induced by toxic chemicals, overexercising, pain, trauma or malnutrition.

Your stress hormone levels will rise with every kind of psychological stress—from being busy and meeting deadlines to emotional suffering and unhappiness. How high your hormones go and how long they remain elevated depends on several factors: the cause of the stress, how long it lasts, how much control you have over the stressful event and how you learn to deal with the stress. Although the ideal would be to eliminate as many psychological stresses as you can, sometimes the only real control you have is learning how to better manage or cope with them.

Everyone Needs Downtime

When your brain is working overtime, so are your major hormones. Therefore, when your brain is at rest it is not sending stress signals to your adrenal glands, and this allows them time to heal. It also keeps your insulin levels from staying high from the secretion of adrenaline and cortisol.

For the purposes of this book, the process of dealing with stress will be known as downtime. Downtime is when your brain is *not* being bombarded with 1,001 different thoughts or tasks. It is important to have downtime because this is one of the times that your brain rests and rebuilds neurotransmitters.

Making Downtime a Daily Practice

Do you have enough downtime? It is important to plan downtime every day and to use it well. There are many ways to achieve downtime. Everyone will have their own way of putting their brain to rest and filling themselves with joy. Some patients tell me that their brain rests while they are doing household chores; others rest their brains by taking baths or getting bodywork done such as a massage or a facial. Others read mindless books. Some play a musical instrument or sing. Get to know yourself and what it takes to rest your brain. Nothing is a waste of time if it puts your brain to rest.

Doing the right amount and kinds of exercise for your current metabolism type is beneficial and may be used for downtime. However, do not confuse putting your brain to rest with the mindless time you spend while overexercising. Overexercising results in the opposite of what you want to do—rest your brain—because it causes you to use your neurotransmitters as energy. It also raises your insulin levels and is a factor in adrenal gland burnout.

If it is hard for you to achieve downtime, you will need to learn a stress management technique such as deep breathing, visualization or meditation. Or use these techniques in addition to your other down-time methods.

Relax Those Muscles

Most of us become tense when we are under stress, so it is impor-tant to learn to release the tension from your body. Practice the muscle relaxation technique below to ease the effects of a tense day. As you relax, you will lower your adrenaline, cortisol and insulin levels.

Muscle Relaxation Technique

This exercise is beneficial because it is a way to completely relax your body and put your brain to rest.

- Get comfortable in your favorite chair.
- Breathe deeply, in through your nose and out through your mouth, and concentrate on your body and how it feels as you sit in the chair. Notice any tension you may feel in your neck, shoulders or back.
- Continue breathing and concentrating this way for a few minutes.
- Begin to contract your muscles, starting with your toes and feet; keep your muscles contracted for a few seconds and then slowly relax them. Focus on the feeling of contracting and relaxing your muscles.
- Work your way up your body, continuing to contract and relax your muscles as you go from your feet, to your calves, to your thighs, to your stomach, to your buttocks, to your arms and to your neck—ending with your facial muscles.
- When you are finished, take a few more deep breaths. You will notice how much tension you have released and how much better you feel.

Get Quiet, Relax and Breathe

Another way to relieve stress, lower your major hormone levels and put your brain to rest is by meditating. It allows you to get quiet and relax. When you begin practicing meditation, you can start by doing it for five minutes and then work up to whatever length of time feels comfortable for you. It has been proven that setting aside even five minutes each day for meditation will benefit you emotionally and physically.

Here are five different methods to try.

Meditation Exercise One

Find your favorite quiet space. Get comfortable in any position you like. Breathe deeply* a few times. Repeat a short and simple word that is meaningless to you. Let whatever thoughts you have drift in and out of your mind. Continue to allow your thoughts to drift in and then use your chosen word to help you push those thoughts away. Repeat this exercise until you feel sufficiently relaxed.

Meditation Exercise Two

Focus on your breathing* by counting slowly from one to ten as you breathe in and out. Continue until you feel calm and relaxed.

Meditation Exercise Three

Sit quietly in a favorite spot, close your eyes and visualize your thoughts as they drift in and out of your mind, observing them as if they were not your own. Do not let your mind wander to the past or future.

Meditation Exercise Four

Focus on an object of beauty and breathe deeply in and out.* As your thoughts wander, recognize that your brain is thinking and then quietly focus on your object again.

---

*Inhale deeply through your nose, hold for a few seconds and then exhale deeply through your mouth. You should exhale for twice as long as you inhale. For example, if you inhale for one count, exhale for two counts and so on.

Meditation Exercise Five

Prayer can be a form of meditation. Breathe deeply* in and out and relax as you pray.

Putting Your Life in Perspective

Another way to manage stress is by putting your life in perspective. Perhaps you have lost sight of the important people and things in your life that give you love and joy. This exercise will help you keep your life in perspective and decrease feelings of worry, hostility, anxiety, guilt and anything else that may contribute to a stressed emotional state. As you practice these six steps, your stressful thoughts and emotions will be replaced by positive, loving ones that help restore emotional and physical balance. By putting your life in perspective and changing your negative thoughts to positive ones, you can put your brain to rest. Positive thoughts will also calm your adrenal glands and lower your insulin levels.

Positive Thinking Exercise

- Stop what you are doing and become aware of your feelings.
- Identify what is disturbing you. If need be, jot it down to clarify what is bothering you.
- Place your hand over your heart to center your emotions.
- Think of a positive, humorous or joyful event, person or place. For the next few minutes, imagine yourself back in that event, or spending time with that person, or being in that place.
- Next, think of something that you absolutely love and cherish, such as an infant or a baby animal. Focus on that loving feeling for a few minutes.
- Lastly, reflect on something that you are thankful for in your life.

Inhale deeply through your nose, hold for a few seconds and then exhale deeply through your mouth. You should exhale for twice as long as you inhale. For example, if you inhale for one count, exhale for two counts and so on.

Do You Overreact to Daily Stresses?

Do you find yourself overreacting to daily stresses? If you do, then you may have another issue. Your daily nutrition and lifestyle habits may be elevating your stress hormone levels as well. When you encounter a small problem, the added release of even more stress hormones sends your hormone levels even higher, and you boil over very easily. In this case, stress management techniques may not be the answer. Improving your habits may be the best way to deal with this type of stress reaction because it addresses the root cause of your stress. If improving your habits does not help you to stop overreacting, try stress management techniques or consult a mental health professional who can help determine why you are overreacting.

Irritation List

Make a list of the things that really bother you and the feelings you experience when they happen. Are you sad, angry, mad, frustrated? Are you overreacting?

Things That Bother Me: **How I Feel When They Happen:**

_____   _____

_____   _____

_____   _____

_____   _____

_____   _____

_____   _____

_____   _____

_____   _____

_____   _____

Keeping Track of Stress Signals

Things happen every day that can make you angry, nervous and upset, and cause your adrenaline, cortisol and insulin levels to increase. It is important to learn what upsets you and to notice how your body reacts when you are upset. The chart below will be useful for understanding your body's reactions to stress. When you find yourself reacting to stress, it is time to practice your stress management techniques.

It is important to identify your body's reaction to stress so that you can break the stress cycle. When you are angry, frustrated, sad or upset, your brain sends signals to your body that you are under stress. This stress manifests itself through tightening of the muscles, excessive sweating and/or a faster heartbeat. Check the physical, behavioral, emotional and psychological symptoms you experience under stress. These are *your* stress warning signs.

What are your stress warning signals?

Physical Symptoms
- ☐ Back pain
- ☐ Dizziness
- ☐ Fatigue
- ☐ Grinding of teeth at night
- ☐ Headaches
- ☐ Indigestion
- ☐ Racing heart
- ☐ Ringing in ears
- ☐ Sleep difficulties
- ☐ Stomachaches
- ☐ Sweaty palms
- ☐ Tight neck, shoulders

Behavioral Symptoms
- ☐ Bossiness
- ☐ Compulsive eating
- ☐ Compulsive gum chewing
- ☐ Critical attitude
- ☐ Excessive smoking
- ☐ Overuse of alcohol

Emotional Symptoms
- ☐ Anger
- ☐ Boredom, no meaning to things
- ☐ Constant worry
- ☐ Crying
- ☐ Easily upset
- ☐ Edginess, feeling ready to explode
- ☐ Feeling powerless to change things
- ☐ Loneliness
- ☐ Nervousness, anxiety

Psychological Symptoms
- ☐ Forgetfulness
- ☐ Inability to get things done
- ☐ Inability to make decisions
- ☐ Lack of creativity
- ☐ Loss of sense of humor
- ☐ Memory loss
- ☐ Overwhelming sense of pressure
- ☐ Restlessness
- ☐ Thoughts of running away
- ☐ Trouble thinking clearly
- ☐ Unhappiness for no reason

Are there any other stress warning signals that you experience which are not listed? If so, be sure to list them in the space provided below so that you can learn to measure and manage your stress better.

My Personal Stress Warning Signals

Record your personal warning signals below.

The things I notice about my body when I get upset are:

_____

_____

_____

_____

_____

_____

_____

_____

_____

Tips for Measuring and Managing Your Stress

To measure how you are dealing with stress, take your pulse rate or note how fast your heart is beating during a stressful situation and evaluate your sleep patterns. If your pulse is higher than ninety beats a minute and/or if you cannot fall asleep or you wake up in the middle of the night or in the early-morning hours, your stress hormones are high. Another measure of your stress is how joyful you are on a daily basis. A lack of joy is a marker for depression. Although stress is not the only reason for depression, the hormonal responses to chronic stress can lead to depression.

Here are some techniques that may help you manage your stress better.

- Learn to manage your time effectively. Poor time-management skills lead to unnecessary stress.

- Decide what is important. Instead of prioritizing your schedule, learn to schedule your priorities.

- Learn to breathe deeply. Breathing deeply lowers stress hormones. Shallow breathing is an indication that you are tense and stressed.

- Find an exercise you enjoy. Exercise is a good way to relieve tension after a hard day at work. (See chapter 14.)

- Develop a positive mental attitude. Look for the bright side of situations instead of dwelling on the negative. Studies have shown that negative thinking raises stress hormones.

- Do not take life too seriously. Learn to laugh at yourself and find the humor in every situation. Laughter is very healing.

- Pick your battles carefully. Not all causes are worth fighting for. If a point is not important in the long run, let it go. Don't sweat the small stuff.

- Get a massage. Massage helps relieve muscle tension and relaxes the brain.

- Engage in an activity that allows your brain to rest.

- Allow yourself enough time to sleep each night. This will help lower your stress hormones. A good night's rest helps give you a new perspective on life.

- Do not make several life changes at one time (if you can avoid it). Ending a relationship, moving to a new house or city, changing jobs or losing loved ones are very stressful situations. You compound your stress when several life changes occur at one time. Stress hormone levels are cumulative. If you cannot avoid such a situation, realize how extremely stressed you are and make other changes in your life to help you counter the stress.

- Take a vacation. If you do not have the time or cannot afford a long vacation, plan a short getaway. Even a picnic at the beach, in the mountains or in your own backyard can be a relaxing getaway that helps you reduce your stress.

- Take up yoga. Yoga stretches your muscles and relaxes your body and brain. Another benefit to yoga is that you will learn to breathe deeply.

- Learn to meditate. Meditation is an opportunity for your body to obtain quality rest while you are awake.

- If you believe in God, pray. Put your life into perspective by connecting with God.

- Set realistic goals for yourself and others. If you can learn to do this, you will not be continually disappointed when those goals are not met. Disappointment raises stress hormones.

- Take a long, hot bubble bath!

- Surround yourself with beauty, such as flowers, scented candles, artwork and anything else that appeals to your senses.

- Organize your environment to unclutter your mind. Tidy up the house, clean your desk, pay your bills and respond to correspondence. This will provide you with an organized base from which to handle the other stresses in your life.

- Make a To Do list and cross off each item as you complete it. This will give you a visual sense of accomplishment and helps to eliminate the "I've got too much to do" feeling.

- Attend a stress management seminar, read a good book or listen to tapes on the subject of stress. There are several good courses, books and audiotapes available to help you get a handle on your stress.

- Ask for help. It is not a shameful thing to seek advice from professionals. After all, your health is at stake!

Recommended Reading and Listening for Managing Stress

There are many good books and tapes available to help you learn to manage your stress. I have listed a few of them to help you get started.

Books

A Manual for Living, Epictetus. Harper San Francisco.
Being Peace, Thich Nhat Hanh. Parallax Press.
Find a Quiet Corner, Nancy O'Hara. Warner Books.
One Day My Soul Just Opened Up, Iyanla Vanzant. Simon & Schuster.
Peace Is Every Step, Thich Nhat Hanh. Bantam Books.
Succulent Wild Woman: Dancing with Your Wonder-Full Self, Sark. Simon & Schuster.

Recommended Reading and Listening for Managing Stress

The Artist's Way, Julia Cameron. G. P. Putnam's Sons.

The Creative Journal: The Art of Finding Yourself, Lucia Capacchione, Ph.D. New Page Books.

Little Book of Joy: An Interactive Journal for Thoughts, Prayers, and Wishes, Bill Zimmerman. Hazelden Information Education.

The Power of Optimism, Alan Loy McGinnis. HarperCollins

The Quieting Reflex, Charles Stroebel, M.D., Ph.D. Putnam Publishing Group.

The Relaxation Response, Herbert Benson, M.D. Avon Books.

The Simple Abundance Companion, Sarah Ban Breathnach. Warner Books.

The Woman's Book of Courage: Meditations for Empowerment and Peace of Mind, Sue Patton Thoele. Conari Press.

You Must Relax, Edmund Jacobson. McGraw-Hill.

The Taming of the Chew: A Holistic Guide to Stopping Compulsive Eating, Denise Lamothe, Psy.D., H.H.D. Penguin Books. (This book is important for anyone who is stressed from his or her eating disorder.)

Audiotapes (available from Image Paths, 1-800-800-8661)

Affirmations, Belleruth Naparstek. Health Journeys.

For People Experiencing Stress, Belleruth Naparstek. Health Journeys.

General Wellness, Belleruth Naparstek. Health Journeys.

Taking the time to take care of yourself on a daily basis is essential to balancing your body's hormones. Stress management techniques work to help keep you regenerating efficiently. But you are not completely managing your stress unless you are also getting enough sleep. The next section will help you understand the importance of getting a good night's rest and show you how to achieve it.

Getting Enough Sleep

Sleep is antiaging and more important than you realize because while you are sleeping, your body does most of its rebuilding. Also, all three levels of the major hormones—insulin, adrenaline and cortisol—are higher when you are sleep-deprived. Therefore, if you do not get enough quality sleep, you may end up with a degenerative disease of aging at an early age.

What Is Enough Sleep?

When you were a baby, you needed to sleep around the clock. During childhood you needed to sleep more than you were awake. In puberty you needed around ten to twelve hours of sleep. As an adult, you should get between eight and ten hours of sleep a night. For those of you who meditate, meditation can take the place of some hours of sleep.

The different seasons also affect sleep patterns. Light and dark dictate the normal circadian rhythm of the wake-and-sleep cycle. When it is light, you produce more serotonin and are awake. When it is dark, you produce more melatonin to sleep. It is easier to make serotonin in the summer and harder to make it in the winter. You need less sleep in the summer than you do in the winter because more sunlight increases serotonin production.

You need to honor these daily and seasonal cycles by resting when it is dark and being active when it is light. If you constantly overstimulate yourself at night to stay up longer, you will disrupt this normal sleep rhythm. Overstimulation can occur for many reasons, such as using alcohol or stimulants, forcing yourself to stay awake late to read, do household chores, watch TV, study or party, or because of a nightshift job. Once your sleep pattern is disrupted, it needs to be healed.

Teens Need to Sleep!

Teenagers need a lot of sleep—ten to twelve hours a night. Some parents believe that their teenagers are just lazy when they sleep in, and I have had many parents tell me that they wake their kids up and make them do chores or get out of the house and run around. This is a mistake. This creates sleep deprivation. One of the highest mortality rates is seen in teenagers because of accidents related to sleep deprivation with or without drugs. Just be aware that sleeping a lot is normal during the teen years and is a requirement for good health.

Myths About Sleep Deprivation

It is a myth that you need less sleep as you age. The truth is that you need just as much sleep when you are older as you did when you were younger. The problem is that you lose the ability to sleep well as you age, and thus lose the ability to rebuild as efficiently. Alternatively, you lose the ability to rebuild efficiently as you age, and therefore lose the ability to sleep as much as your body needs. In either case, you are not sleeping enough, and this leads to sleep deprivation.

Another myth is that you are getting enough sleep if you are not tired when you wake in the morning. This is not always true because you might be running on higher levels of stress hormones, which gives you a false sense of having energy. This situation can go on for many years until you crash and burn out. In fact, it happened to me after my residency program. However, because I had already healed my metabolism, I was able to recover quickly.

My Own Crash and Recovery

For almost five years during my medical training, I was awake for thirty-six hours at a time while I was "on call" every three to five days. I thought I was handling this schedule because I had the energy that I needed to get through my days. I should have realized, however, by the end of those five years, that the lapses in my short-term memory about social events were a warning that something was not quite right.

But it was not until I completely finished training and started my endocrinology fellowship that I crashed. There are no "on-call" nights in endocrinology, and the days are filled with more research and less urgent patient contact. I was able to relax because my days were not as stressed as they had been during my residency. This is when I began to sleep ten to twelve hours a night.

At first I thought I was ill because the more I slept the more fatigued I became during the day. And in fact, after the first month when I did not regain my energy, I really was worried that I had caused irreversible damage to my adrenal glands.

In the past I was always able to stay awake to meet the demands of my residency program. After I slept for a few days, I would regain my energy. But now I was the walking dead. No matter how many hours I slept, my body was asking for more.

I cannot describe to you how scared I was when I first started feeling tired all the time again. Then I attended a lecture about sleep deprivation. The professor said that you must always catch up on sleep after being deprived. He said that sleep would restore the body's energy. I trusted that he was right. Although I was not happy that I would feel tired until I caught up with my sleep, I was relieved to know that I would regain my energy again. And I did.

Miraculously, almost six months to the day after I started sleeping regularly, I was back to feeling better than ever and requiring only eight hours a night again. I healed faster because I ate well, exercised moderately and did not self-medicate with stimulants to stay awake or with sedatives (alcohol or sleeping pills) to fall asleep. I acknowledged that I was sleep-deprived and that I needed to catch up on my sleep. I simply slept to heal myself.

I had crashed after five years of running on adrenaline and cortisol to keep me going. I was able to heal in six months. This may seem like a long time, but in reality, I got off easy. I was fortunate that I stopped having to be up all night on call before I completely burned out my adrenal glands. Otherwise, it would have taken me much longer to regain my energy because I would also have had to fully heal my adrenal glands. If this had been the case, I don't believe I would have been able to finish my endocrinology fellowship at that time.

Sleep Deprivation Leads to Poor Habits

I cannot emphasize enough the importance of getting enough sleep since it is extremely difficult to change poor nutrition and lifestyle habits when you are sleep-deprived.

For example, if you are sleep-deprived, you may start comfort eating. Comfort foods usually contain or are carbohydrates, and the more carbohydrates you eat, the more carbohydrates you will want. Alternatively, you may go completely in the opposite direction and not want to eat enough because eating makes you more tired. In both cases, you become malnourished. This makes it harder to sleep at night, and the cycle continues.

Here is another example. When you are sleep-deprived and cannot afford to be tired during the day, you may try to raise your energy by consuming more stimulants. After consuming stimulants to stay awake during the day, you may find yourself consuming alcohol at night to fall asleep. Unfortunately, ingesting alcohol can both cause you to wake up in the middle of the night around 2 to 4 A.M. *and* make it harder to fall back to sleep. So when you get up in the morning, you are so tired that you start consuming stimulants again. It becomes a vicious cycle.

Sleep deprivation also makes it difficult to start or stay on an exercise program.

Finally, if you are sleep-deprived, you can forget about handling other stresses well. It is not going to happen.

The bottom line is that one of the most important risk factors for accelerated aging *that you have control over* is getting enough quality sleep. The term "beauty sleep" is more than just words. You will feel more beautiful after a good night's rest because your body will rebuild during that time.

You may not feel beautiful, however, until you have caught up on *all* your sleep. Hang in there and trust that you will heal.

Catching Up on Sleep Takes Time and Patience

If you have been sleep-deprived, it can be hard adjusting to sleeping again because of the initial feeling of fatigue that you can experience when your body is trying to catch up with sleep. When you relax long enough to let yourself catch up on sleep, deep fatigue sets in until your body catches up completely. This happens because your adrenal glands realize that the stress is gone. They then go into shut-down mode and do not secrete a lot of adrenaline and cortisol—the wake-up hormones. Another example of this "let-down phenomenon" occurs when you force yourself to stay awake to study for finals or to meet a deadline. After the test or project is finished, you relax and feel tired—and catch a cold.

Most people do not like to feel tired and will blame their tiredness—incorrectly—on their new sleeping habits when in fact their fatigue is a normal response to catching up on sleep. Unfortunately, if you are sleep-deprived, you will not be able to bypass the healing process. You will have to be tired for a while before you can be re-energized. This is the healing phase, the time in your transition when you are healing from the damage caused previously by years of poor nutrition and lifestyle habits.

Give Yourself Permission to Be Tired

If you are insulin-sensitive or insulin-resistant with healthy adrenal glands, getting enough sleep at night will make you feel good in the morning. This positive feeling will make you want to sleep more. However, if your adrenal glands are burned out, sleep will probably make you feel more tired the next day. Subconsciously, you may sabotage getting a good night's rest because you do not like to feel this tired.

Therefore, you need to consciously think of sleep as restorative and give yourself permission and time to be tired so that you can heal. It is also important to understand *why* you are so tired, so that you can try to avoid becoming sleep-deprived in the future. A tired feeling is your body's way of signaling to you that it is not able to keep up with rebuilding. Your body is trying to keep you from being more active because activity requires you to use up your biochemicals. Fatigue is your body's way of telling you that it needs more time to rest and heal.

It is very important to heed this fatigue because your body is sending signals that it has been overworking for a long time. Give your body and yourself a break. If you start using a lot of sugar and stimulants to give you "energy," your body will continue to use up its biochemicals by raising adrenaline and cortisol levels higher than insulin levels and you will "crash" harder.

Do not be discouraged. Your body will catch up with sleep, and you will heal your adrenal glands. Once this happens, your adrenal glands will again be able to secrete enough adrenaline and cortisol to give you good, balanced energy throughout the day.

When Catching Up on Sleep Is Impossible

If your adrenal glands are severely burned out, it may be impossible for you to fall or stay asleep. This is the time to take a prescription medication such as desyrel to help reset your sleep clock. You may also need to take an antidepressant medication called a selective serotonin reuptake inhibitor (SSRI) in the morning for energy. Consult with your physician if you feel you need to take desyrel and an SSRI. As long as you are working on your nutrition and lifestyle habits to heal your metabolism, these drugs are not the worst thing you can do for your health. If you need to take these medications to get you through your transition, you should take them. However, if you use these types of medicines to make yourself feel better *and* ignore your nutrition and lifestyle habits, you will get worse over time by using them.

What Normal Sleep Looks Like

Sleep deprivation occurs when you do not get enough hours of quality sleep. If you do not get enough sleep, your body will not be able to regenerate from the previous day. Sleep deprivation is caused by many different things. To better determine if you need to work on your sleeping habits, consider the following example of an ideal sleep pattern:

1. You should be asleep within fifteen minutes of your head touching the pillow.
2. Over the next eight hours, you should cycle through the various stages of sleep, including REM (dream) sleep.
3. You should not get up to urinate or for any other reason, even if it is easy for you to fall back to sleep.
4. When you wake up you should feel rested.

Is this what you do every night? If not, you have a sleep disturbance.

Sleep disturbances come in every shape and size. Some people get up one or two times a night to urinate and then go back to sleep easily. Others, on the opposite end of the spectrum, stay up all night once they are awakened. Wherever you fall in this sleep disturbance pattern, you need to work on your sleeping conditions and habits so that they do not get progressively worse. Any sleep disturbance creates a deficiency, and your deficiency will continue to increase until you catch up on your sleep again.

Check Out Your Sleeping Conditions

There are many reasons for not getting a good night's sleep. If you do not sleep well, check your sleeping conditions first.

Is the room quiet enough?

Stimulation will make it hard to fall asleep. Being woken up by sound may make it difficult to get back to sleep. If you cannot get rid of external noises, consider earplugs. Soft, expandable foam-type earplugs that are less irritating are now available. If a snoring partner is keeping you awake, make sure that he or she is evaluated for sleep apnea (see page 352). If the snoring issue is not resolved, you may have to sleep in another room.

Is the room dark enough?

Sunlight and moonlight disturb sleep hormones. If you cannot make the room absolutely dark, consider sleep eyeshades.

Is your bed comfortable?

If you have not tried rotating the mattress, do so now. If it does not help, consider buying a new bed. It is worth the investment.

Is the room too cold or too hot?

Being too cold or too hot can keep you from getting a good night's rest. Make sure you know what temperature you need in order to fall and stay asleep all night. You may need a temperature that is different from the person you are sleeping with. Discuss a way to get the correct temperature for both of you. Will it be an open window? The heater? A comforter that is used on half the bed but not the other? Sleeping with or without pajamas?

Evaluate Your Nighttime Habits

Next, evaluate your habits right before bed.

Are you waking up in the night with a full bladder?

Watch your bedtime fluid intake. If you do not drink fluids before bed and still wake up in the night to urinate, you may have a hormone problem such as diabetes or menopause that needs to be addressed.

Are you running around finishing chores and staying busy right before bedtime?

This activates the stress hormones that are also known as the wake-up hormones. Do something relaxing before bed like taking a warm bath, reading or deep breathing.

Are you giving yourself enough hours in bed?

You must make the time for at least eight hours of sleep. Try not to wake up to alarm clocks, but get to bed early enough that you will wake up naturally eight hours later.

Examine Your Nutritional and Chemical Habits

You also need to examine your nutritional and chemical habits.

Are you eating enough food during the day?

If you do not eat enough food throughout the day, you will end up with low blood-sugar levels. However, since low blood-sugar levels are not compatible with life, the body releases the stress hormones adrenaline and cortisol to counter the drop in blood-sugar levels. Your blood-sugar levels never get too low, but your stress-hormone levels, which are also your wake-up hormones, get too high. You will have both a hard time falling asleep and staying asleep if this occurs.

Are you eating enough carbohydrates at dinner?

Not enough carbohydrates for dinner can lead to the inability to fall or stay asleep. Again, this is related to high adrenaline and cortisol levels. This is one of the most important factors I ask patients to check for on my eating program because it is just as harmful to eat too few carbohydrates as it is to eat too many.

Are you eating refined sugars?

Eating foods high in refined sugar may also keep you from falling and/or staying asleep. Refined white sugar products are very potent triggers of insulin secretion. When you eat sugary foods, your insulin levels go very high. The excess sugar is diverted into your cells, leaving you with low blood-sugar levels. Since low blood-sugar levels are incompatible with life, the stress hormones—adrenaline and cortisol—are secreted in high amounts to overcome the stress. This will keep you awake or cause you to wake up in the middle of the night.

Are you drinking too many caffeinated beverages?

If you drink caffeinated beverages at bedtime, you may not be able to fall asleep because of the higher adrenaline effect. If you drink them during the day, you may fall asleep at bedtime, but then wake up in the middle of the night. Some people experience the opposite effect with stimulants. They get sleepy because the stimulant is causing the release of serotonin between their brain cells. With time this extra secretion will lead to less serotonin and the need for stimulants will increase. Sometime during this process, sleep disorders can occur.

Are you drinking alcohol in the evening?

Alcohol consumption at night usually helps to relax people, and they fall asleep readily. However, it is very common for them to wake up between 2 and 4 A.M. because of the hypoglycemic effects of alcohol. While you are sleeping, your brain still needs a constant supply of sugar to survive, but alcohol blocks the liver's ability to supply enough sugar to the brain during this time. This is a stressful situation for the body; therefore, stress hormones are released to help bring sugar levels back up. Remember, it is the stress hormones that keep you awake or cause you to wake up in the middle of the night.

Are you using tobacco products?

The use of tobacco in any form can disrupt your sleep. Although people use these types of products to calm down, nicotine in fact mimics the effects of adrenaline. Though you will not be able to stop this habit overnight, it must be addressed if you want a good night's sleep. (See chapter 13.)

Are you taking B vitamins too late in the day?

The B vitamins are stimulating because they help your adrenal glands make adrenal-gland hormones. If you take them too late in the day, you may not sleep well at night.

Look at Health, Lifestyle and Social Situations That Prevent Good Sleep

Last, but not least, look over the following *other* reasons for not sleeping well, and see if any pertain to you.

Stress

Stress is another common reason that people have trouble falling asleep or staying asleep. To help with this problem, work on stress management techniques. One technique you can try is to keep a pad and paper by your bedside and write down all the thoughts that are in your head that may be keeping you from relaxing. Sometimes by writing your list down, you can get it to stay out of your brain for the night. The same applies to waking up in the middle of the night with 101 worries and "to do" thoughts. Write them down so that you may fall back to sleep.

Power napping

Power napping during the day is a very common reason that many people cannot sleep well through the night. Ironically, power napping leads to sleep deprivation because it interferes with your normal circadian rhythms.

Overexercising

Overexercising is another cause for sleep deprivation. When you overexercise, your stress hormones are higher, and they can keep you from falling or staying asleep. You also are more likely to be calorie-deprived when you overexercise, another reason for having a hard time sleeping. Additionally, injuries from overexercising can cause pain that keeps you tossing and turning throughout the night.

Pain

Pain from any cause is another reason people do not sleep well at night. Initially, the pain itself will keep you awake, but later it is the hormone imbalances that occur from chronic pain that keep you from getting a good night's rest. Acute pain causes the release of adrenaline and cortisol; chronic pain causes the depletion of serotonin, leading to lower melatonin levels, and melatonin is necessary for falling and staying asleep.

Perimenopause/Menopause

Perimenopausal or menopausal women are usually able to fall asleep easily, but because of the low levels or lack of the hormone estradiol, they may wake up in the middle of the night. This is one reason you might belong to the 2 to 4 A.M. club. Check with your physician to see if you need to start taking HRT or have your estradiol prescription adjusted or changed. You may need more or sometimes even less, because fluctuating high to normal levels of estradiol can also wake you. Fluctuating estradiol levels are not just associated with being hot or having hot flashes.

If you are not on an estradiol preparation, ask your physician to prescribe one. There are estradiol pills, patches, topical and vaginal creams, sublingual troches (tablets or lozenges) and sublingual drops. Not every delivery system works the same for every woman. Trial and error will help you find the system that works best for you.

Diabetes

If you have poorly controlled diabetes manifested by high blood-sugar levels, you may be waking up at night to urinate. You need to get your blood-sugar levels back down to normal so that you can sleep through the night. Frequent nighttime urination can be a symptom of diabetes. You may want to have yourself screened for high blood-sugar levels.

Hyperthyroidism

Any thyroid condition causing hyperthyroidism (an overactive thyroid) can keep you from falling or staying asleep. This includes taking a dose of prescription thyroid replacement therapy that is too high for you. Having high thyroid hormone levels makes adrenaline more potent.

Sleep apnea

Sleep apnea is another very common cause of interrupted sleep. Sleep apnea is a medical condition where you stop breathing for an extended time interval when you are sleeping. Have a significant other check to see that you do not stop breathing during the night. People at high risk for this are usually extremely overweight and insulin-resistant, but not always. It is important to make sure that sleep apnea is not your reason for sleep disturbances because it is highly associated with depression, heart disease and death if left untreated.

Antidepressant medications

Some of the antidepressants are known to cause sleep problems. Consult with your physician regarding these medications if you are not sleeping well.

Prescription and over-the-counter medications

Many prescription and over-the-counter medications disrupt the normal sleep cycles. If you are not sleeping well, ask your physician or pharmacist whether anything that you are taking, including herbal products, contains any chemical that may disturb sleep.

Antianxiety and sleeping pills

The long-term use of diazepam, lorazepam and alprazolam (antianxiety drugs), and other drugs of this class disrupt REM sleep.

Many people use these types of drugs to relax. The irony is that these types of drugs are known to disrupt the normal sleep cycle. Taking these medications for a long period of time can actually worsen sleep and cause more anxiety.

One of the most common reasons for sleep problems is the chronic use of sleeping pills, both over-the-counter and prescription. Sleeping pills cause sleep disturbances because they do not cure the reason that you are not sleeping well. All they do is knock you out. They do not reset your sleep cycle or get you into REM sleep. If you do not get into REM sleep, you will never heal.

Acid reflux

If you have acid reflux, you may wake up in the night from the pain of heartburn or the spasm of coughing.

Allergies

If you have allergies, you may wake up in the night because your nose is stuffed up, your throat is scratchy and dry, or you are coughing.

A new baby

Getting up at night to feed a baby is an obvious reason for sleep deprivation—ask any new mother or father. There is not much that can be done about this one except to share the nighttime duties with your partner. Also, hope and pray that your baby starts to sleep well soon so that you can, too. Napping is a good way to catch up on some of the missed sleep. However, as soon as you can, you should resume your normal sleep habits because over the long-term, napping disrupts your circadian rhythm.

Note: If you do not get enough hours of sleep during the week, make sure to make it up during the weekend, though this is not as ideal as sleeping enough hours every night.

Short- and Long-Term Effects
of Chronic Sleep Deprivation

Research shows that you have to catch up with sleep deprivation or you will stay chronically sleep-deprived, which can lead to some or all of the following symptoms and/or disease states:

Short-Term Effects

- Achy joints and/or sore muscles
- Acne
- Change in bowel habits—constipation or loose bowels
- Fatigue
- Hair loss
- Headaches
- Intestinal bloating
- Loss of memory and/or concentration
- Mood disorders such as anxiety, irritability, being excessively weepy or disoriented
- Weakness
- Weight gain

Long-Term Effects

- Anxiety disorders, depression or psychosis
- Cancers
- Cholesterol abnormalities
- Chronic fatigue syndrome
- Fibromyalgia
- Heart attacks
- High blood pressure
- Irritable bowel syndrome (IBS)
- Migraines
- Obesity
- Osteoarthritis
- Osteoporosis
- Stroke
- Type II diabetes
- Ulcers

Tips for Getting a Good Night's Sleep

Here are some special tips for getting a good night's sleep.

Use Your Bed Only for Sleeping!

If you are awake, get up out of bed and go to a place where you can sit and relax. Do not read or watch TV. These activities can be too stimulating. Instead, try a stress management technique such as deep breathing or meditation.

Do not try to fall asleep out of bed. When you feel you may be able to fall sleep again, get back in bed. It is important to associate your bed with a place to sleep and not a place where it is okay to toss and turn.

Add Calcium and Magnesium to Your Bedtime Regimen

Try calcium and magnesium at bedtime. Take anywhere between 500 and 1,500 mg of calcium and 250 to 750 mg of magnesium together with as little water as needed to swallow. Calcium can be constipating, and magnesium can promote loose bowels. If this regimen constipates you, add more magnesium to the mix or lower the calcium content. If you are having loose bowel movements, either increase calcium or lower magnesium.

Supplement with Tryptophan

Try supplementing with tryptophan or 5-hydroxy-tryptophan (5-HTP), if calcium and magnesium alone do not help. Tryptophan becomes 5-HTP, which becomes serotonin, and serotonin becomes melatonin—one of the most important sleep hormones.

Start with 500 mg of tryptophan or 50 mg of 5-HTP at bedtime and work your way up to 2,000 mg or 200 mg respectively, as needed. Do not use tryptophan or 5-HTP if you are on an antidepressant.

Whatever you do, do not use melatonin supplements to help you sleep every night. This may help your sleep in the short-term but can lead to depression and even worse sleep disruption over time. (Although I do not usually recommend it, melatonin may be used short-term for jet lag.)

Note: Tryptophan can be obtained by prescription only. 5-HTP can be bought over-the-counter, but you should be extremely cautious of the brand because of possible contaminants. It is better to buy a pharmaceutical-grade 5-HTP supplement from a medical practitioner's office. A note of caution: Do not take tryptophan or 5-HTP if you are on an antidepressant.

Make Sure You Are Getting Enough of the B Vitamins

Inositol is a B vitamin that has been shown to be helpful with sleep because it improves REM (dream) sleep. Try 1,000 to 3,000 mg at bedtime.

Many of the other B vitamins are important for sleep. Make sure you are getting enough of them in your foods. If not, take a B-complex supplement in the morning. Taken too late in the day, a B-complex can keep you awake.

Consider Taking GABA

Try taking gamma-aminobutyric acid or GABA (an inhibitory neurotransmitter) to help you sleep, especially if you have a hard time relaxing before bed. Take 300 mg to 500 mg. Make sure you buy a good brand of GABA because this chemical crosses into your brain. As with 5-HTP, consider buying a pharmaceutical-grade GABA supplement from a physician's office.

Try Herbal Remedies

Valerian root, lemon balm, passionflower, skullcap and chamomile are all helpful for overcoming sleep disturbances. Use these herbal preparations cautiously and for a short period of time only because herbs are drugs, too. Always consult with your physician for any possible contraindications or side effects before taking any herbs. **Caution:** Valerian root and alcohol should never be used together.

Lavender oil helps relieve stress and depression. Lavender-scented sachets and handkerchiefs (placed in your pillowcase) or lavender pillows can be helpful. **Caution:** Do not use lavender if you are pregnant and never take it orally.

Seek Professional Help if Needed

If you suffer from post-traumatic stress disorder, you need to work with a psychotherapist who specializes in this syndrome. There are many techniques to help you overcome the effects of trauma—and these are being updated continuously. Seek expert advice.

The Last Resort

If nothing else works, try a sleep "resetting" medication such as desyrel for a few months. In general, I do not prescribe many drugs. But using this class of drugs for resetting sleep is very important. Sometimes taking as little as 25 mg at night is enough to do the trick. You will have to work with your physician on this one.

Note: There are many sleep disorders—far too many to cover in this chapter. If you feel you have a sleep disorder, consider being evaluated at a sleep disorder clinic or consult your physician.

Can I Sleep Too Much?

People generally get too little sleep, not too much. However, if you feel you are sleeping too much, it may be due to any of the following reasons:

- You may have a glandular-based endocrine disorder
- You are catching up from past sleep deprivation
- You are healing your adrenal glands
- You are going through a growth spurt
- You are depressed
- You are taking medication that affects your sleep
- You have been overexercising
- You have an infection or more serious illness
- You want to escape from responsibilities
- You are tired
- You ingested too much alcohol or other toxic chemicals the night before

If you continue to require a lot of sleep and do not know why, get evaluated by your physician.

Common Excuses for Not Getting Enough Sleep

Below, in italics, are some of the excuses or comments in relation to sleep that I have heard from patients throughout my years of practice. My responses follow. All the practices listed below cause sleep deprivation and can lead to premature metabolic aging.

I do not need to sleep more because I have enough energy to get my daily work done. You are using up your biochemicals more than rebuilding them, and this will eventually catch up with you.

I do not want to sleep more because I feel like I am missing out on life. If you do not get enough sleep, you will shorten your life span or decrease your quality of life by ending up with a degenerative disease of aging.

There aren't enough hours in the day to get done what I need to do, so I will give up some hours of sleep. You are doing too much if you cannot find the time to get enough sleep.

I work long hours, and because I want to see my family and spend more time with my friends, I am willing to give up sleep time. If I am tired I will just drink more caffeinated beverages. Drinking caffeine to keep you going will lead to adrenal gland burnout.

I feel more tired if I sleep longer than six hours. This may be an indication that you are already sleep-deprived.

I catch up on my sleep during the weekends. It is better to get the right amount of sleep each night.

I catch up on my sleep during my yearly vacation. You cannot possibly make up a year of sleep deprivation during one yearly vacation.

I don't have time to sleep; my job is very important and demanding. You need to put your health before your career or it will happen anyway when you crash from your poor sleeping habits.

I cannot fall asleep if I do not drink alcohol at dinner. Your adrenal glands are burned out. You may have to use desyrel to reset your sleep clock.

I feel better when I don't sleep. The fact that you are not letting your body shut down and rest at night indicates that you are staying awake to squeeze adrenaline and cortisol out of your burned-out adrenal glands.

I would rather go out with my friends and party and get up the next day and drink coffee rather than get enough sleep. As an adult you need to learn how to take better care of yourself.

If I eat more food, I will be more tired and I do not have time to sleep more. If eating makes you tired, you are either not eating balanced meals or you have burned-out adrenal glands. If you do not start eating now, you will never heal.

If I sleep too much I am not creative. Many creative and innovative thinkers got their ideas through dreams.

Sleep is for sissies. Real men and women understand the need for adequate sleep.

Sleep is boring. As boring as sleep may seem to you, it is necessary for good health and longevity.

Getting enough hours of sleep each night is important for keeping your hormones balanced. This will keep you regenerating efficiently, which in turn will keep your metabolism working at its optimum level. Make sure to put aside enough hours in the night to sleep—and have fun regenerating!

Eating well and managing stress, including getting enough sleep, are only two of the five steps in the SPII program. Step three is about tapering off toxic chemicals or avoiding them completely.

Thirteen

Step Three: Tapering Off or Avoiding Toxic Chemicals

S tep Three of the SPII program involves tapering off or avoiding toxic chemicals, such as tobacco, alcohol, refined sugars, caffeine and other products. These chemicals stimulate the release or increase or mimic the action of adrenaline and/or cortisol, so eliminating or avoiding them completely is an important step in healing your metabolism. Remember, adrenaline and cortisol are the stress hormones, and they cause your body to use up its biochemicals faster. Also remember that healing can only occur when the rate of rebuilding exceeds the rate of utilization. These chemicals also block the action of insulin, causing further insulin resistance. In addition, some toxic chemicals, such as alcohol, refined sugar and tobacco, damage your cells directly.

Toxic Chemicals and Aging

As discussed throughout this book, your body uses up its biochemicals on a daily basis and then needs to rebuild them. Unfortunately, as you grow older, it becomes harder for your body to rebuild its biochemicals. This is part of the normal aging process. However, when you add the stress of toxic chemicals to the normal aging process, they compound the problems your body already has in regenerating efficiently, which leads to accelerated metabolic aging.

Note: The term "biochemicals" is being used to describe chemicals that your body needs for regeneration, and the term "toxic chemical" is being used in reference to chemicals that are not needed for regeneration and have the potential to cause cellular damage.

Toxic Chemicals Are Addicting

You will not necessarily recognize that these chemicals are toxic because you will initially achieve a sense of well-being from using or ingesting them. Since they all cause a release of hormones and other biochemicals—such as neurotransmitters and endorphins—they make you feel good. Anything that makes you feel that good can become addicting. The problem is first recognized only after you use up these "feel good" chemicals or damage the cells that make them, and then you cannot get the same chemical high unless you use more and more toxic chemicals. Or you will find that you do not feel better even when you use more of these toxic chemicals because your brain biochemicals have been depleted.

If you are using toxic chemicals on a daily basis to get you through the day, you are either doing too much or you already have a damaged metabolism. If you are doing too much, you need to work on stress-management techniques and stop using these chemicals as soon as possible. (Refer to chapter 12.)

If you have a damaged metabolism, you will not be able to get off these toxic chemicals until you have begun to eat well first. You are using them to cope both mentally and physically because you have depleted your biochemicals through years of poor nutrition and lifestyle habits. So do not taper off before you begin to eat well, or you will not be able to maintain good eating habits.

However, you may not be able to get off your toxic chemicals completely until your metabolism has done a significant amount of healing. The idea is to use food to rebuild your biochemicals and only small amounts of the toxic chemicals to access your newly built functional biochemicals, so that you achieve a small sense of well-being and stay in your transition process.

As stated previously, you are healing only if your insulin levels are higher than your adrenaline/cortisol levels. This causes you to rebuild the biochemicals you used up previously. However, if this ratio of insulin over adrenaline/cortisol gets too high, you will not be able to use up your biochemicals very well. Although you are healing when this happens, you will feel as if you are not. This is the time that a *small* amount of toxic chemicals, which helps narrow the gap between your insulin and adrenaline/cortisol levels, becomes important. This is not an endorsement for using toxic chemicals all day long. If you overuse these chemicals, your adrenaline/cortisol levels will become higher than your insulin levels, and you will be further damaging, not healing, your metabolism.

What If I Have a Healthy Metabolism?

If you are insulin-sensitive and have healthy adrenal glands, consuming a small amount of sugar, caffeine and alcohol will not destroy your health, but it is best to stay away from all toxic chemicals because they accelerate the aging process. However, if you enjoy a cup of tea daily, a homemade dessert occasionally, or a glass of wine sporadically, you will not destroy your health if the other aspects of your life are under control—that is, if you eat real and healthy foods, manage your stress consistently, sleep enough hours, do a moderate amount of cross-training exercises and take HRT, if needed.

Getting Off Toxic Chemicals: Cold Turkey or Gradually?

If you are insulin-sensitive with healthy adrenal glands, or you are insulin-resistant with healthy adrenal glands, you will not have any problems coming off toxic chemicals quickly. You may stop using them cold turkey. (This does not mean you should stop your prescription medication.) If you have burned-out adrenal glands, however, you will have to taper off your toxic chemicals. If you have not yet determined your metabolism type, refer back to chapter 8. If you are still undecided about whether you have burned-out adrenal glands or not, err on the side of caution and taper off your toxic chemicals.

If you stop ingesting toxic chemicals too quickly, you may reveal underlying hormonal imbalances that can cause a myriad of symptoms, including achy joints, depression, fatigue, general aches and pains, headaches, increased infections, irritability, mental exhaustion, mood swings, sleep disorders, sugar cravings and worsening of allergies and asthma.

Good Nutrition, Stress Management and Patience Are Keys to Success

Once you realize that these chemicals are harmful, you may want to get off them as soon as possible. But try to be patient. If your adrenal glands are burned out, you first must be eating at least three balanced meals a day and beginning to control your stress.

You are more likely to be successful in staying off toxic chemicals if you do not taper off them too quickly. A few more weeks or months of using them is not going to ruin your overall health program. Tapering off them more slowly will keep you from feeling like a "failure" and giving up.

If you have already stopped cold turkey and are not having any symptoms, you probably do not have burned-out adrenal glands. Do not go back on your toxic chemicals just so that you can taper off them. However, if you are experiencing withdrawal symptoms after having stopped cold turkey, try drinking green tea to self-medicate before resuming your other toxic chemicals, and then taper off them as described below. Caffeine is less harmful than refined sugar, tobacco and alcohol, so it is the best choice to use as self-medication. Green tea is healthier than sodas, coffee or black teas. Green tea has antioxidants and other good phytochemicals; therefore, it has more beneficial effects than other caffeinated drinks. However, if you do not like green tea, black tea is a good second choice.

The first step to successfully getting and staying off a toxic chemical is to be sure that you are eating well and not skipping meals. You will also need to start drinking more water. Next, you need to work on stress management techniques.

Once you are eating well and managing your stress, start by cutting down on the amount of toxic chemicals you are consuming, but keep the frequency of consumption the same—as described under each toxic chemical discussion.

If You Have Burned-Out Adrenal Glands

The best way to come off toxic chemicals if your adrenal glands are burned out is to replace all your toxic chemicals with green or black tea and then taper off the tea as described below. This is not always possible, however. Always keep in mind that getting off toxic chemicals is not the first step in healing your metabolism. Eating well comes first, and if you need to self-medicate to eat well, you need to stay on some of your chemicals a while longer.

In the meantime, come off all the other toxic chemicals you do not need to taper off, such as artificial sugars, fake fats, carbohydrate and fat blockers, monosodium glutamate (MSG) and other preservatives and additives.

If You Are Insulin-Resistant

For those of you who are insulin-resistant, getting off nicotine, alcohol and refined sugar is a priority. Use stevia as your artificial sweetener and stop all other artificial sugars, fake fats, carbohydrate and fat blockers, MSG, and other preservatives and additives. Caffeinated beverages can be eliminated last.

Nicotine

Nicotine products include but are not limited to cigarettes, cigars, pipes and chewing tobacco. You probably use nicotine to calm yourself and for energy and concentration; therefore, you will have a better chance of tapering off tobacco products if you have first improved your eating habits and learned to manage your stress.

Eating well is difficult when you use tobacco products because the nicotine in them mimics adrenaline action and causes your body to use up its structural and functional proteins and fats to be used as food. You will have a false sense of satiation and therefore believe you are not hungry. Do not be fooled; you are just "eating" yourself. While you are using tobacco products, you may have to force-feed yourself to overcome your increased adrenaline effects. Besides burning out your adrenal glands, nicotine increases your risk of becoming insulin-resistant.

Tapering Off or Eliminating Tobacco

Any of the following suggestions can help you eliminate tobacco.

- Taper off by decreasing the amount of tobacco products you use on a predetermined schedule. There is no right or wrong way to do this. If you can cut your intake in half right away, do so. If you can only taper off one cigarette at a time, that is also good. The idea is to continuously try to taper off tobacco products. First acknowledge that you need to do so and then make a conscious choice to taper off and then quit.

- Switch to nicotine patches, inhalers, nasal sprays or gum*, and then taper off these nicotine products on a predetermined schedule. If all you ever do is switch from tobacco products to nicotine products, you have done a lot because you are no longer inhaling the damaging hydrocarbons found in smoke. Ultimately, the ideal is to taper off tobacco and nicotine products completely so that you can heal. Remember, do not use nicotine substitutes and tobacco products together. This can cause nicotine poisoning, leading to increased risk of stroke and heart attacks.

- Stop cold turkey if your adrenal glands are healthy.

- Try hypnosis, acupuncture or any other stop-smoking program. Consult the American Lung Association and American Cancer Society for programs they may offer through schools, hospitals or your local YMCA.

———————
*Discuss the safety of these nicotine products in relation to your health with your personal physician.

- Use any of the prescription antismoking medications that contain the chemical bupropion hydrochloride. You will need to consult with your physician on this one.

- Substitute one high-adrenaline lifestyle habit for another that is not as harmful as tobacco, such as drinking caffeinated beverages or overdoing cardiovascular exercises. Although this is not ideal, it is better for you than if you continued with the more harmful habit. Drinking a regular cola or running for several miles is better than smoking! When you are ready, you can taper off the caffeinated beverages as described later in this section, or taper off the excessive exercise in such a way that you do not get an increased craving for tobacco. Make sure that you get clearance from your physician before you start an exercise program. Smoking increases your risk for stroke and heart disease as well as cancer.

- Supplement with vitamins. A good vitamin protocol can both help you get off tobacco products and protect you from their harmful effects. (See chapter 11, page 317.)

Alcohol

Alcohol can raise blood pressure, triglyceride and sugar levels, and cause fat-weight gain. People with high blood pressure, high triglyceride levels, morbid obesity, known plaque buildup in the heart or brain arteries, or diabetes should not drink alcohol at all.

If your adrenal glands are burned out, your cortisol levels may be low and you may want to drink alcohol to try to raise them back up again. You will be drinking to self-medicate—to make yourself feel better—which may make tapering off more difficult.

Menopausal women also need to be aware that it can be hard to give up alcohol completely if their estradiol levels are too low. Since alcohol helps keep estradiol levels in the bloodstream higher, women will unknowingly be self-medicating with alcohol to keep their low estradiol levels a little higher. If you are in menopause, discuss your HRT regimen with your physician to see if it may be contributing to your cravings.

If you are alcohol-dependent or have trouble tapering off alcohol following the schedule outlined below, you should consider seeking professional help.

Tapering Off or Eliminating Alcohol

Follow this schedule to taper off alcohol.

- Start by cutting your alcohol intake in half. If you drink two glasses of wine every night with dinner, taper off to one glass of wine. If you drink eight beers with your friends on a weekend night, cut back to four beers. *There is no room for hard liquor on this program.* If you are using it, switch to red wine or beer and then taper off it as previously noted.

- Continue tapering off your intake by one-half at a pace you are comfortable with.

- Taking supplements that help heal your adrenal glands and reduce anxiety, stress and alcohol cravings can also help you taper off alcohol. (See chapter 11, page 318.)

Ideally, you should not drink at all. However, if alcohol is something you thoroughly enjoy and just the thought of never being able to drink it again causes you increased stress, taper off to one-half of a glass of wine a night or one beer a night. But remember, any alcohol makes you more insulin-resistant and burns out your adrenal glands even more.

Note: This is not an endorsement to drink alcohol! Furthermore, although drinking one beer or one-half of a glass of white wine is equivalent to one-half of a glass of red wine in terms of alcohol content, researchers do not report the same benefits to drinking white wine and beer that they attribute to drinking small amounts of red wine.

Refined Sugars

Refined white or brown sugars include sucrose, fructose, maltose, dextrose, maltodextrin, polydextrose, corn syrup and molasses. If you are addicted to refined sugars, you will have a very difficult time stopping sugary foods cold turkey. The first step to tapering off sugary foods is *not* to skip your balanced meals—*and* to continue eating sugary foods if you are still craving them. (Do not, however, substitute sugary foods for balanced meals.) In the beginning, it is more important for you to eat balanced, healthy meals than it is to worry about stopping sugary foods. Do remember, though, that your ultimate goal is to taper off all refined sugar products. As impossible as this may sound right now, as you heal your metabolism your sweet tooth will go away.

Tapering Off or Eliminating Refined Sugars

There are three ways to taper off and/or eliminate refined sugars. The third method is only an option if you are insulin-sensitive.

1. Begin eating balanced meals and snacks with your designated complex carbohydrate count. Refer to the personal program for your current metabolism type. (See chapter 17, 18, 19 or 20.) Eat real complex carbohydrates such as legumes, whole grains and starchy vegetables. If you have uncontrollable cravings for sugar, give in to them by eating fruit instead. By eating this way, the worst that can happen to you is that you end up eating too much fruit in addition to your balanced meals and snacks. Since you need healthy food to heal, eating balanced meals will heal your metabolism and you will notice your carbohydrate cravings

subsiding with time. Try to eat only fruits with the lowest glycemic index (GI). (See chapter 11, page 269.) If you still have sugar cravings, try eating higher glycemic index fruits or a small amount of dark unsweetened chocolate.

2. Initially, replace all your sugary foods with fruit, and then decrease your fruit intake by five grams per meal per week. For example, replace all of the candy, cookies, cakes, desserts, fruit juices and regular sodas that you consume with fruit. If the amount of carbohydrates in fruit you are now eating exceeds your recommended carbohydrate count, gradually reduce the amount of fruit you eat until you reach your carbohydrate goal. Then substitute other complex carbohydrates such as legumes, whole grains and starchy vegetables—you should not be eating fruit as your only carbohydrate. If you are eating fruit as a snack, try to balance your fruit snack with a protein because this will help get your hormones into balance sooner. (See snack recommendations in chapter 11, page 308.)

   If you can decrease your fruit intake more quickly, do so. However, if you find yourself getting tired, depressed or irritable, or you are having an increased craving for sugars, or you are waking up at night, slow down your tapering process.

3. The following is not the best method, and you should only consider this way of tapering off sugary foods if you are *insulin-sensitive*. Decrease your refined sugar intake by five grams per meal per week. Once your refined sugar intake is equal to your target carbohydrate amount per meal, start replacing your sugary foods with real complex carbohydrates such as legumes, whole grains and starchy vegetables until you have eliminated sugary foods. You also can incorporate some fruit.

Note: If you must have refined sugars, or you are having a hard time getting off refined sugars, or you want to bake with the best type of sugar, using honey is better than using white or brown sugar. And unsweetened dark chocolate is better than most sweets. (This is not an endorsement to eat sugar, however!)

You will find your sweet tooth disappearing on the SPII program as your adrenal glands heal. You will not need to use willpower on this program because your cravings will go away. Supplements that help reduce sugar cravings can be found in chapter 11, pages 315–317.

Artificial Sweeteners

You can stop these chemicals cold turkey because they do not affect your adrenal glands like refined sugars do. The only alternative sugar that I recommend is a product called Stevia because it is not a toxic chemical. I do not endorse or recommend that you use any type of artificial sweetener. I do not like aspartame, acesulfame K, sorbitol, sucralose or saccharine because they are harmful. Alternatively, use a small amount of real honey instead of artificial sweeteners. Although honey causes a rise in insulin levels, it is always better to ingest real food.

Illicit Drugs and Narcotics

These should not be used because of the damage that they do to brain cells. Illicit drugs such as marijuana, cocaine and ecstasy deplete your neurotransmitters and damage the brain cells that make them. If you are addicted to any of these drugs, you may need to get into a detoxification program. Check with your physician or local hospital for programs near you. If you can just stop using them because you are not addicted to them, then do so. There is nothing good about these drugs.

MSG and Other Preservatives and Additives

Avoid or eliminate these chemicals from your diet. Your body cannot use them to help you rebuild, and they are harmful to your health. You do not need to taper off. Just stop them completely.

Fake Fats

Avoid or eliminate fake fats such as Olestra from your diet. Your body cannot use these chemicals for energy or rebuilding, and they may cause a deficiency in your fat-soluble vitamins (A, D, E and K) and in your essential fatty acids. You do not need to taper off. Just stop them completely.

Carbohydrate and Fat Blockers

Avoid or eliminate these toxic chemicals because they disrupt the absorption of real food. You do not need to taper off. Just stop them completely.

Caffeine

Caffeine products include but are not limited to coffee, teas and sodas. Taper off one caffeinated beverage at a time, starting with sodas, then coffee, then tea. Start by going to three-quarters caffeine and one-quarter decaffeinated for each caffeinated beverage you normally consume. Do not taper off the number of beverages that you drink in a day. If you do not feel any ill effects from this after a week, then it is time to cut back to one-half caffeine and one-half decaffeinated for each beverage. After a week, assuming you feel okay, taper off to one-quarter caffeine and three-quarters decaffeinated for each beverage. Following this tapering schedule, you should be completely off the caffeinated form of this beverage by the fourth week.

If you feel lousy after cutting back your caffeine intake at any point in the tapering schedule, either try to continue on this amount of caffeine for another week and reevaluate how you feel, or resume the same amount of caffeine as the prior week when you felt well. You will have to make the call depending on how poorly you feel. If you have to start over, do not despair. This is perfectly normal. Just follow the guidelines, but taper off caffeine over longer intervals.

An alternative way to get off caffeine is to drink green tea, which is healthier than sodas, coffee or black teas, though black tea is a good second choice. Try switching all your caffeinated beverages to green or black tea and then taper off from caffeinated to decaffeinated green or black tea. If you need to continue with caffeinated green or black tea for a long time, at least this is better for you than coffee or sodas.

Instant coffee has less caffeine than brewed coffee. However, most brands are filled with chemicals, so it is best to avoid it.

Remember, if you need to self-medicate through your transition, tea is the best choice. This may not be the time to taper off it.

Prescription Medications to Avoid or Eliminate if Possible

The prescription drugs listed below should be avoided or eliminated if possible. However, *do not stop taking* any of these medications on your own. Stopping these medications requires supervision. Work with your physician.

Cholesterol-Lowering Drugs—HMG CoA Reductase Medicines

If you are diabetic or insulin-resistant, this class of cholesterol-lowering drugs (statins) may increase your blood-sugar or triglyceride levels. If you have to be on this type of medication*, pravastatin sodium or simvastatin, in my opinion, are the better ones to use because studies have shown them to be effective in reducing heart attack events.

Furthermore, if your cholesterol levels get too low, you can end up with burned-out adrenal glands, among other health problems, because the body uses cholesterol to make most of your adrenal gland hormones.

---

*You should take CoEnzyme Q-10 if you are taking a statin drug because these drugs deplete your body of CoEnzyme Q-10. CoEnzyme Q-10 has been shown to decrease the risk of heart disease.

Beta-Blockers

These medicines block the action of adrenaline (see chapter 4). If you are insulin-resistant or have burned-out adrenal glands, these drugs are not a good choice for you. They can increase your insulin resistance and make the symptoms of adrenal gland burnout worse because they block the action of adrenaline. If you are taking this class of medicines for heart disease, ask your physician if there is another drug that would work just as well for your condition. Since adrenaline improves blood flow to your lungs and increases the release of neurotransmitters, beta-blockers can also make asthma worse and cause depression by blocking the action of adrenaline.

Diuretics

Diuretics get rid of excess body water and salt. Unfortunately, most of them get rid of magnesium and potassium, too. The loss of magnesium and potassium makes you more insulin-resistant and decreases your production of adrenaline and cortisol. Do not stop these drugs if you need them for heart disease, but make sure you are receiving enough magnesium and potassium. This can be checked by routine lab tests. Additionally, if you are diabetic and take a class of diuretics known as the thiazide diuretics, ask your physician to switch you to a different class of diuretic since these drugs are contraindicated.

However, you may also be able to switch to another class of drugs (that are not diuretics) if you are using a diuretic for high blood pressure. Ask your primary-care physician.

The long-term use of diuretics for non-cardiac leg swelling also is not a good idea. If you are just using diuretics for this purpose, then get off them and work on your hormone balance. You may want to try natural diuretics, such as the amino acid taurine along with vitamin B_6, together with lowering your salt intake to less than two grams a day. (See the Two-Gram Sodium Diet in chapter 11, page 312.)

Sulfonylurea or Meglitinide Drugs

These two classes of drugs are used to treat the high blood-sugar levels in people with Type II diabetes. They cause the pancreas to increase its output of insulin. So, they really do not "work" because your body exchanges higher blood-sugar levels for higher insulin levels—and neither one is good for you.

Early on in Type II diabetes, the pancreas secretes high amounts of insulin. Prescribing a drug to *increase* insulin secretion further is therefore not the solution. Although these types of drugs will lower your blood-sugar levels, over time, however, you will have secondary drug failure: The drugs will partially deplete your body of insulin, and you will need more drugs or will be put on insulin injections.

In early-stage Type II diabetes, it would be preferable to use insulin-sensitizing drugs such as Glucophage (metformin), Actos (pioglitazone) and Avandia (rosiglitazone), because they help the cells respond to insulin better, and by doing so, lower insulin and blood-sugar levels. Ideally you would not need any medication and could keep your blood-sugar and insulin levels under control with changes in your nutrition and lifestyle habits. This will depend on how damaged your current metabolism is.

Furthermore, as Type II diabetes progresses, pancreatic beta cell function becomes increasingly lower because of damage to the pancreas from high blood-sugar levels. When this happens, the pancreas is unable to secrete high enough levels of insulin to handle the high blood-sugar levels caused by insulin resistance.

Therefore, prescribing drugs that increase insulin levels in order to lower blood-sugar levels is analogous to beating down the door to get it to open versus using the key. If you have progressed this far into diabetes, insulin replacement by injections, if needed, is a better choice because it gives the pancreas a chance to recover and may increase insulin production on its own over time.

Antidepressants

Please do *not* stop taking an antidepressant because you are reading this book. If you have a reversible form of depression, you may be able to taper off your antidepressant(s) after you have worked on healing your metabolism. This takes time. However, if you are in the middle of a stressful time or are not eating well, do not start to taper off your antidepressant. If your adrenal glands are burned out, stay on or start taking an antidepressant to help you through your healing phase. You may need to continue or use these medications even if you are not depressed to keep you from self-medicating with alcohol, nicotine, refined sugars and large amounts of caffeine. As long as you are in your transition process and are healing your metabolism, these types of drugs used for a short period of time are not necessarily bad for you. However, as with all drugs, they do have potential side effects.

When you feel that you are ready to come off your medication, make sure that you discuss this with your physician. The worst time of the year to try to stop this type of medicine is in the middle of the winter when serotonin production is naturally at its lowest.

Steroids

Steroids are cortisol derivatives. They are used as anti-inflammatory drugs for many disorders, including asthma, soft tissue injuries, connective tissue disorders and autoimmune problems.

If you have been taking steroids for a long period, you need to taper off them very slowly. Always check with your physician first. It is very dangerous to come off these medications if you still need them. If your physician feels that it is time for you to stop taking them, and you taper off them too quickly, the disease you took them for will likely flare up again, or your own adrenal gland production of cortisol will not have sufficient time to recover and you will end up with the problems of too little cortisol. This can be a life-threatening situation.

It is important, however, to still try to taper off steroids *when you can* because the long-term use of these drugs may cause Type II diabetes, osteoporosis, suppressed immune system problems, destruction of connective tissues, osteoarthritis and heart disease, to name just a few disorders.

Birth Control Pills

Women are not receiving the correct information about how dangerous birth control pills (BCPs) really are. Do not get me wrong; I do believe in a woman's right to birth control as long as she has made an informed decision. However, you can never achieve complete hormonal balance while taking BCPs because they disrupt the sex hormone system, and, because all hormones are connected, the body's entire hormone system is disrupted, too. Long-term use of BCPs can lead to many problems such as obesity, infertility, fibroid tumors, chronic fatigue, headaches, insomnia, high blood pressure, pulmonary embolisms, strokes, heart attacks and Type II diabetes.

You can stop using BCPs without supervision as long as you have healthy adrenal glands. But be aware that if you have been taking BCPs for a long time, you may experience numerous hormonal imbalance symptoms until your body starts producing the sex hormones again.

If you feel lousy after stopping BCPs, get your estradiol and progesterone levels checked. You may require short-term hormone replacement therapy (HRT) with real hormones until your body starts cycling on its own again. See the four rules for HRT in chapter 15.

If you have burned-out adrenal glands, you will have to improve your nutrition and lifestyle habits before coming off BCPs, or you may end up with any or all of the symptoms of low adrenaline and cortisol. (See chapters 4 and 6.)

Alternative birth control methods are safer and can be just as effective if used correctly. Discuss the different barrier-method options with your health-care practitioner.

Continuous Combined Therapy for Menopause

Continuous combined therapy is when you take any form of estrogen combined daily with a very high dose of any form of progestogen. This combination form of HRT increases adrenaline, cortisol and insulin levels and therefore increases your risk for the degenerative diseases of aging (see chapter 15 pages 400–402 for an in-depth discussion of the harm of taking continuous combined therapy). Discuss the option of cycling your hormones with your personal physician. If possible, get your doctor to put you on real estradiol and progesterone preparations as well. Be very careful when switching from continuous combined therapy to cycling therapy if you have been on this method for more than a few months. Since continuous combined therapy raises adrenaline and cortisol levels, it can be "addicting." You may have to taper off as you would any "addictive" drug, especially if you have burned-out adrenal glands.

Other Prescription Drugs

There are many prescription drugs too numerous to mention here that cause numerous side effects. If you are taking various prescription drugs, discuss with your physician the option of stopping or lowering the dose of any of your medications, or switching to another medicine with fewer side effects. Also, be aware that you may be taking a medicine because of another drug's side effects. Be sure you know the reasons why you are taking your specific drugs.

You have now learned about the first three steps of the SPII program. Healthy nutrition, stress management and tapering off/avoiding toxic chemicals are all-important steps to healing or maintaining your metabolism. However, your program would not be complete without a balanced exercise program. It is time to move on to Step Four and learn about setting up a cross-training exercise program.

Fourteen

Step Four: Cross-Training Exercise Program

A sensible cross-training exercise program helps you balance your hormones, maintain coordination, and strengthen bones and supporting tissues such as cartilage, ligaments and tendons. Exercise also improves your mental functioning and increases your sense of well-being. Therefore, it is important in keeping you strong, happy and healthy.

However, if you are not eating well or enough to rebuild your biochemicals, exercise does just the opposite. It causes you to have hormone imbalances, injuries and depression, and makes you feel lousy.

The Three Components of a Cross-Training Program

There are three types of activities you should include in any cross-training exercise program: flexibility/calming exercises, resistance/

adaptive training and cardiovascular/stimulating exercises.* In general, flexibility/calming exercises lower your adrenaline and cortisol levels, resistance/adaptive exercises raise your human growth hormone (HGH) levels, and cardiovascular/stimulating exercises raise your adrenaline and cortisol levels. All exercise initially lowers your insulin levels; however, if you only do cardiovascular/stimulating exercises, you will eventually raise your insulin levels. So a cross-training exercise program helps you keep your hormones balanced.

Flexibility/calming exercises focus on elongating the muscles and/or calming you down, and include yoga, stretching exercises, easy walking and Pilates.**

Resistance/adaptive exercises are those that involve working your muscles against a force. Each of the following are resistance/adaptive forms of exercise with the force they are working against in parentheses. Weight training (weights), swimming (water), yoga (floor), recumbent bicycling (the amount of resistance you choose), resistance bands (the bands) and Pilates (the reformer springs and pulleys). But you must keep your heart rate below 90 beats per minute for these to be pure resistance/adaptive exercises. If your heart rate remains higher than 90 beats per minute throughout the duration of your workout, you are doing both cardiovascular/stimulating and resistance/adaptive training at the same time. An exception is weight training or any other exercise where you are doing repetitions and sets. As long as you are getting your heart rate over 90 beats per minute for short amounts of time (fifteen to thirty seconds) and your heart rate recovers quickly (under 90 beats) in between sets, you are still doing resistance/adaptive exercises.

Cardiovascular/stimulating exercises are those that elevate and sustain your heart rate above 90 beats per minute, such as walking at a fast pace, running, playing soccer, volleyball or tennis, and dancing.

---

*For the exercise physiologists who are reading this book, I am modifying the terms flexibility, resistance and cardiovascular to flexibility/calming, resistance/adaptive and cardiovascular/stimulating for the purpose of explaining a workout program that will help balance the hormones of the body.

**Pilates is a full-body exercise program designed by Joseph Pilates in the 1930s that improves strength, flexibility, balance and muscular symmetry. It was orginally used by ballet dancers to keep them strong and has recently been introduced to the public by private gyms across the U.S.

Some exercise workouts are naturally a combination of two forms of exercise. For example, walking uphill quickly is both a cardiovascular/stimulating and a resistance/adaptive exercise; Pilates works on resistance/adaptive and flexibility/calming. A form of yoga called Ashtanga yoga involves both cardiovascular/stimulating and flexibility/calming training. If you do a form of exercise that is a combination of cardiovascular/stimulating and resistance/adaptive training, then consider it a cardiovascular/stimulating exercise. Any combination with flexibility/calming exercises included can be considered both.

The American Exercising Myth

As with everything else in the American culture, people think exercise is something that they should be doing fast and furiously. And most Americans believe that the more cardiovascular/stimulating exercise they do, the longer they will live, the better their heart will function and the more fat they will burn.

All of these beliefs are 180 degrees off the mark. The more cardiovascular exercise you do, the faster you will age and the more heart attacks you can expect. And the only type of weight loss you will "successfully" achieve is the loss of your functional and structural proteins and fats. Consider this fact: a Tibetan monk who does yoga and meditates lives longer than an American athlete who is involved in some type of running sport.

However, exercising in a moderate way is beneficial. See the following page for the benefits you can derive from following a good cross-training program.

Benefits of *Moderate* Exercise

- Exercise helps you retain your independence as you age. Starting in your twenties you can lose a pound of muscle each year if you do not exercise to maintain muscle tone and strength. You may become more dependent on those around you to help with daily chores such as opening jars or lifting empty boxes up to a higher shelf if you do not keep physically fit.
- Exercise helps you reduce the risk of the degenerative diseases of aging such as arthritis, cancers, coronary heart disease, dementia, depression, high blood pressure, osteoporosis, stroke and Type II diabetes.
- Exercise helps keep your body composition ideal: more lean body tissue and less stored fat around your midsection.
- Exercise helps with your coordination and balance. If your balance is better, you decrease the risk of falling. Therefore, exercise helps decrease the risk of bone fractures and other injuries.
- Exercise helps boost your energy and improves your sense of well-being.
- Exercise helps lower your blood pressure and improve heart function.
- Exercise lowers your cholesterol and blood-sugar levels.
- Exercise boosts your self-esteem. This sense of self-esteem is a by-product of being independent and obtaining realistic goals.
- Exercise improves your bowel movements and sleep patterns.
- Exercise usually decreases the cost of your medical care.
- Keep in mind that all these benefits will not occur if you are overexercising.

Exercising Smarter, Not Harder

A popular saying about exercise in the 1980s was "No pain, no gain." The popular belief was and still is that if you just exercised long and hard enough, your health and body composition would improve. The irony, of course, is that overexercising damages your metabolism.

Instead of working out to the point of physical exhaustion or pain, be smart about your exercising—do the right types of exercises for your current metabolism type and be aware that you do not have to exercise several hours each day to achieve your goals.

In general you should not be exercising more than five days a week. Golf and short walks should not be considered part of your exercise routine; therefore, you can do them on the two days when you are not doing your program. You can also stretch daily without worrying about overexercising.

The Dangers of Overexercising

Do you think you have not exercised if you do not sweat? If you do, you may be overexercising, and that is a problem. You are also overexercising anytime you exercise but do not eat enough food to match your current metabolism and activity level, or if you do too much cardiovascular/stimulating exercise when you have burned-out adrenal glands.

Some signs of overexercising are pain in your joints; painful, sore muscles to the touch for several days afterwards; a few days or more of swelling, stiffness and/or loss of range of motion; or any obvious injury. If you are only doing cardiovascular/stimulating exercises daily—even if you do not have any of the above signs—you are still overexercising.

Overexercising leads to the hormonal imbalances that direct your body to use up its functional and structural biochemicals more than rebuild them. You may feel that you are doing what is best for you, but in reality, you are aging faster.

Here's why.

When you overexercise, you raise adrenaline and cortisol levels. If adrenaline is higher than cortisol, you will use up fat, protein and sugar biochemicals. If cortisol is higher than adrenaline, you may use up protein and sugar biochemicals, but store more fat around your midsection because cortisol causes a redistribution of fat from your arms and legs to your middle. Either way, you are destroying your metabolism.

In addition, overexercising can lead to insulin resistance. Your insulin levels rise too high when you overexercise in order to keep you from completely using up your structural and functional biochemicals and also to help you rebuild them again.

Finally, overexercising leads to injuries. Your soft tissues are made up of protein, and overexercising causes protein wasting, which leads to tissue breakdown.

Any way you look at it, overexercising leads to the degenerative diseases of aging.

Profile of an *Over*exerciser

Do you recognize yourself in any of the following scenarios? If so, you are overexercising.

- **The Weekend Warrior** Overexercising once a week causes a buildup of lactic acid in your muscles. This causes stiffness, pain and swelling that may keep you from exercising throughout the week. This also leads to an increased risk of injuries.
- **The Marathoner** Continuous daily overtraining leads to protein wasting. Some signs and symptoms of this are decreased memory and concentration, sleep disturbances, depression and/or emotional mood swings, frequent injuries and bone loss. Exercising in this manner is a good way to burn out your adrenal glands and end up with a lowered metabolism.
- **The Enthusiastic Beginner** Overexercising at the beginning of a new workout program may lead to fatigue, stiffness and pain. These in turn may keep you from following through with your good intentions.
- **The Dieter** Exercising as a way to lose body fat quickly will lead to the loss of structural and functional proteins and fats, too. You will end up destroying your metabolism this way— and getting very frustrated with exercising.

Profile of an *Under*exerciser

Underexercising is also a problem. Do you recognize yourself in any of the following scenarios? If so, you are underexercising.

- **The Couch Potato** You come home and sit on the couch after a long hard day at work. You drink alcohol to relax you while you are watching TV. You may grab a few chips and wait for dinner to be delivered.

Profile of an *Under*exerciser (cont'd)

- **The Procrastinator** You think about what a good idea it would be to get into a routine exercise program. But every time that thought enters your mind, you come up with a million and one reasons why it cannot happen today. There is always tomorrow.
- **The Good-Intention Exerciser** You make a real effort to join a gym, and you think daily about what exercise you will do when you get home that night. But when you get home you are tired, and you decide to start your program tomorrow.
- **The Intermittent Exerciser** You follow a good exercise program for a few weeks at a time, but then you get busy with work, kids and/or travel, and you quit. You end up starting all over again in a few weeks.

Helpful Exercise Tips

In order to have a good workout, follow these helpful tips:

- Get plenty of sleep every night. Do not exercise if you are sleep-deprived. This will only lead to more injuries because adrenaline and cortisol levels are higher if you have not slept well.
- Drink plenty of water to keep hydrated. When you are dehydrated, your heart has to pump harder to get blood to carry oxygen to your tissues. This means your body needs more adrenaline and cortisol, and exercising with higher adrenaline and cortisol levels for a sustained period of time causes your body to use up its biochemicals faster.
- Do light stretching for five minutes before you start exercising; stretch for at least ten minutes at the end of your exercise routine.
- Remember to breathe. Your breathing should be regular and deep—from the abdominal area. You should breathe out during the strenuous part of your exercise—such as lifting a weight or hitting a tennis ball—and breathe in during the recovery phase. Breathing properly helps keep oxygen flowing to the cells. It also helps decrease muscle tension and tightness, which improves performance without increasing strain.
- Eat well. Do not lower your caloric intake, eliminate food groups or skip meals. The purpose of eating and exercising is to regenerate. If you exercise and do not eat, your body will use up its biochemicals more than it rebuilds them.
- The best time to exercise is first thing in the morning because it will make you feel good the rest of the day. Also, studies show that exercising first thing in the morning increases the chance that you will be consistent with exercise over the years. It is too easy to come up with an excuse not to exercise at the end of a long day. However, do not change your exercise routine or think that exercising later is bad for you if you already exercise at night.

> ## Helpful Exercise Tips (cont'd)
>
> - Vary your exercise routine to keep it interesting. For example, you may want to vary your cardiovascular exercises by playing a sport, taking a dance class or riding a bike instead of always doing the same activity.
> - Keep your workout schedule the same. This will ensure that you build time into your day to exercise and guarantees a higher rate of consistency.
> - Work out with friends or a personal trainer if you have a hard time keeping to a schedule. Accountability really helps consistency.
> - Make sure you have the proper shoes and equipment for the activity you have chosen.
> - Be consistent and have fun! Just do it.

Eating and Exercising

It is very important to match your energy input with your energy output. Any amount of exercise is too much if you are not eating well. If you do not eat enough food, your adrenaline/cortisol levels will be higher. Be careful not to fall into the trap of feeling good when you are using up your biochemicals because of adrenaline and cortisol. You will feel good initially and even feel stronger because of your higher adrenaline/cortisol levels. Eventually, however, you will burn out.

Getting Medical Clearance

If you are insulin-resistant, have burned-out adrenal glands, are malnourished, have multiple health issues, or are out of shape and over the age of fifty, consult your physician for clearance to exercise. If you have multiple health problems, consider starting your program at an exercise rehabilitation center. Your physician can advise you about facilities in your area.

Training Program: Insulin-Sensitive with Healthy Adrenal Glands

If you are insulin-sensitive with healthy adrenal glands, a realistic and sufficient cross-training program should consist of the following:

- flexibility/calming exercises: 15 to 30 minutes, five to seven days a week
- resistance/adaptive training: 45- to 60-minute sessions, three times a week
- cardiovascular/stimulating exercises: 30- to 60-minute sessions, at least two times a week at 75 to 85 percent maximum heart rate*

The ratio of exercise types done should be resistance(adaptive)/flexibility(calming)/cardiovascular(stimulating) at two-to-one-to-one—especially if you are over the age of forty. Since there is a natural decline in human growth hormone as you age, you need to do more resistance/adaptive than cardiovascular/stimulating exercises as you get older.

Alternate between cardiovascular/stimulating and resistance/adaptive exercises every other day, but do not exercise seven days a week.

Flexibility/calming exercises should be done along with your cardiovascular/stimulating and resistance/adaptive program.

If you do not have time for a full cross-training program, the most important exercise components to incorporate first are flexibility/calming and resistance/adaptive training exercises.

---

*To estimate your maximum heart rate, subtract your age from 220. Next, to calculate your target heart rate range, multiply the result by 0.75 first and then by 0.85. For example, a 40-year-old would have a target heart rate of 220 − 40 or 180. Seventy-five percent of his/her maximum heart rate is 135; 85 percent is 153. Target heart rate is therefore 135 to 153.

Training Program: Insulin-Resistant with Healthy Adrenal Glands

If you are insulin-resistant with healthy adrenal glands, you first need to be cleared by your physician before beginning or continuing your exercise program.

After clearance, you should first do mostly flexibility/calming and resistance/adaptive training exercises. Too much cardiovascular/stimulating exercise raises adrenaline and cortisol levels and causes more insulin resistance.

Your initial cross-training goal should be as follows:

- flexibility/calming exercises: 15 to 30 minutes, five to seven days a week

- resistance/adaptive training: 45- to 60-minute sessions, three times a week

- cardiovascular/stimulating exercises: 15-minute sessions, two to three times a week at 70 to 80 percent maximum heart rate.*

Alternate between cardiovascular/stimulating and resistance/adaptive exercises every other day but do not exercise seven days a week.

As you get into better shape, you may increase your cardiovascular/stimulating exercise time to 20 to 25 minutes two to three times a week. While you are healing your metabolism, it is better to spread out your cardiovascular/stimulating workout to three times a week. However, when you have healed your metabolism, you will be able to increase the amount of cardiovascular/stimulating exercises that you do to 30- to 60-minute sessions on two separate days.

---

*To estimate your maximum heart rate, subtract your age from 220. Next, to calculate your target heart rate range, multiply the result first by 0.70 and then by 0.80. For example, the maximum heart rate for a 40-year-old is 220 – 40 or 180. Seventy percent of his/her maximum heart rate is 126; 80 percent is 144. Target heart rate is therefore 126 to 144.

Training Program: Insulin-Sensitive with Burned-Out Adrenal Glands

If you are insulin-sensitive with burned-out adrenal glands, you first need to be cleared by your physician before beginning or continuing your exercise program.

After clearance, you should do mostly flexibility/calming and resistance/adaptive exercises. Too much cardiovascular/stimulating exercise raises adrenaline and cortisol levels, and your adrenal glands will burn out more.

If you are extremely exhausted and do not exercise, do not start an exercise program at this time. If you are extremely exhausted *and* are exercising, stop your exercise program at this time. After you have been eating well and resting for a minimum of one month, you may resume exercising again.

Start slowly with resistance/adaptive and flexibility/calming exercises first. Your initial cross-training goal should be to build up to the following levels of exercise:

- flexibility/calming exercises: 15 to 30 minutes, five to seven days a week

- resistance/adaptive training: 30- to 60-minute sessions, three times a week

Note: If you do not feel well enough to start or continue the above exercise program, try to incorporate 5 minutes of stretching in the morning and in the evening, and add in 5 minutes of walking twice a day. This is a small but important start to get you ready to do resistance/adaptive exercises again.

When you have partly healed your adrenal glands, add cardiovascular/stimulating exercises to your program. Start with 5- to 10-minute sessions, two to three times a week at 65 to 75 percent maximum heart rate,* on the days when you are not doing resistance/adaptive training. Slowly build yourself up to 20- to 25-minute sessions, two to three times a week. (**Note:** You will know when your adrenal glands are "partly healed" because you will begin to feel better and doing 5 to 10 minutes of exercise will make you feel better and not worse.)

While you are healing your metabolism, it is better to spread out your cardiovascular/stimulating workout to three times a week. However, when you have completely healed, you may do 30 to 60 minutes of cardiovascular/stimulating exercises two times a week.

Alternate between cardiovascular/stimulating and resistance/ adaptive exercises every other day, but do not exercise seven days a week.

Training Program: Insulin-Resistant with Burned-Out Adrenal Glands

If you are insulin-resistant with burned-out adrenal glands, you first need to be cleared by your physician before beginning or continuing your exercise program.

After clearance, you should do mostly resistance/adaptive and flexibility/calming exercises. Too much cardiovascular/stimulating exercise raises adrenaline and cortisol levels. This causes more insulin resistance and further burns out your adrenal glands.

If you are extremely exhausted and do not exercise, do not start an exercise program at this time. If you are extremely exhausted *and* are exercising, stop your exercise program at this time. After you have been eating well and resting for a minimum of one month, you may resume exercising again.

Start slowly with resistance/adaptive and flexibility/calming

---

*To estimate your maximum heart rate, subtract your age from 220. Next, to calculate your target heart rate range, multiply the result by 0.65 first and then by 0.75. For example, the maximum heart rate for a 40-year-old is 220 – 40 or 180. Sixty-five percent of his/her maximum heart rate is 117; 75 percent is 135. Target heart rate is therefore 117 to 135.

exercises first. Your initial cross-training goal should be to build up to the following levels of exercise:

- flexibility/calming exercises: 15 to 30 minutes, five to seven days a week

- resistance/adaptive training: 30- to 60-minute sessions, three times a week

Note: If you do not feel well enough to start or continue the above exercise program, try to incorporate 5 minutes of stretching in the morning and in the evening, and add in 5 minutes of walking twice a day. This is a small but important start to get you ready to do resistance/adaptive exercises again.

When you have partly healed your adrenal glands, add cardiovascular/stimulating exercises to your program. Start with 5- to 10-minute sessions, two to three times a week at 60 to 70 percent maximum heart rate,* on the days when you are not doing resistance/adaptive training. Slowly build yourself up to 20- to 25-minute sessions, two to three times a week. (**Note:** You will know when your adrenal glands are "partly healed" because you will begin to feel better and doing 5 to 10 minutes of exercise will make you feel better and not worse.)

While you are healing your metabolism, it is better to spread out your cardiovascular/stimulating workout to three times a week. However, when you have completely healed, you may do 30 to 60 minutes of cardiovascular/stimulating exercises two times a week.

Alternate between cardiovascular/stimulating and resistance/adaptive exercises every other day, but do not exercise seven days a week.

---

*To estimate your maximum heart rate, subtract your age from 220. Next, to calculate your target heart rate range, multiply the result by 0.60 first and then by 0.70. For example, the maximum heart rate for a 40-year-old is 220 – 40 or 180. Sixty percent of his/her maximum heart rate is 108; 70 percent is 126. Target heart rate is therefore 108 to 126.

Walking-for-Resistance Exercise

In general, walking quickly is cardiovascular/stimulating and walking slowly is good for your soul. However, you can use walking as a resistance/adaptive form of exercise if you walk slowly, go up and down hills, keep your heart rate below 90 beats per minute and walk at least five miles at a time.

If you are insulin-sensitive or insulin-resistant, you may use the walking-for-resistance exercise.

If you have burned-out adrenal glands, walking for five miles at a stretch is too much. You can use walking as exercise for your soul by walking slowly and limiting your walk to 15 to 30 minutes. Or you can start with a 15-minute walk and build up slowly over time to a five-mile walk.

In summary, there are many benefits to a cross-training exercise program. That is why it is a must in the SPII program.

The first four steps of the SPII program help you balance your hormones, heal your metabolism and achieve optimal health. However, if your body can no longer make a hormone in sufficient quantities, you will never be in total balance unless you replace the missing hormone (or hormones) through hormone replacement therapy (HRT). Step Five is all about HRT.

Fifteen

Step Five: Hormone Replacement Therapy

ecause the systems of the human body are interconnected and
because one imbalance creates another imbalance, if one hormone is missing, all your hormones are out of balance. If the
missing hormone is a minor hormone, you may not feel the loss of
this hormone. Therefore, you may not feel that it is important to
replace it. But as stated throughout this book, all hormones play a role
in the quality and quantity of your life.

Balancing All Your Hormones

The purpose of the first four steps of the SPII program is to balance
your body's hormones through improving your nutrition and lifestyle
habits. When you improve nutrition and lifestyle habits, your hormone levels that are too high will be brought down to normal levels,
and your hormone levels that are too low will be brought up to

normal levels. Therefore, the first four steps of the SPII program will be all you need to do to balance all your hormones unless one of your hormone systems is not functioning. For example, you can eat well, manage your stress better, taper off toxic chemicals and do a moderate cross-training exercise program and still be out of balance if your body can no longer produce a hormone. This is when you need hormone replacement therapy (HRT).

If a hormone needs to be replaced, it is important to replace it with the same hormone and to try to replace it in the identical way that your body used to make and secrete it. This can be accomplished by mimicking normal physiology as much as possible.

The Four Rules of Hormone Replacement Therapy

Here are four rules for HRT that I strongly believe should be followed to balance not only the missing hormone(s), but also *all* your hormone systems.

Rule One: You Must Qualify for Hormone Replacement Therapy

The first rule of HRT is that you must qualify for it. You never want to replace a hormone that is not low or missing. Too much of a hormone is no better than too little. Balance is always the key. First, identify the hormone system or systems that have failed by having lab work done. Once the loss of a hormone has been identified, it is time for rule 2.

Rule Two: Replace a Missing Hormone with a Bioidentical Hormone

The second rule of HRT is to replace the missing hormone(s) with a bioidentical hormone(s). Bioidentical hormones are the same in chemical structure as the hormones your body makes whether they are found in nature or made in a lab (synthetic). Everything else is a drug to your body. Do not substitute one hormone for another, and do not take drug hormones instead of bioidentical ones. This rule may seem straightforward and filled with common sense, but it is broken every day. An example is when Premarin, a drug estrogen made from pregnant mare's urine, is prescribed instead of an estradiol preparation (estradiol is the human estrogen made in the ovaries).

Do not confuse hormones found in nature with natural hormones. The term "natural hormones" includes synthetic hormones as long as the synthetic hormone is bioidentical in structure to the one your body used to make. For example, the T4 and T3 preparations used in the treatment of hypothyroidism are mostly made in a laboratory, but they are bioidentical in structure to the T4 and T3 found in the human body and therefore are natural hormones. Hence, switching the terminology to "bioidentical" is less confusing than the word "natural." Once you have been given a prescription for a bioidentical hormone, it is time to move on to rule 3, the hardest component of HRT to accomplish—but one that is achievable.

Rule Three: Match the Replaced Hormone's Normal Production and Secretion

The third rule of HRT is to match the normal production and secretion of the hormone that needs to be replaced. This is difficult, and often inconvenient, to do. For example, a person who has Type I diabetes needs to take insulin shots. To exactly mimic the way the pancreas makes and secretes insulin is impossible because there are too many variables, so we try to match insulin dosing to food intake only. This is good enough—but not perfect—and requires the person with diabetes to take multiple shots of differing amounts of insulin throughout the day. This is what I mean by mimicking normal physiology. It would be more convenient for this person to take one big shot of insulin a day. However, this will not work because the body does not secrete insulin in one big dose every day. The body secretes different amounts of insulin all day long at different times of the day.

Following are discussions of some popularly prescribed drugs that do *not* mimic normal physiology.

Prepackaged T4 and T3

An example of a drug that does not mimic normal physiology is the prepackaged T4 and T3 preparations such as Armour thyroid. Although these preparations contain the bioidentical thyroid hormones, they are not good for you because they do not contain the right ratio of these two hormones for most individuals. Taking these types of preparations does not mimic normal physiology. If you need both T4 and T3, it is important to take them as separate pills and adjust the levels of each individual hormone as needed.

Progesterone for Premenstrual Syndrome

Another example of HRT taken incorrectly is the use of progesterone for premenstrual syndrome (PMS). Many over-the-counter progesterone creams come with instructions for using them three out of four weeks of the month. This practice goes against the body's natural production of this hormone. In the normal menstrual cycle, progesterone is secreted in very low amounts during the first part of the cycle, followed by higher amounts at the end. If you need to replace progesterone because you no longer make this hormone in sufficient amounts during the second half of your menstrual cycle, you should use progesterone only during the last fourteen days of your cycle. Do not use progesterone during the first half of the menstrual cycle because this does not mimic normal physiology and causes a hormone imbalance.

Combined Estrogen/Progestin for Menopause

The final example of HRT taken incorrectly is the use of small doses of an estrogen (synthetic or bioidentical) taken together daily with a large dose of a progestogen/progestin (synthetic or bioidentical). This is known as continuous combined therapy. The purpose of combined therapy was to give a woman the advantage of HRT after menopause without the messy withdrawal period. Women were actually told they had a choice! Take HRT and have monthly uterine bleeding or take HRT and have no uterine bleeding. Who wouldn't want the benefits of HRT after menopause without a menstrual flow?

As appealing as this sounds, this type of therapy actually is very harmful because taking hormones this way does not mimic the way your body used to make them. In fact, instead of decreasing the risks of certain diseases that are known to be helped by estradiol, taking HRT the wrong way increases the risks for them. For example, women who take combined therapy are at risk for more not fewer heart attacks, strokes and breast cancer. The only way to mimic the normal menstrual cycle is to take HRT and have monthly withdrawal bleeding. Taking combined therapy mimics your body's hormone balance during pregnancy (higher levels of progesterone than estradiol on a continuous basis). Postmenopausal women should not be mimicking pregnancy since the risks associated with pregnancy, such as heart attacks, strokes, Type II diabetes and breast cancer, increase exponentially as a woman ages.

In terms of hormones, combined therapy causes high adrenaline, cortisol and insulin levels. The longer a woman takes HRT this way, the greater her chance of either causing adrenal gland burnout, burning out her adrenal glands further, becoming insulin-resistant or making preexisting insulin resistance worse. If a woman's adrenal glands burn out, she increases her risk for depression, allergies and headaches. If she becomes insulin-resistant, she will increase her risk for breast cancer, blood clots, stroke and heart attacks.

Combined Therapy Is Bad Medicine

The science that supports that taking combined HRT is harmful has been around for a long time. The study* that supports the science was published in July 2002. Even with this news, many medical practitioners are still not warning their patients of the risks of taking HRT this way. Some are even downplaying the results. What is it going to take to get everyone to understand that taking HRT incorrectly is harmful? For those who think that this study, which was done on PremPro, applies to synthetic HRT only, you are wrong. Bioidentical hormones given in a continuous combined way (daily low doses of estradiol, daily high doses of progesterone) will also cause the same increased risk because they will still cause adrenaline, cortisol and insulin to rise higher than normal. The real choice for women now is to take HRT correctly, by mimicking the menstrual cycle with bioidentical hormones, or not to take HRT at all.

Once you are taking your bioidentical hormone(s) in such a way as to mimic normal physiology, you are ready for rule 4.

Rule Four: Take Hormone Replacement Therapy Seriously

The fourth rule of HRT is that it needs to be taken seriously. HRT needs to be tracked with lab tests and physician follow-up visits. This may seem obvious if you have Type I diabetes or thyroid disease, but this rule is usually ignored in menopause.

It is important to follow every parameter available for each hormone deficiency state. With diabetes, this involves the patient doing home blood-glucose monitoring and then having more intensive lab work and physician follow-up visits on a regular basis. Menopausal women need to have their estradiol and progesterone levels measured by a good lab and reviewed by their physician. They should also track their withdrawal periods and keep up with breast self-exams, Pap

---

*Women Health Initiative Investigators. "Risks and Benefits of Estrogen Plus Progestin in Healthy Postmenopausal Women." Journal of the American Medical Association. 288. (July 14, 2002): 321–333.

smears, bone mineral density studies and uterine ultrasound evalua-
tions, if indicated.

In summary, since the hormones of the body are interconnected
and one hormone imbalance leads to all hormones being imbalanced,
it is very important to replace a hormone if it is low or missing and
cannot be made by your body.

You have now learned about the five basic steps of the SPII program. It is time to individualize the program to fit your current
metabolism type. Chapter 16 introduces the personal programs for
the four different metabolic types.

Sixteen

The SPII Personal Programs for Your Current Metabolism

I n the next four chapters you will learn about your personal SPII program for your current metabolism type and what you need to do to heal a badly damaged metabolism or maintain a healthy one.

Your Personal Health Goal

Your goal is to improve your nutrition and lifestyle habits so that you can become insulin-sensitive and have healthy adrenal glands again—this is the best current metabolism to have and the one you were born with. However, if you are already insulin-sensitive with healthy adrenal glands, you still can improve your nutrition and lifestyle choices to balance your hormones and ensure you stay healthy.

Although everyone should end up following the "insulin-sensitive with healthy adrenal glands program," you cannot start with this program if you have a badly damaged metabolism. You first need to go through your transition in order to heal your metabolism. You need to know your current metabolism type* to begin your healing process, and you need to remember that these types are acquired and not genetic. By going through your transition, you can acquire the best metabolism no matter how damaged your current metabolism is. Success is only a matter of time.

The four different current metabolism types all have slight modifications to the basic SPII program, which includes:

- Healthy nutrition, including supplementation with vitamins, antioxidants, minerals, and amino and fatty acids, if needed

- Stress management, including getting enough sleep

- Tapering off or avoiding toxic chemicals

- Cross-training exercises

- Hormone replacement therapy (HRT), if needed

To ensure a successful transition you need to follow the recommendations for your current metabolism type and then switch to the correct SPII program as your metabolism heals. Your individual program (which you will read about later in the book) will indicate when you should change over to a program for a different current metabolism type.

General Program Guidelines

Insulin-Sensitive with Healthy Adrenal Glands

If you are insulin-sensitive with healthy adrenal glands, you can incorporate all five steps of the program into your life at the same time.

If you do not know your type, you may begin your transition by following the insulin-sensitive with burned-out adrenal gland program until you get tested.

Follow the recommended meal plans, manage your stress, stop all toxic chemicals, begin or continue a moderate cross-training exercise program and start HRT, if needed.

Insulin-Resistant with Healthy Adrenal Glands

If you are insulin-resistant and have healthy adrenal glands, you can incorporate all five steps of the program into your life at the same time—with modifications.

Follow the recommended meal plans, manage your stress and/or address stress management techniques, stop all toxic chemicals, begin or continue a slightly modified cross-training exercise program and start HRT, if needed.

Insulin-Sensitive with Burned-Out Adrenal Glands

If you are insulin-sensitive with burned-out adrenal glands, you have to incorporate the five steps of the program into your life more slowly. This will minimize the symptoms of your healing phase. You also may need to self-medicate to get through your transition.

Follow the recommended meal plans and start managing your stress and/or implementing stress management techniques immediately. Do not stop ingesting all toxic chemicals at this time.

If your adrenal glands are very worn out, you may have to stop cardiovascular/stimulating exercises and focus only on resistance/adaptive training and flexibility/calming exercises. Or you may have to stop exercising all together in order to give your adrenal glands time to rest and heal.

If you need HRT, work with a medical professional who is well-versed in using HRT with patients who have burned-out adrenal glands.

Insulin-Resistant with Burned-Out Adrenal Glands

If you are insulin-resistant with burned-out adrenal glands, you have to incorporate the five steps of the program into your life more slowly. This will minimize the symptoms of your healing phase. You also may need to self-medicate to get through your transition.

Follow the recommended meal plans and start managing your stress and/or implementing stress management techniques immediately. Do not stop ingesting all toxic chemicals at this time, but taper off nicotine, alcohol and refined sugar as soon as possible.

If your adrenal glands are very burned out, you may have to stop cardiovascular/stimulating exercises and focus only on resistance/adaptive training and flexibility/calming exercises. Or you may have to stop exercising in order to give your adrenal glands time to rest and heal. If you need HRT, work with a medical professional who is well-versed in using HRT with patients who have burned-out adrenal glands.

It is now time for you to refer to the current metabolism type program that is right for you. To avoid confusion, *only read* about the program that pertains to your current metabolism type.

- For the insulin-sensitive with healthy adrenal glands program, go to chapter 17.

- For the insulin-resistant with healthy adrenal glands program, go to chapter 18.

- For the insulin-sensitive with burned-out adrenal glands program, go to chapter 19.

- For the insulin-resistant with burned-out adrenal glands program, go to chapter 20.

Seventeen

Personal Program: Insulin-Sensitive with Healthy Adrenal Glands

If you are insulin-sensitive with healthy adrenal glands, your transition will happen quickly. You have not damaged your metabolism; therefore, it will respond immediately to your improved nutrition and lifestyle habits. You just need to be consistent. By following the recommended meal plans and the other steps of the SPII program, your hormones should become balanced very quickly, and you can achieve your ideal body composition easily.

Step One: Healthy Nutrition, Including Supplementation with Vitamins, Antioxidants, Minerals, and Amino and Fatty Acids

Why It Is Best to Eat Smaller Meals More Frequently

It is always better to eat smaller meals more frequently because eating too much food at any given moment raises insulin levels too high; eating too little food raises adrenaline and cortisol levels too high.

Initial Meal and Carbohydrate Guidelines

You need to eat a minimum of 30 to 35 grams of carbohydrates with each meal and ideally two 15-gram carbohydrate snacks. If you are not a person who likes to eat snacks, you can eat 40 to 45 grams of carbohydrates three times a day. For food suggestions, refer to the meal plans on pages 302–307 and see snacks on pages 308–311 in chapter 11.

Why You May Need Fewer or More Carbohydrates Per Meal

Because you are insulin-sensitive, you will have high-insulin levels if you eat more carbohydrates than needed for your activity level. Because your adrenal glands are healthy, you should not eat *less* than 30 grams of carbohydrates three times a day or your adrenaline/ cortisol levels will get too high and you will increase the risk of burning out your adrenal glands.

Note: You must eat more carbohydrates if you are more active, but make sure you are also eating enough protein, healthy fats and non-starchy vegetables.

The Best Carbohydrate Choices, Including Fruit

Eat more whole grains, legumes, fruits and starchy vegetables as your carbohydrate choices. I highly recommend that you do not eat white flour or processed refined foods because they are non-nutritious.

Count your fruit intake as a carbohydrate unless it is a low GI fruit, and you are eating less than or equal to 45 grams or three servings a day. However, do not eat fruit as your only carbohydrate.

Protein Requirements

You do not have to monitor your protein consumption—just listen to your body. Your feedback mechanisms are working because you have healthy adrenal glands. As long as you are following the carbohydrate guidelines and eating enough of the healthy fats and non-starchy vegetables, your body will let you know when you have had enough. If you like guidelines, however, follow this regimen:

- Eat at *least* two to three ounces of protein with each meal and one to three ounces per snack if you eat five times a day.

- Eat at *least* two to four ounces of protein with each meal and snack if you eat four times a day.

- Eat at *least* three to five ounces of protein with each meal if you eat only three times a day.

These are your estimated *minimum* daily requirements. Refer to the protein portions guidelines in chapter 11 for more information on how to calculate your minimum daily protein requirement range.

Supplements

Your minimal vitamin regimen should include a pharmaceutical-grade multivitamin and mineral, extra calcium and magnesium and a stress B-complex vitamin. You will also need to add in an omega-3 supplement if you do not eat enough foods high in omega-3 fatty acids, such as fish, walnuts, cooked soybeans or ground flaxseeds. See chapter 11 for more on omega-3 foods, (page 251) as well as general information on nutrition and supplements (pages 314–319).

Step Two: Stress Management, Including Getting Enough Sleep

When to Begin Stress Management Techniques

You do not have to begin stress management techniques immediately. However, because stress causes an imbalance in your major hormones, I highly recommended that you begin as soon as possible to learn how to manage stress better—and thus achieve balance in your life.

Getting Enough Sleep

If you are not getting at least seven to eight hours of uninterrupted sleep every night, you are not sleeping enough. See chapter 12 for more on stress management and how to ensure you get enough sleep.

Step Three: Tapering Off Toxic Chemicals or Avoiding Them Completely

What to Eliminate First

You can eliminate all refined sugars, nicotine, caffeine, alcohol and any other stimulant you use at this time because you will not need to self-medicate. *This does not include your prescription medications.* Do *not* eliminate your prescription drugs without discussing it with your physician first.

If you find eliminating these toxic chemicals extremely difficult to do or your cravings for carbohydrates and/or sweets increases when off of them, you have incorrectly categorized yourself as having healthy adrenal glands. You are, in fact, insulin-sensitive with burned-out adrenal glands. Refer to your new program in chapter 19.

Note: Ingesting a small amount of sugar, caffeine and/or alcohol will not destroy your health, but it is best to stay away from all toxic chemicals because they cause your body to use up its biochemicals. Anything that causes your body to use itself up also accelerates your aging process. However, if you enjoy a cup of green tea daily or an occasional glass of wine or homemade dessert, you will not destroy your health if the other aspects of your life are under control—that is, if you are eating real and healthy foods, managing your stress well, sleeping enough, following a moderate cross-training exercise program and taking HRT, if you need to.

See chapter 13 for more information on toxic chemicals.

Step Four: Cross-Training Exercise Program

When to Start a Cross-Training Program

You can continue or begin cross-training exercises. Your minimum goal is to work up to the following exercise regimen:

- Flexibility/calming exercises: 15 to 30 minutes, five to seven days a week

- Resistance/adaptive training: 45- to 60-minute sessions, three times a week

- Cardiovascular/stimulating exercises: 30- to 60-minute sessions, two times a week at 75 to 85 percent of your maximum heart rate* (alternate days with resistance/adaptive training)

To estimate your maximum heart rate, subtract your age from 220.

Always try to keep the ratio of resistance/adaptive training to cardiovascular/stimulating exercises between one-to-one or two-to-one.

Make Sure That You Are Not Overexercising

Your adrenaline/cortisol levels rise and your body uses up its biochemicals when you overexercise. Since it feels good when this happens, it is easy to overexercise. Be aware, however, that too much exercise will destroy your metabolism. See chapter 14 for more information on exercise.

Step Five: Hormone Replacement Therapy, If Needed

When to Take HRT

You should take HRT if you need it. Since all hormones communicate with each other, it is important to make sure that all your hormones are present—this will ensure your metabolism has a chance to stay healthy. Work with a medical professional who understands how all hormones interact with one another. See chapter 15 for more information on hormone replacement therapy.

Summary: Insulin-Sensitive with Healthy Adrenal Glands

General

- You can follow all five steps of the SPII program at the same time.

Transition Time

- Your transition will not last very long.

Step One

- Minimum carbohydrate requirement: 30 to 35 grams with each meal and two 15-gram carbohydrate snacks. Count your fruit as carbohydrates.
- Need to measure protein portions: No.
- Need for low-salt diet: No.
- Need for low-saturated fat diet: No, unless you cannot exercise consistently.
- Minimum supplements requirement: Pharmaceutical-grade multivitamin and mineral, extra calcium and magnesium, and a stress B-complex vitamin.

Step Two

- Stress: Manage stress better.
- Sleep: Strive for seven to eight hours of uninterrupted sleep.

Step Three

- It is ideal and easy to stop all toxic chemicals immediately. This does not include prescription medications.

- Sugar, alcohol and caffeine in small amounts will not break your program.

Step Four

- Cross-training exercise program: Continue or begin.
- Minimum amount of exercise: flexibility/calming—work up to 15 to 30 minutes daily; resistance/adaptive—work up to 45- to 60-minute sessions three times a week; cardiovascular/stimulating—work up to 30-minute to 60-minute sessions on two different days a week.
- Avoid overexercising—it destroys your metabolism.

Step Five

- Take HRT if needed.
- If you end up with a glandular-based endocrine disorder that is left untreated or treated inappropriately, you can become insulin-resistant and/or burn out your adrenal glands.
- Work with a medical professional who understands how all hormones interact with one another.

Eighteen

Personal Program: Insulin-Resistant with Healthy Adrenal Glands

If you are insulin-resistant with healthy adrenal glands, it will take time to heal your metabolism. But do not get discouraged. By following the recommended meal plans and the other steps of the SPII program, you can become insulin-sensitive again. It will probably take you a few years to complete your transition, but you should be able to begin losing fat weight slowly. You should also feel better throughout the process and notice improvements in your health along the way.

You probably became insulin-resistant from years of yo-yo dieting and eating high-carbohydrate, low-fat foods.

There are other paths besides yo-yo dieting that can lead to insulin resistance, but they all include eating too many carbohydrates for your personal metabolism and activity level. You may have become insulin-resistant through a combination of poor nutrition and overworking, excessive exercise, and use of stimulants and/or alcohol. Or you may have consumed too many carbohydrates in conjunction with a glandular-based endocrine disease such as Grave's that was not diagnosed or treated in a timely matter. Or you may be in menopause and have been treated with combined therapy for too many years. (Refer to chapter 15.) If you have burned out your adrenals from one of these paths, you need to heal from your previous habits or take hormone replacement therapy correctly.

It is never too late to improve your nutrition and lifestyle habits. By doing this, you will balance your hormones, thereby healing your metabolism and achieving your ideal body composition.

Note: You need to heal your metabolism to become healthy and to lose fat weight, *not* lose weight to become healthy.

Step One: Healthy Nutrition, Including Supplementation with Vitamins, Antioxidants, Minerals, and Amino and Fatty Acids

Why You Should Eat Smaller Meals More Frequently

It is important that you eat enough healthy food to heal your metabolism again. The best way to get enough food into your body without causing further hormone imbalances is to eat smaller meals more frequently. It is always better to eat this way because eating too much food at any given moment raises insulin levels too high; eating too little food raises adrenaline and cortisol levels too high. If you eat too much, you will stay insulin-resistant. If you eat too little, you will cause your adrenal glands to burn out. Here's why.

Because you are insulin-resistant, you will keep your insulin levels too high if you eat too much food or carbohydrates at any given moment. If you do not eat enough food or carbohydrates during a meal or throughout the day, you will not be able to heal your metabolism. If you skip meals, your adrenaline and cortisol levels rise and your insulin level falls. However, this is a very short-term response. As soon as you eat the next meal, your insulin levels rise even higher. Your body secretes more insulin to overcome your higher adrenaline/cortisol levels and match your incoming food. Skipping meals keeps your hormones out of balance. The only way to rebuild your functional and structural biochemicals (made from proteins and fats) and become insulin-sensitive again is by eating enough of the right types of healthy foods.

Because your adrenal glands are healthy, your adrenaline and cortisol levels will rise and you may initially feel better if you do not eat enough carbohydrates or food per meal. This feeling of well-being may be accompanied by signs of improvement in your health such as decreased triglyceride and blood-sugar levels, lowered blood pressure, and fat-weight loss.

Do not be fooled, however. When you do not eat enough food or carbohydrates for your current metabolism and activity levels, your body uses up more than it rebuilds its functional and structural proteins and fats. The same applies to skipping meals. Although you may be losing weight—you are not just losing fat weight; you are losing functional (hormones, neurotransmitters, enzymes) and structural (muscles and bones) biochemicals as well. You will never be able to heal your metabolism this way.

In fact, you are digging yourself into a deeper metabolic hole, and over time you will end up burning out your adrenal glands. You will then acquire a new current metabolism type—insulin-resistant with burned-out adrenal glands. If this happens, you will have higher triglyceride and blood-sugar levels, worsening of your blood pressure and more fat-weight gain than ever before.

In summary, in order to prevent your insulin levels from staying too high or your adrenaline/cortisol levels from becoming too low, you need to eat smaller meals more frequently, and you must eat the right amount of carbohydrates for your current metabolism type and activity level. If you eat this way, you will heal faster and minimize the amount of potential fat weight you may gain during your transition.

Initial Meal and Carbohydrate Guidelines

Your initial meal and minimum carbohydrate guideline is to eat five times a day: three meals a day, each containing 20 grams of carbohydrates, and two 20-gram carbohydrate snacks.

As your metabolism heals, you must increase your carbohydrate intake to 30 grams per meal, three times a day, along with two 15-gram carbohydrate snacks; *or* eat 35 grams of carbohydrates per meal, three times a day, along with one 15-gram carbohydrate snack. As you increase your carbohydrate consumption, decrease your saturated fat consumption unless you are already following a lower-saturated fat plan. See the Saturated Fats section in chapter 11 page 244.

You will know that it is time to increase your carbohydrate consumption when you notice an abrupt change in symptoms. For example, you lose weight too quickly (more than one to two pounds a week), you start to wake up in the night from hunger, you are extremely tired or you are getting irritable. If you are not completely sure if you should increase your carbohydrates, try eating 5 more grams of carbohydrates a meal without increasing the amount of carbohydrates per snack, and see if you feel better. (See more carbohydrate guidelines in the following section.)

For food suggestions, refer to the meal plans on pages 295–298 and snacks pages 308–311.

Note: It is important for you to eat smaller meals more frequently. If you only succeed in eating three meals a day, you may gain more fat weight, and you may never fully heal your metabolism.

Why You May Need Fewer or More Carbohydrates Per Meal

You may initially require fewer carbohydrates if your triglyceride levels or blood-sugar levels are extremely high and do not improve within three months of following this program. But *never* eat less than 15 grams of carbohydrates per meal along with two snacks containing 7.5 grams of carbohydrates each. If you eat less, you will never heal.

By eating too few carbohydrates you may cause an initial drop in your blood-sugar and triglyceride levels, but you are only temporarily treating the problem. If you do not eat enough carbohydrates for your current metabolism and activity level, you will burn out your adrenal glands.

Alternatively, you must eat more carbohydrates if you become more active. Monitor your carbohydrate needs carefully because eating too few carbohydrates is just as damaging as eating too many.

The most common symptoms of eating too few carbohydrates are fatigue, rapid weight loss, irritability, heart palpitations, disrupted sleep, nausea, headaches and light-headedness. If you are on medication for diabetes, you may experience low blood-sugar reactions. However, you may not experience any of these symptoms, so it is important to count your carbohydrate intake.

Special Considerations About Your Carbohydrate Count

If you have Type II diabetes, are taking blood-sugar-lowering medication *and* your blood-sugar levels are dropping too low, you must increase your carbohydrate intake or ask your physician to adjust your medication.

The Best Carbohydrate Choices, Including Fruit

Because you are insulin-resistant, you *must* eat whole grains, legumes and starchy vegetables as your carbohydrate choices. Do not eat white flour or processed refined foods because they are non-nutritious and their glycemic index (GI) is too high.

You must count your fruit intake as a carbohydrate, limit your fruit choices to the lowest GI fruits, and have the equivalent of one serving or less of fruit a day. The best time to eat fruit is for your mid-afternoon snack.

Protein Requirements

You do not have to monitor your protein consumption—just listen to your body. Your feedback mechanisms are working because you have healthy adrenal glands. As long as you are following the carbo-hydrate guidelines and eating enough healthy fats and nonstarchy vegetables, your body will let you know when you have had enough. If you like guidelines, however, follow this regimen:

Eat at *least* two to three ounces of protein with each meal and one- to three-ounce per snack if you eat five times a day.

Eat at *least* two to four ounces of protein with each meal and snack if you eat four times a day.

These are your estimated *minimum* daily requirements. Refer to the protein portions guidelines in chapter 11 page 232 for more informa-tion on how to calculate your minimum daily protein requirement range.

When to Use the Low-Salt Diet

If you find yourself bloating or retaining a lot of fluid, or your blood pressure is rising, incorporate the Two-Gram Sodium Diet found on page 312 in chapter 11, and re-evaluate your meal plans. You may need to eat more frequently to avoid too many carbohydrates at a given time. As your metabolism heals, you can add in some naturally saltier foods, but do not add salt to your food.

If you are already taking a diuretic because you have high blood pres-sure or fluid retention, follow the Two-Gram Sodium Diet but notify your physician first that you are going to do so. By working with your physician and eating less salt, you may be able to reduce your blood pressure medication. Remember that thiazide diuretics are contraindicated if you have Type II diabetes, and they also make insulin resistance worse.

Special Considerations on Fat Consumption

If you have been insulin-resistant for a long time, you may already have plaque buildup in your arteries, very high triglyceride levels, high blood pressure, morbid obesity and/or Type II diabetes. Although saturated fats in theory are not bad for you, they will keep your triglyceride and blood-sugar levels higher and cause your insulin levels to be high as well if you do not need them and cannot burn them off for energy.

Ideally you will be able to switch all your excess carbohydrates, including refined sugars, to saturated, monounsaturated and polyunsaturated fats. However, if you find this difficult to do, you will need to reduce your saturated fat intake and eat more monounsaturated and polyunsaturated fats until you have tapered off your excess carbohydrates.

Additionally, if there is any reason that you are unable to maintain an adequate exercise program, or you are not responding well to a normal saturated-fat intake, you need to follow the lower saturated-fat meal plans listed in chapter 11. Refer to the Saturated Fats section in chapter 11 starting on page 244 to learn what foods to avoid or eat sparingly.

This does not mean you are going on a low-fat diet nor does it mean you are eliminating all saturated fats from your meals. You will need to eat plenty of monounsaturated and healthy polyunsaturated oils in place of your saturated fats. Make sure your ratio of omega-3 to omega-6 fatty acid intake is at least 1-to-3. Read more about omega-3 and omega-6 fatty acids in chapter 11 pages 247–252.

Supplements

Your minimal vitamin regimen should include a pharmaceutical-grade multivitamin and mineral, extra calcium and magnesium, a stress B-complex vitamin, omega-3 fatty acids, and extra vitamin E and vitamin C. Additionally, consider adding in a few of these other supplements that help with insulin sensitivity, such as alpha lipoic acid, carnitine, chromium, CoEnzyme Q-10, garlic, glutamine, taurine, conjugated linoleic acid, vanadium and zinc.

See chapter 11 (pages 314–319) for more information about nutrition and supplements.

Eating for Your Current Metabolism Type

When you have completely healed your metabolism, follow the insulin-sensitive with healthy adrenal glands program (see chapter 17). The only way to know if you are insulin-sensitive again is by testing your fasting insulin and lipid levels. Ask your physician to test you or visit my Web site, *www.SchwarzbeinPrinciple.com*, to find out how you can be tested.

Step Two: Stress Management, Including Getting Enough Sleep

When to Begin Stress Management Techniques

You need to work on managing your stress better or begin to use stress management techniques. Stress raises adrenaline and cortisol levels, which makes you more insulin-resistant.

Getting Enough Sleep

If you are not getting at least seven to eight hours of uninterrupted sleep, you are not sleeping enough. Sleep deprivation also causes you to become more insulin-resistant. Because you are insulin-resistant, you may have sleep apnea. Ask your physician about getting tested for this condition.

See chapter 12 for more on stress management and how to ensure you get enough sleep.

Step Three: Tapering Off Toxic Chemicals or Avoiding Them Completely

What to Eliminate First

You need to eliminate refined sugars, nicotine, caffeine, alcohol and any other stimulant you use as soon as possible because you will not need to self-medicate, and these chemicals all cause insulin resistance. *Do not eliminate your prescription medications.*

If you find eliminating these toxic chemicals difficult to do, you have probably incorrectly categorized yourself as having healthy adrenal glands. At this point you should have your metabolism tested. Discuss this with your physician or visit my Web site at *www.SchwarzbeinPrinciple.com* for information on how to get tested. If it turns out that you do have burned-out adrenal glands and you are not insulin-resistant, follow the insulin-sensitive with burned-out adrenal gland program in chapter 19. If you are, in fact, insulin-resistant with burned-out adrenal glands, refer to your new program in chapter 20.

See chapter 13 for more information on toxic chemicals.

Step Four: Cross-Training Exercise Program

When to Start a Cross-Training Program

Because you are insulin-resistant, you need to be cleared by your physician before beginning or increasing your exercise program. You should initially do mostly resistance/adaptive and flexibility/calming exercises. Because your adrenal glands are healthy, too much cardiovascular/stimulating exercise will raise adrenaline and cortisol levels and cause more insulin resistance. Your initial goal is to work up to the following exercise regimen:

- Flexibility/calming exercises: 15 to 30 minutes, five to seven days a week

- Resistance/adaptive training: 45- to 60-minute sessions, three times a week

- Cardiovascular/stimulating exercises: 15-minute sessions, two times a week at 70 to 80 percent of your maximum heart rate* (alternate days with resistance/adaptive training).

Always try to keep your ratio of resistance/adaptive training to cardiovascular/stimulating exercises around two-to-one or greater until you have completely healed your metabolism. As you heal your metabolism, you will be able to increase the amount of cardiovascular/stimulating exercises that you do to 20- to 25-minute sessions. When you have completely healed, you can do 30- to 60-minute cardiovascular sessions.

Make Sure That You Are Not Overexercising

Your adrenaline/cortisol levels rise and your body uses up its bio-chemicals when you overexercise. Since it feels good when this happens, it is easy to overexercise. Be aware, however, that too much exercise will destroy your metabolism further because overexercising causes more insulin resistance. If you are overexercising, you will also notice that you are unable to lose fat weight.

See chapter 14 for more information on exercise.

---

*To estimate your maximum heart rate, subtract your age from 220.

Step Five: Hormone Replacement Therapy, If Needed

When to Take HRT

You should take HRT if you need it. Work with a medical professional who understands how all hormones interact with one another.

Replacing Missing Hormones Will Help You Become Insulin-Sensitive

If you have hypothyroidism (an underactive thyroid), you need thyroid hormone replacement therapy. Having hypothyroidism will make you more insulin-resistant. However, you must be careful not to take too much thyroid hormone because any type of *hyper*thyroidism (an overactive thyroid) also causes insulin resistance.

Too little DHEA or testosterone also causes insulin resistance. You should take these if you need them, but be aware that too much DHEA or testosterone will also make you insulin-resistant.

The loss of estradiol and progesterone in menopause also makes you more insulin-resistant. Take HRT for menopause, but make sure you take it correctly. If the balance between these two hormones is off, you can become more insulin-resistant.

The use of birth control pills (BCPs) is not hormone replacement therapy. These types of drugs make you more insulin-resistant—you should not be on them.

See chapter 15 for more information on hormone replacement therapy.

Summary: Insulin-Resistant with Healthy Adrenal Glands

General

- You can follow all five steps of the SPII program at the same time, but keep cardiovascular/stimulating exercises to a minimum.

Transition Time

- It takes a few years to become insulin-sensitive again.

Step One

- Minimum carbohydrate requirement: 20 grams with each meal and two 20-gram carbohydrate snacks. Eat only low GI fruits and count them as carbohydrates.

- Need to measure protein portions: No.

- Need for low-salt diet: Maybe.

- Need for low-saturated fat diet: Maybe.

- Minimum supplement requirement: pharmaceutical-grade multivitamin and mineral, extra calcium and magnesium, a stress B-complex and omega-3 fatty acids. Consider other supplements that help with insulin sensitivity, such as alpha lipoic acid, carnitine, chromium, CoEnzyme Q-10, garlic, glutamine, taurine, conjugated linoleic acid, vanadium and zinc.

Step Two

- Stress: Manage stress better and/or use stress management techniques.

- Sleep: Strive for seven to eight hours of uninterrupted sleep.

Step Three

- Stop all toxic chemicals immediately. This does not include prescription medications.

Step Four

- Cross-training exercise program: You need to get medical clearance.

- Minimum amount of exercise: flexibility/calming—work up to 15 minutes daily; resistance/adaptive—work up to 45-minute sessions three times a week; cardiovascular/stimulating—work up to 15-minute sessions on two different days a week. Increase as tolerated. Keep resistance/adaptive to cardiovascular/stimulating ratio approximately two-to-one or greater.

- Avoid overexercising: It leads to further insulin resistance.

Step Five

- Take HRT if needed: Work with a medical professional who understands how all hormones interact with one another.

Nineteen

Personal Program: Insulin-Sensitive with Burned-Out Adrenal Glands

---

If you are insulin-sensitive with burned-out adrenal glands, you must slowly incorporate all five steps of the program into your life in order to minimize your transition symptoms and to keep you from overwhelming yourself with too many changes. You are in a group that is likely to require self-medication in your healing phase, and you are most likely to gain fat weight before losing fat weight. However, you can still expect to increase lean body mass, such as muscles and bones, at the same time.

You have burned out your adrenal glands because you are someone who does too much! You will feel that you do not have time to change your habits, and you are part of the current metabolism-type group that will be the most frustrated, angry and in denial about having to change your nutrition and lifestyle habits. Your years of hard work and overachieving have brought you here. It is time to take better care of yourself.

There are other paths besides overworking that can lead to adrenal gland burnout. You may have burned out your adrenal glands through yo-yo dieting, excessive exercise, and use of stimulants and/or alcohol. Or you may have had a glandular-based endocrine disease such as Grave's that was not diagnosed or treated in a timely matter. Or you may be in menopause and untreated or taking HRT incorrectly (refer to chapter 15). If you burned out your adrenals from one of these paths, you probably are not in denial and understand that you need to heal from your previous habits or take hormone replacement therapy as needed. You also need to be careful about trying to make too many changes at once because this will only make you feel worse.

You also need to understand that as you begin to heal your adrenal glands, you will experience higher energy levels. When this happens, try not to get so enthusiastic about having more energy again that you go out and immediately expend all your newly found energy reserves. You will only have to start all over again. As hard as it seems, you need to treat yourself with kid gloves for at least a year so that at the end of that year some healing will have taken place. If you do not monitor yourself closely, you can heal a little bit, overuse the energy and burn out again, heal a little bit and so on. It can be a vicious cycle from which you may never fully recover if you are not careful.

By following the recommended meal plans and the other steps of the SPII program, you will be able to balance your hormones to heal your adrenal glands and achieve your ideal body composition. But this will take time. You can expect to be a lot healthier after one year of following this program.

Note: You need to heal your metabolism to become healthy and to lose fat weight, *not* lose weight to become healthy.

Step One: Healthy Nutrition, Including Supplementation with Vitamins, Antioxidants, Minerals, and Amino and Fatty Acids

Why You Should Eat Smaller Meals More Frequently

It is important that you eat enough healthy food to heal your metabolism again. The best way to get enough food into your body without causing further hormone imbalances is to eat smaller meals more frequently. It is always better to eat smaller meals more frequently because eating too much food at any given moment raises insulin levels too high; eating too little food raises adrenaline and cortisol levels too high. Here's why.

Because you are insulin-sensitive, you have the potential to put on fat weight easily, especially if you are eating too many carbohydrates for your current activity levels. However, because your adrenal glands are burned out, you must eat enough carbohydrates or your body will send signals to your adrenal glands to release more adrenaline and cortisol. This will lead either to further adrenal gland burnout or the inability to heal them.

Furthermore, if you eat too much food at any given time, your adrenaline and cortisol levels will go even lower and your insulin levels will go even higher. Consequently, you will experience many troublesome symptoms such as increased fatigue, bloating, fat-weight gain and mental fogginess. This will make you want to go back to your past poor eating habits again, but you will never heal your metabolism if you do.

However, if you do not eat *enough* at each meal or throughout the day, or if you skip meals, you will not be able to heal your metabolism. By not eating enough food, you increase the demand of adrenaline and cortisol production by the adrenal glands, and your adrenal glands will not get a chance to heal. Also, healthy food is what you need to restore the health of your adrenal glands.

Therefore, you need to eat smaller meals more frequently. If you eat this way, you will be able to stay in the healing phase of your transition and heal faster, feel better and minimize the amount of potential fat weight you may gain.

Initial Meal and Carbohydrate Guidelines

Your initial meal and minimum carbohydrate guideline is to eat five times a day: three meals a day, each containing 20 to 25 grams of carbohydrates, and two 20-gram carbohydrate snacks.

As your metabolism heals, you must increase your carbohydrate intake to thirty grams per meal, three times a day, along with two fifteen-gram carbohydrate snacks; or eat 35 grams of carbohydrates per meal, three times a day, along with one 15-gram carbohydrate snack. As you increase your carbohydrate consumption, decrease your saturated-fat consumption, unless you are already following a lower-saturated fat plan. See Saturated Fats in chapter 11 page 244.

You will know that it is time to increase your carbohydrate consumption when you notice an abrupt change in symptoms. For example, you lose weight too quickly (more than one to two pounds a week), you start to wake up in the night from hunger, you are extremely tired or you are getting irritable. If you are not completely sure if you should increase your carbohydrates, try eating 5 more grams of carbohydrates a meal without increasing the amount of carbohydrates per snack, and see if you feel better. (See more carbohydrate guidelines in the following section.)

For food suggestions, refer to the meal plans on pages 295–301 and snacks on pages 308–311 in chapter 11.

Note: If you make the effort to eat smaller meals more frequently, you will heal and feel better faster.

Why You May Need More Carbohydrates Per Meal

You must eat more carbohydrates if you are more active or you will never heal your adrenal glands. The most common symptoms of eating too few carbohydrates are fatigue, rapid weight loss, irritability, heart palpitations, disrupted sleep, nausea, headaches and light-headedness. If your adrenal glands are severely burned out you may not experience any symptoms and may even feel better on low to no carbohydrates. Therefore, it is important to make sure you are eating enough carbohydrates.

The Best Carbohydrate Choices, Including Fruit

You need to eat whole grains, legumes, fruits and starchy vegetables as your carbohydrate choices. The goal is to eliminate white flour and processed refined foods because they are non-nutritious, raise your adrenaline and cortisol levels, and cause further adrenal gland burnout.

Count your fruit intake as a carbohydrate and read below for ways to use fruit if you have a sugar addiction.

What to Do If You Are Addicted to Refined Sugars

Because your adrenal glands are burned out, you may be addicted to refined sugars, or you may eat too few real complex carbohydrates in order to make yourself feel better.

If you are eating more refined sugars than your target carbohydrate grams per meal, eliminate your sugary foods slowly. Here are three ways to do this, ordered from the best to the worst method.

- Begin eating balanced meals and snacks with your designated complex carbohydrate count. Eat real complex carbohydrates such as legumes, whole grains and starchy vegetables. If you have uncontrollable cravings for sugar, give in to them by eating fruit. Try to eat fruits with the lowest glycemic index (GI) first, such as berries and grapefruit. But eat any type of fruit if these lowest GI fruits do not satisfy your cravings. By eating this way the worst that can happen to you is that you end up eating too much fruit in addition to balanced meals and snacks. Since you need healthy food to heal, eating balanced meals will heal your adrenal glands, and you will notice your carbohydrate cravings subsiding. If fruit does not work for you, you can try a small amount of dark chocolate. You should only do this if you are having a very hard time getting off sugars.

- Initially replace all your sugary foods with fruit and then decrease your fruit intake by 5 grams per meal per week. Once your fruit intake is equal to your target carbohydrate amount per meal, start replacing the fruit with other real complex carbohydrates such as legumes, whole grains and starchy vegetables. If you can decrease faster, do so. However, if you find yourself getting tired, depressed or irritable, having an increased craving for sugars, or waking up at night, slow down your tapering process.

- Decrease your refined sugar intake by 5 grams per meal per week. Once your refined sugar intake is equal to your target carbohydrate amount per meal, start replacing your sugary foods with real complex carbohydrates such as legumes, whole grains and starchy vegetables until you have eliminated sugary foods. You also can incorporate some fruit.

What to Do If You Are Not Eating Enough Carbohydrates

If you are eating less than your target carbohydrate grams per meal, slowly increase your carbohydrate intake by 5 grams per meal per week. If you find yourself gaining weight quickly, getting tired, bloating, having increased ankle swelling and/or getting depressed, try adding fruit as your real carbohydrate first, or decrease your carbohydrate consumption and add carbohydrates back into your diet more slowly.

After you have reached your target carbohydrate count per meal—and if you achieved your carbohydrate count by adding fruit—start switching to complex carbohydrates such as legumes, whole grains and starchy vegetables slowly until most of your fruit has been replaced with them.

Another alternative to cutting back on your carbohydrate intake or adding fruit is to add in green tea to self-medicate. Green tea has caffeine in it and will help keep your adrenaline levels from going too low as you increase your carbohydrate consumption and improve your eating habits. Drink as many cups of green tea as needed to keep you eating well. Black tea is a good second choice. If you continue to experience intestinal bloating after eating, try taking digestive enzymes with each meal.

Note: It is important to eat well first before worrying about coming off caffeinated beverages, because eating healthy food is essential to healing your adrenal glands.

What Else You Can Do to Balance Your Meals and Have Fewer Symptoms

If you continue to have difficulty cutting back on *or* increasing your carbohydrate intake, you can take supplements to help your carbohydrate cravings or minimize your specific symptoms. (See the supplements section in chapter 11 on pages 314–319.) If the supplements do not help, you have really burned out your adrenal glands. You may need a prescription for a selective serotonin reuptake inhibitor (SSRI), an antidepressant medication that can help get you through your transition.

Note: As long as you are working on your nutrition and lifestyle habits to heal your metabolism, taking SSRI drugs for a short period of time is not a problem. It is when you use these types of medicines to make yourself feel better and ignore your nutrition and lifestyle habits that you create a problem—you will get worse over time by using them.

Protein Requirements

Because your adrenal glands are burned out, you also have to monitor your protein intake.

- Eat at *least* two to three ounces of protein with each meal and one to three ounces of protein per snack if you eat five times a day.

- Eat at *least* two to four ounces of protein with each meal and snack if you eat four times a day.

These are your estimated *minimum* daily requirements. Refer to the protein portions guidelines in chapter 11 pages 232–233 for more information on how to calculate your minimum daily protein requirement range.

If you are a visual person, two ounces of protein is approximately half the size of your palm and as thick as a deck of cards. Three ounces of protein is approximately the size and thickness of a deck of cards. Four ounces of protein is approximately the size of your palm and as thick as a deck of cards.

The bigger you are or the more active you are, the more ounces of protein you may eat. If you find it difficult to abruptly decrease your protein consumption at this point, you can also taper down on your protein intake. Try decreasing your protein intake by one ounce per meal per week. If you still are having a difficult time, try adding in another meal with the same amount of proteins and carbohydrates in order to distribute your protein intake throughout the day.

If you find it difficult to eat enough proteins, you may need hydrochloric acid and/or digestive enzymes.

When to Use the Low-Salt Diet

If you find yourself bloating and retaining a lot of fluid, or your blood pressure is rising, incorporate the Two-Gram Sodium Diet found on page 312 in chapter 11 and reevaluate your meal plans. You may need to eat more frequently to avoid eating too much food at a given time. As your metabolism heals, you can add in some naturally saltier foods, but do not add salt to your food.

If you are already taking a diuretic because you have high blood pressure or fluid retention, follow the Two-Gram Sodium Diet, but notify your physician first that you are going to do so. By working with your physician and eating less salt, you may be able to reduce your blood pressure medication.

Caution: If your adrenal glands are extremely burned out, you may need more salt. If you find yourself getting light-headed or dizzy, increase your salt intake to 3 to 4 grams daily. Do not restrict your salt intake just to lose one or two pounds of water weight.

Special Considerations on Fat Consumption

Both carbohydrates and saturated fats are used for energy. If you have extremely burned-out adrenal glands, your ability to use up energy biochemicals is very limited. Therefore, until your adrenal glands start functioning better, you may need to eat fewer saturated fats. Although saturated fats in theory are not bad for you, you will gain a lot of fat weight if you do not need them and cannot burn them off for energy.

Ideally you will be able to switch all your excess carbohydrates, including refined sugars, to saturated, monounsaturated and poly-unsaturated fats. However, if you find this difficult to do, you will need to reduce your saturated fat intake and eat more monounsaturated and polyunsaturated fats until you have tapered off your excess carbohydrates.

Additionally, if there is any reason that you are unable to maintain an adequate exercise program or you are not responding well to a normal saturated-fat intake, you need to follow the low-saturated fat meal plans listed in chapter 11. Refer to the Saturated Fats section on page 244 of chapter 11 to learn what foods to avoid or eat sparingly.

Note: This does not mean you are going on a low-fat diet nor does it mean you are eliminating all saturated fats from your meals. You will need to eat plenty of monounsaturated and healthy polyunsaturated oils in place of your saturated fats. Make sure your ratio of omega-3 to omega-6 fatty acid intake is at least one-to-three. Read more about omega-3 and omega-6 fatty acids in chapter 11, pages 247–252.

Supplements

Your minimal vitamin regimen should include a pharmaceutical-grade multivitamin and mineral, extra calcium and magnesium, a stress B-complex vitamin, extra vitamin E and vitamin C, and extra pantothenic acid. Additionally, you should take a few of the supplements that help your adrenal glands function better, such as CoEnzyme A, CoEnzyme Q-10 and L-tyrosine.

See chapter 11 for more information about nutrition and supplements.

Eating for Your Current Metabolism Type

When you have completely healed your metabolism, follow the insulin-sensitive with healthy adrenal glands program (see chapter 17). The best way to know if your adrenal glands have healed is through testing. Ask your physician to test your adrenal glands or visit my Web site at *www.SchwarzbeinPrinciple.com* to find out how you can be tested.

Step Two: Stress Management, Including Getting Enough Sleep

When to Begin Stress Management Techniques

Because you usually are an overachiever and stress raises adrenaline and cortisol levels—which burns out your adrenal glands even more—you need to manage your stress and learn some stress management techniques immediately. Sleep deprivation also causes your adrenal glands to burn out.

When to Use Sleep Medication

If you are not getting at least seven to eight hours of uninterrupted sleep, you are not sleeping enough. Because your adrenal glands are burned out, it is very likely that you are *not* getting enough sleep. You may need a medication such as desyrel to reset your sleep cycle. If you are unable to sleep well despite improving your nutrition and lifestyle habits, and you have been following the sleep suggestions in chapter 12, discuss taking desyrel with your physician. Do not use antianxiety drugs or sleeping pills for this problem because in the long term they will disrupt your sleep cycle further.

See chapter 12 for more on stress management and how to ensure you get enough sleep.

Step Three: Tapering Off Toxic Chemicals or Avoiding Them Completely

What to Eliminate First

Because your adrenal glands are burned out, you cannot eliminate all your toxic chemicals at the same time or you will "crash." If you are using a lot of different toxic chemicals, including refined sugar, make sure you are eating balanced meals before you begin to taper off any toxic chemical. Alcohol and nicotine are more damaging than refined sugar. Work on eliminating them first. *Do not eliminate your prescription medications* without discussing it with your physician first.

An alternative to tapering off nicotine, alcohol and refined sugar is to replace them with green tea as a means to self-medicate. Green tea has caffeine in it and will help keep your adrenaline levels from getting too low as you improve your habits. Drink as many cups of green tea as needed to keep you feeling well. Black tea is a good second choice.

Because you have burned-out adrenal glands, you may need a prescription for a selective serotonin reuptake inhibitor* (SSRI), an antidepressant medication that will help you get off toxic chemicals.

See chapter 13 for more information on how to taper off toxic chemicals.

Note: If you have chosen to replace your refined sugars with fruit, begin tapering off another toxic chemical before you start to replace your fruit with complex carbohydrates such as whole grains, legumes and starchy vegetables. However, do not start tapering off caffeine before switching to more complex carbohydrates. It is important to be eating well before tapering off all your stimulants.

Step Four: Cross-Training Exercise Program

When to Start a Cross-Training Program

Because your adrenal glands are burned out, you need to be cleared by your physician before beginning or continuing your exercise program. You should initially do flexibility/calming and resistance/adaptive exercises. Any amount of cardiovascular/stimulating exercise raises adrenaline and cortisol levels, and your adrenal glands will burn

---

*You can first try the natural serotonin supplements found in chapter 6 on page 135.

out more if you do too much. Your initial goal is to *slowly* work up to the following exercise regimen:

- Flexibility/calming exercises: 15 to 30 minutes, five to seven days a week

- Resistance/adaptive training: 30- to 60-minute sessions, three times a week

As you begin to heal your metabolism, you will be able to add 5 to 15 minutes of cardiovascular/stimulating exercises three times a week at 65 to 75 percent of your maximum heart rate* (alternate days with resistance training).

As you heal your metabolism, you may slowly increase your cardiovascular/stimulating exercises per session from 15 minutes to 20 minutes and then from 20 minutes to 25 minutes. While you are healing your metabolism, it is better to spread out your cardiovascular/stimulating workout to three times a week. However, when you have completely healed your metabolism, you will be able to increase the amount of cardiovascular/stimulating exercises that you do at each session to 30 to 60 minutes, two times a week. Keep resistance/adaptive to cardiovascular/stimulating ratio approximately two-to-one or greater.

When *Not* to Exercise

If you are extremely exhausted and do not exercise, do not start an exercise program at this time. If you are extremely exhausted and are exercising, stop your exercise program at this time. After you have been eating well and resting for a minimum of one month, you may resume exercising again.

Start slowly with flexibility/calming and resistance/adaptive exercises. The initial goal is to slowly work up to 15 minutes of flexibility/calming exercises daily and 30 minutes of resistance/adaptive exercises three

*To estimate your maximum heart rate, subtract your age from 220.

times a week. Start by incorporating 5 minutes of stretching in the morning and in the evening and add in 5 minutes of walking twice a day. This is a small but important start to get you ready to do resistance/adaptive exercises again. No amount of movement is too little.

As you improve, follow the recommendations listed under "When to Start a Cross-Training Program."

Note: You may initially use walking as a form of resistance/adaptive exercise to get you started with your exercise program again. However, you must limit your walk to 30 minutes and switch to a true resistance/adaptive exercise such as weight training, Pilates or slow swimming when you are consistently and comfortably walking for 30 minutes at a time.

Make Sure That You Are Not Overexercising

Your adrenaline/cortisol levels rise and your body uses up its biochemicals when you overexercise. Since it can feel good when this happens, it is easy to overexercise. But if you overexercise, you will "crash" with time, and if you have extremely burned-out adrenal glands, you may crash right afterwards. You will have gone two steps forward but three steps backward if you crash. Be aware that too much exercise will slow your healing process because overexercising when your adrenal glands are already exhausted causes further burnout.

See chapter 14 for more information on exercise.

Step Five: Hormone Replacement Therapy, If Needed

When to Take HRT

You should take HRT if you need it. You need to know, however, that when you begin taking a hormone that has been low for quite some time *and* your adrenal glands are burned out, you may experience adverse effects. Work with a medical professional who is well versed in prescribing HRT to patients who have burned-out adrenal glands.

Note: Because you have burned-out adrenal glands, you may need a prescription for a selective serotonin reuptake inhibitor (SSRI),* an antidepressant medication to help you tolerate a minor hormone that is missing. This is because some minor hormones affect the action of adrenaline, and if adrenaline is already low, it may be difficult for you to tolerate replacing the missing hormone. After your hormones are in balance and your metabolism is healed, you will be able to come off the SSRI medication.

Replacing Missing Hormones Will Help Heal Your Adrenal Glands

If you have hypothyroidism (an underactive thyroid), you need thyroid hormone replacement therapy. If you do not make enough thyroid hormone, you will not be able to heal your adrenal glands. However, you must be careful not to take too much thyroid hormone because any type of *hyper*thyroidism (an overactive thyroid) causes further burnout of your adrenal glands.

Too little DHEA or testosterone also leads to an inability to heal your adrenal glands. You should take these if you need them, but be aware that too much DHEA or testosterone will cause further burnout of your adrenal glands.

The loss of estradiol and progesterone in menopause also causes further burnout of your adrenal glands. Take HRT for menopause, but make sure you take it correctly. If the balance between these two hormones is off, you can further burn out your adrenal glands.

The use of birth control pills (BCPs) is not hormone replacement

---

*You can first try the natural serotonin supplements found in chapter 6 on page 135.

therapy. These types of drugs cause your adrenal glands to burn out; you should not be on them. Since most BCPs also act as stimulants, you may "crash" if you come off them without addressing your underlying adrenal gland problem. Work with your physician to get off BCPs.

See chapter 15 for more information on hormone replacement therapy.

Summary: Insulin-Sensitive with Burned-Out Adrenal Glands

General

You must slowly incorporate all five steps of the program into your life to minimize your transition symptoms. Address nutrition and stress issues first before tapering off toxic chemicals. Go slowly. Start by doing flexibility/calming and resistance/adaptive exercises only.

Transition Time

It will take at least one year or more to fully heal your adrenal glands.

Step One

- Minimum carbohydrate requirement: 20 to 25 grams with each meal and two 20-gram carbohydrate snacks. You may eat all types of fruits to satisfy your sugar cravings, but try eating the low GI fruits first and count all fruit as carbohydrates.
- Need to measure protein portions: Yes.
- Need for low-salt diet: Maybe.
- Need for lower-saturated fat diet: Probably not, but it can be used to help minimize the amount of fat-weight gain or if you cannot or do not follow a moderate exercise program.

- Minimum supplement requirement: Pharmaceutical-grade multivitamin and mineral, extra calcium and magnesium, a stress B-complex vitamin, extra vitamin E and vitamin C, extra pantothenic acid, and a few of the supplements that help your adrenal glands function better, such as CoEnzyme Q-10, CoEnzyme A and L-tyrosine.

Step Two

- Stress: You are usually an overachiever. You need to manage stress better and/or use stress management techniques immediately.
- Sleep: Strive for seven to eight hours of uninterrupted sleep.
- Need for desyrel for sleep: Probably, but try sleep suggestions in chapter 12 first.

Step Three

- Taper off toxic chemicals one at a time; this does not include prescription medications.
- Nicotine is worse than alcohol, alcohol is worse than sugar and sugar is worse than caffeine.
- Stop using artificial sugars and other nonaddicting chemicals now.
- Use caffeine to self-medicate: Most likely.
- Need for an SSRI antidepressant: Most likely, but try serotonin supplements first.

Step Four

Cross-training exercise program: you need to get medical clearance. Minimum amount of exercise: flexibility/calming—slowly work up to 15 minutes daily; resistance/adaptive—slowly work up to 30- to 60-minute sessions three times a week; cardiovascular/stimulating—over time, add in 15-minute session three times a week (alternate days with resistance/adaptive training). Keep resistance/adaptive to cardiovascular/ stimulating ratio approximately two-to-one or greater.

Avoid overexercising; it leads to further burnout.

Step Five

Take HRT if needed: Work with a medical professional who is well versed in prescribing HRT to patients who have burned-out adrenal glands.

Twenty

Personal Program: Insulin-Resistant with Burned-Out Adrenal Glands

If you are insulin-resistant with burned-out adrenal glands, your healing phase will take the longest time because your metabolism is badly damaged. You have to incorporate all five steps of the program into your life more slowly to minimize your transition symptoms.

Because you have both insulin resistance and burned-out adrenal glands, you are likely to require self-medication in your healing phase, and you are more than likely to gain more fat weight before you begin to slowly lose your current fat weight. However, you can still expect to increase lean body mass, such as muscles and bones, as this happens.

You have more than likely become insulin-resistant and burned out your adrenal glands by trying to "improve" your health by losing weight through repeated yo-yo dieting and eating high-carbohydrate, low-fat foods. Now is the time to learn about how you dug your metabolic hole so that you can climb out of it.

There are other paths besides yo-yo dieting that can lead to insulin resistance and adrenal gland burnout. You may have become insulin-resistant and burned out your adrenal glands through overworking, excessive exercise, use of stimulants and/or alcohol. Or you may have had a glandular-based endocrine disease such as Grave's that was not diagnosed or treated in a timely matter. Or you may be in menopause and untreated or taking HRT incorrectly (refer to chapter 15). If you have become insulin-resistant and burned out your adrenals from one of these paths, you need to heal from your previous habits or take hormone replacement therapy as needed. You need to be careful about trying to make too many changes at once because this will only make you feel worse.

You also need to understand that as you begin to heal, you will experience higher energy levels. When this happens, try not to get overly enthusiastic about it and use up all your newly found energy reserves. If you do, you will only be starting all over again. As hard as it seems, you need to treat yourself with kid gloves for at least a year or two so that at the end of that time period some healing will have taken place. If you do not monitor yourself closely, you can heal a little bit, overuse the energy and be back where you started from, heal a little bit and so on. It can be a vicious cycle from which you may never fully recover if you are not careful.

Do not expect to achieve your ideal body composition within the first year of your healing program. You have to balance all your hormones, heal your adrenal glands and become insulin-sensitive again for this to happen. As upsetting as this may be, the good news is that you can make yourself better. By following the recommended meal plans and the other steps of the SPII program, you can start healing today.

Note: You need to heal your metabolism to become healthy and to lose fat weight, *not* lose weight to become healthy.

Step One: Healthy Nutrition, Including Supplementation with Vitamins, Antioxidants, Minerals, and Amino and Fatty Acids

Why You Should Eat Smaller Meals More Frequently

It is important that you eat enough healthy food to heal your metabolism again. The only way for you to get enough food into your body without causing further hormone imbalances is to eat smaller meals more frequently. Here's why.

Because you are insulin-resistant with burned-out adrenal glands, if you eat too much food or carbohydrates at a given time, you will keep your insulin levels too high and your adrenaline and cortisol levels will go even lower. You will experience many troublesome symptoms, such as increased fatigue, bloating, fat-weight gain and mental fogginess. Feeling this poorly and gaining weight this rapidly may make you want to go back to your past poor eating habits again; however, you will only dig yourself into a deeper metabolic hole if you do.

If you skip meals or you do not eat enough food or carbohydrates during a meal or throughout the day, you will not be able to heal your metabolism. The only way to rebuild your functional and structural proteins and fats to become insulin-sensitive again is by eating enough—and the right types of—healthy foods.

Because your adrenal glands are burned out, you must eat enough food including carbohydrates or you will send signals to your adrenal glands to release more adrenaline and cortisol. This will lead either to further adrenal gland burnout or the inability for them to heal. You will need to eat healthy foods to restore the health of your adrenal glands.

Because you are insulin-resistant and your adrenal glands are burned out, you must eat smaller meals more frequently. If you eat this way, you will be able to stay in the healing phase of your transition and heal faster, feel better and minimize the amount of potential fat weight you may gain.

Initial Meal and Carbohydrate Guidelines

Your initial meal and minimum carbohydrate guideline is to eat five times a day: three meals a day, each containing 15 grams of carbohydrates, and two 15-gram carbohydrate snacks.

As your metabolism heals, you must increase your carbohydrate intake to 20 grams per meal, three times a day, along with two 20-gram carbohydrate snacks. As your metabolism continues to improve, further increase your carbohydrates to 25 grams per meal, three times a day, along with two 25-gram carbohydrate snacks. As you increase your carbohydrate consumption, decrease your saturated-fat consumption unless you are already following a lower-saturated fat plan. See the Saturated Fats section beginning on page 244.

You will know that it is time to increase your carbohydrate consumption when you notice an abrupt change in symptoms. For example, you lose weight too quickly (more than one to two pounds a week), you start to wake up in the night from hunger, you are extremely tired or you are getting irritable. If you are not completely sure if you should increase your carbohydrates, try eating 5 more grams of carbohydrates a meal without increasing the amount of carbohydrates per snack, and see if you feel better. (See more carbohydrate guidelines in the following section.)

For food suggestions, refer to the meal plans in chapter 11 on pages 291–294 and the snack suggestions on pages 308–311.

Note: If you do not eat smaller meals more frequently, you may never fully heal your metabolism. You will also feel much better by eating this way and can minimize your potential fat-weight gain.

Why You May Need Fewer or More Carbohydrates Per Meal

You may initially require fewer carbohydrates if your triglyceride levels or blood-sugar levels are extremely high and do not improve within three months of following this program. But *never* eat less than 15 grams of carbohydrates per meal (three times a day), together with two snacks containing 7.5 grams of carbohydrates each. If you eat less, you will never heal. By eating too few carbohydrates you may cause an initial drop in your blood-sugar and triglyceride levels, but you are only temporarily treating the problem. If you do not eat enough carbohydrates for your current metabolism and activity level, you will burn out your adrenal glands even further.

Alternatively, you must eat *more* carbohydrates if you become more active at any time. Monitor your carbohydrate needs carefully because eating too few carbohydrates is just as damaging as eating too many.

The most common symptoms of eating too few carbohydrates are fatigue, rapid weight loss, irritability, heart palpitations, disrupted sleep, nausea, headaches and light-headedness. If you are on medication for diabetes, you may experience low-blood-sugar reactions. However, if you are extremely insulin-resistant or your adrenal glands are severely burned out, you may not experience any symptoms. Therefore it is important to make sure you are eating enough carbohydrates.

Special Considerations About Your Carbohydrate Count

If you have Type II diabetes, are taking blood-sugar lowering medication *and* your blood-sugar levels are dropping too low, you must increase your carbohydrate intake or ask your physician to adjust your medication.

The Best Carbohydrate Choices, Including Fruit

Because you are insulin-resistant with burned-out adrenal glands, you *must* eat whole grains, legumes and starchy vegetables as your carbohydrate choices. Do not eat white flour or processed refined foods because their glycemic index (GI) is too high, they are non-nutritious and they raise your adrenaline and cortisol levels.

You must count your fruit intake as a carbohydrate; however, because you are insulin-resistant, you must limit your fruit choices to the lowest GI fruits (see list in chapter 11). Your goal is to taper down to the equivalent of one serving or less of fruit a day. Read below for ways to use fruit to help if you have a sugar addiction.

What to Do If You Are Addicted to Refined Sugars

Because you are insulin-resistant, you need to get off refined sugars as quickly as possible (see the supplements section in chapter 11 on pages 314–319 for supplements that can help reduce carbohydrate cravings). However, because your adrenal glands are burned out, this may be very difficult to do. Here are two ways to do this.

- The best way for you to get off refined sugars is to begin eating balanced meals with your designated complex carbohydrate count. Eat real complex carbohydrates such as legumes, whole grains and starchy vegetables. If you have uncontrollable cravings for sugar, give in to them by eating low GI fruits. By eating this way the worst that can happen to you is that you end up eating too much fruit in addition to balanced meals. Since you need healthy foods to heal, eating balanced meals will heal your metabolism and you will notice your carbohydrate cravings subsiding with time. If fruit does not work for you, you can try a small amount of dark chocolate. You should only do this if you are having *a very hard time* tapering off sugars.

- The second best way to taper off refined sugars is to initially replace all your sugary foods with fruit, and then decrease your fruit intake by 5 grams per meal per week. Once your fruit intake is equal to your target carbohydrate amount per meal, start replacing the fruit with other real complex carbohydrates such as legumes, whole grains and starchy vegetables. If you can decrease faster, do so, but if you find yourself getting tired, depressed, irritable, having an increased craving for sugars or waking up at night, slow down your tapering process.

What to Do If You Are Not Eating Enough Carbohydrates

If you are eating less than your target carbohydrate grams per meal, slowly increase your intake by 5 grams of real complex carbohydrates such as whole grains, legumes and starchy vegetables per meal per week. If you find yourself gaining weight quickly, getting tired, bloating, having increased ankle swelling and/or getting depressed, decrease your carbohydrate consumption and add carbohydrates back into your diet more slowly.

You can also try adding a mixture of fruit and complex carbohydrates to your diet, but remember that you can only eat fruits with the lowest GI. Then, as soon as you are able, replace the fruit in your diet with complex carbohydrates.

Another alternative to cutting back down on your carbohydrate intake or adding fruit is to add in green tea to self-medicate. Green tea has caffeine in it and will help keep your adrenaline levels from going too low as you increase your carbohydrate consumption and improve your eating habits. Drink as many cups of green tea as needed to keep you eating well. Black tea is a good second choice. If you continue to experience intestinal bloating after eating, try taking digestive enzymes after each meal.

Note: It is important to eat well first before worrying about coming off caffeinated beverages, because eating healthy food is essential to healing your adrenal glands and making you insulin-sensitive again.

What Else You Can Do to Balance Your Meals and Have Fewer Symptoms

If you continue to have difficulty cutting back on *or* increasing your carbohydrate intake, you can take supplements to help your carbohydrate cravings or minimize your specific symptoms. (See the supplement section on pages 314–319 in chapter 11.) If the supplements do not help, you are extremely insulin-resistant and/or you have really burned out your adrenal glands. You may need a prescription for a selective serotonin reuptake inhibitor (SSRI), an antidepressant medication that can help get you through your transition.

Note: As long as you are working on your nutrition and lifestyle habits to heal your metabolism, SSRI drugs are not a problem. It is when you use these types of medicines to make yourself feel better and ignore your nutrition and lifestyle habits that you create a problem— you will get worse over time by using them.

Protein Requirements

Because your adrenal glands are burned out, you also have to monitor your protein intake.

Eat at *least* two to three ounces of protein with each meal and at least one to three ounces of protein per snack. This comes out to a total of eight to fifteen ounces of protein a day.

These are your estimated *minimum* daily requirements. Refer to the protein portions guidelines in chapter 11 pages 232–233 for more information on how to calculate your minimum daily protein requirement range.

If you are a visual person, two ounces of protein is approximately half the size of your palm and as thick as a deck of cards, and three ounces of protein is approximately the size and thickness of a deck of cards.

The bigger you are or the more active you are, the more ounces of protein you may eat. If you find it difficult to abruptly decrease your pro-tein consumption at this point, you can also taper down on your protein intake. Try decreasing your protein intake by one ounce per meal per week. If you still are having a difficult time, try adding in another meal with the same amount of protein and carbohydrates in order to distrib-ute your protein intake throughout the day.

If you find it difficult to eat enough protein, you may need hydro-chloric acid and/or digestive enzymes.

When to Use the Low-Salt Diet

Yours is the current metabolism type most likely to need to follow a salt-restrictive diet.

If you find yourself bloating and retaining a lot of fluid, or your blood pressure is rising, incorporate the Two-Gram Sodium Diet found on page 312 in chapter 11 and re-evaluate your meal plans. You may need to eat more frequently to avoid increasing the gap between your insulin and adrenaline/cortisol levels. As your metabolism heals, you can add in some naturally saltier foods, but do not add salt to your food.

If you are already taking a diuretic because you have high blood pressure or fluid retention, follow the Two-Gram Sodium Diet, but notify your physician first that you are going to do so. By working with your physician and eating less salt, you may be able to reduce your blood pressure medication. Remember thiazide diuretics are con-traindicated if you have Type II diabetes, and they also make insulin resistance worse.

Caution: If your adrenal glands are extremely burned out, you may need more salt. If you find yourself getting light-headed or dizzy, increase your salt intake to three to four grams a day. Do not restrict your salt intake just to lose one or two pounds of water weight.

Special Considerations on Fat Consumption

If you have been insulin-resistant for a long time, you may already have plaque buildup in your arteries, very high triglyceride levels, high blood pressure, morbid obesity and/or Type II diabetes. Although saturated fats in theory are not bad for you, they will keep your triglyceride, blood-sugar and insulin levels high if you do not need them or use them as energy.

Because you are both insulin-resistant and have burned-out adrenal glands, you need to follow the low-saturated fat meal plans in chapter 11.

As your metabolism heals and you maintain an adequate exercise routine, you can begin to include more saturated fats in your diet again. However, if for some reason you are unable to maintain an adequate exercise routine, you are unable to lower your carbohydrate intake or stop eating refined sugars, or you are not responding well to a normal saturated-fat intake, you need to continue to follow the lower-saturated fat meal plans.

Refer to the Saturated Fats section in chapter 11 beginning on page 244 to learn what foods to avoid or eat sparingly.

Note: This does not mean you are going on a low-fat diet. You will need to eat plenty of monounsaturated and healthy polyunsaturated oils in place of your saturated fat. Make sure your ratio of omega-3 to omega-6 fatty acid intake is at least one-to-three. Read more about omega-3 and omega-6 fatty acids in chapter 11 on pages 247–252.

Supplements

Your minimal vitamin regimen should include a pharmaceutical-grade multivitamin and mineral, extra calcium and magnesium, a stress B-complex vitamin, omega-3 fatty acids, extra vitamin E and vitamin C, and extra pantothenic acid. Additionally, you will also need to take a few of the supplements that help you become insulin-sensitive and help your adrenal glands function better. These include alpha lipoic acid, carnitine, chromium, CoEnzyme Q-10, garlic, conjugated linoleic acid, glutamine, taurine, vanadium and zinc, CoEnzyme A and L-tyrosine.

See chapter 11 for more information about nutrition and supplements.

Eating for Your Current Metabolism Type

As your metabolism heals, you will either become insulin-sensitive first or heal your adrenal glands first.

If you become insulin-sensitive before your adrenal glands heal, refer to the insulin-sensitive with burned-out adrenal glands program for your new meal plans and program (see chapter 19). The only way to know this is by testing your fasting insulin and lipid levels. Ask your physician to test you or visit my Web site at *www.SchwarzbeinPrinciple.com* to find out how you can be tested.

If your adrenal glands heal before you become insulin-sensitive again, refer to the insulin-resistant with healthy adrenal glands program for your new meal plans and program (see chapter 18). The best way to know if your adrenal glands have healed is through testing. Ask your physician to test your adrenal glands or visit my Web site to find out how you can be tested.

Step Two: Stress Management, Including Getting Enough Sleep

When to Begin Stress Management Techniques

You need to address your stress and learn some stress management techniques immediately because stress raises your adrenaline and cortisol levels, which makes you more insulin-resistant and burns out your adrenal glands further. Sleep deprivation has the same effects.

When to Use Sleep Medication

If you are not getting at least seven to eight hours of uninterrupted sleep, you are not sleeping enough. Because your adrenal glands are burned out, it is very likely that you are *not* getting enough sleep. You may need a medication such as desyrel to reset your sleep cycle.* Do not use antianxiety drugs or sleeping pills for this problem because in the long term they will disrupt your sleep cycle further. Because you are insulin-resistant, you may have sleep apnea. Ask your physician about getting tested for this condition.

See chapter 12 for more on stress management and how to ensure that you get enough sleep.

Step Three: Tapering Off
Toxic Chemicals or Avoiding Them Completely

What to Eliminate First

Because you are insulin-resistant, you need to begin eliminating refined sugars, caffeine, nicotine and/or alcohol as soon as possible. Because your adrenal glands are burned out, coming off these toxic chemicals may be extremely difficult. You must, therefore, taper off them or you will "crash." If you are using a lot of different toxic chemicals, including refined sugar, make sure you are eating balanced meals before you begin to taper off any toxic chemical. *This does not include your prescription medications.* Do not eliminate your prescription drugs without discussing it with your physician first.

Nicotine and alcohol are the worst offenders; sugar is next and caffeine should be tapered off last. All these toxic chemicals cause you to be more insulin-resistant and further burn out your adrenal glands.

An alternative to tapering off nicotine, alcohol and refined sugars is

---

Try the sleep suggestions in chapter 12 first.

to replace them with green tea as a means to self-medicate. Green tea has caffeine in it and will help keep your adrenaline levels from getting too low as you improve your habits. Drink as many cups of green tea as needed to keep you feeling well. Black tea is a good second choice.

Because you have burned-out adrenal glands, you may need a prescription for a selective serotonin reuptake inhibitor* (SSRI), an antidepressant medication that will help you taper off toxic chemicals.

See chapter 13 for more information on how to taper off toxic chemicals.

Note: If you have chosen to replace your refined sugars with fruits, begin tapering off another toxic chemical *before* you start replacing your fruits with complex carbohydrates such as whole grains, legumes and starchy vegetables. However, do not start tapering off caffeine before switching to more complex carbohydrates. It is important to be eating well before tapering off all your stimulants.

Step Four: Cross-Training Exercise Program

When to Start a Cross-Training Program

Because you are insulin-resistant with burned-out adrenal glands, you need to be cleared by your physician before beginning or continuing your exercise program. You should initially do mostly flexibility/calming and resistance/adaptive exercises. Any amount of cardiovascular/stimulating exercise raises adrenaline and cortisol levels. Therefore, too much cardiovascular/stimulating exercise makes you more insulin-resistant and further burns out your adrenal glands. Your initial goal is to *slowly* work up to the following exercise regimen:

- Flexibility/calming exercises: 15 to 30 minutes, five to seven times a week

---

*You can first try the natural serotonin booster supplements found in chapter 6, page 135.

- Resistance/adaptive training: 30- to 60-minute sessions, three times a week

As you begin to heal your metabolism, you will be able to add 5 to 15 minutes of cardiovascular/stimulating exercises three times a week at 60 to 70 percent of your maximum heart rate* (alternate days with resistance/adaptive training).

As you heal your metabolism, you may slowly increase your cardiovascular/stimulating exercises per session from 15 minutes to 20 minutes and from 20 minutes to 25 minutes. While you are healing your metabolism, it is better to spread out your cardiovascular/ stimulating workout to three times a week. However, when you have completely healed your metabolism, you will be able to increase the amount of cardiovascular/stimulating exercises that you do at each session to 30 to 60 minutes, two times a week. Keep resistance/ adaptive to cardiovascular/stimulating ratio approximately two-to-one or greater.

When *Not* to Exercise

If you are extremely exhausted and do not exercise, do not start an exercise program at this time. If you are extremely exhausted and are exercising, stop your exercise program at this time. After you have been eating well and resting for a minimum of one month, you may resume exercising again.

Start slowly with resistance/adaptive and flexibility/calming exercises first. The initial goal is to slowly work up to 15 minutes of flexibility/ calming exercises daily and 30 minutes of resistance/adaptive exercises three times a week. Start by incorporating 5 minutes of stretching in the morning and in the evening and add in 5 minutes of walking twice a day. This is a small but important start to get you ready to do resistance/adaptive exercises again. No amount of movement is too little.

To estimate your maximum heart rate, subtract your age from 220.

As you improve, follow the recommendations listed under "When to Start a Cross-Training Program."

Note: You may initially use walking as a form of resistance/adaptive exercise to get you started with your exercise program again. However, you must limit your walk to 30 minutes and switch to a true resistance/adaptive exercise such as weight training, Pilates or slow swimming when you are consistently and comfortably walking for 30 minutes at a time.

Make Sure That You Are Not Overexercising

Your adrenaline/cortisol levels rise and your body uses up its biochemicals when you overexercise. Since it can feel good when this happens, it is easy to overexercise. But if you overexercise, you will "crash" with time, and if you have extremely burned-out adrenal glands, you may crash right afterwards. You will have gone two steps forward but three steps backward if you crash. Be aware that too much exercise will slow your healing process because overexercising when your adrenal glands are already exhausted causes further burnout. See chapter 14 for more information on exercise.

Step Five: Hormone Replacement Therapy, If Needed

When to Take HRT

You should take HRT if you need it. You need to know, however, that when you begin taking a hormone that has been low for quite some time *and* your adrenal glands are burned out, you may experience adverse effects. Work with a medical professional who is well versed in prescribing HRT to patients who have burned-out adrenal glands.

16

Note: Because you have burned-out adrenal glands, you may need a prescription for a selective serotonin reuptake inhibitor (SSRI), an antidepressant medication to help you tolerate a minor hormone that is missing. This is because some minor hormones affect the action of adrenaline, and if adrenaline is already low, it may be difficult for you to tolerate replacing the missing hormone. After your hormones are in balance and your metabolism is healed, you will be able to come off the SSRI medication. You can try serotonin supplementation first before starting SSRI medication (see page 135).

Replacing Missing Hormones Will Help You Become Insulin-Sensitive and Heal Your Adrenal Glands

If you have hypothyroidism (an underactive thyroid), you need thyroid hormone replacement therapy. Hypothyroidism will make you more insulin-resistant and you will not be able to heal your adrenal glands. However, you must be careful not to take too much thyroid hormone because any type of *hyper*thyroidism (an overactive thyroid) causes insulin resistance and further burns out your adrenal glands.

Too little DHEA or testosterone also causes insulin resistance and the inability to heal your adrenal glands. You should take these if you need them, but be aware that too much DHEA or testosterone will make you insulin-resistant and further burn out your adrenal glands.

The loss of estradiol and progesterone in menopause also causes more insulin resistance and further adrenal gland burnout. Take HRT for menopause, but make sure you take it correctly. If the balance between these two hormones is off, you can become more insulin-resistant and further burn out your adrenal glands.

The use of birth control pills (BCPs) is not hormone replacement therapy. These types of drugs make you more insulin-resistant and cause your adrenal glands to burn out; you should not be on them. Since most BCPs also act as stimulants, you may "crash" if you come off them without addressing your underlying adrenal gland problem. Work with your physician to get off BCPs. See chapter 15 for more information on hormone replacement therapy.

Summary: Insulin-Resistant with Burned-Out Adrenal Glands

General

- You have to incorporate all five steps of the program into your life more slowly to minimize your transition symptoms.

- Address nutrition and stress issues first before tapering off toxic chemicals. Go slowly. Start by doing flexibility/calming and resistance/adaptive training exercises only.

Transition Time

- It will take a few years to become insulin-sensitive again and to heal your adrenal glands. Do not despair. You can still heal, and you will be improving your health all along the way.

Step One

- Minimum carbohydrate requirement: 15 grams with each meal and two 15-gram carbohydrate snacks. Eat only low GI fruits, count them as carbohydrates and use them to satisfy sugar cravings.

- Need to measure protein portions: Yes.

- Need for low-salt diet: Most likely.

- Need for lower-saturated fat diet: Yes. But add saturated fats back in when your metabolism improves.

- Minimum supplement requirement: Pharmaceutical-grade multivitamin and mineral, extra calcium and magnesium, a stress B-complex vitamin, omega-3 fatty acids, extra vitamin E and vitamin C, and extra pantothenic acid. You will also need to take a few of the other supplements that help you become insulin-sensitive and improve your adrenal-gland function, such as alpha lipoic acid, carnitine, chromium, conjugated linoleic acid, CoEnzyme Q-10, garlic, glutamine, taurine, vanadium and zinc, CoEnzyme A, and L-tyrosine.

Step Two

- Stress: You need to manage stress better and/or use stress management techniques immediately.

- Sleep: Strive for seven to eight hours of uninterrupted sleep.

- Need for desyrel for sleep: Probably, but try the sleep suggestions in chapter 12 first.

Step Three

- Taper off of toxic chemicals one at a time; this does not include prescription medications.

- Nicotine is worse than alcohol, alcohol is worse than sugar and sugar is worse than caffeine.

- Stop using artificial sugars and other nonaddicting chemicals now.

- Use caffeine to self-medicate: Most likely.

- Need for an SSRI antidepressant: Probably, but try serotonin supplements first.

Step Four

- Cross-training exercise program: You need to get medical clearance.

- Minimum amount of exercise: Flexibility/calming—slowly work up to 15 minutes daily; resistance/adaptive—slowly work up to

30- to 60-minute sessions three times a week; cardiovascular/stimulating—over time, add in 15-minute sessions three times a week (alternate days with resistance/adaptive training). Keep resistance/adaptive to cardiovascular/stimulating ratio approximately two-to-one or greater.

- Avoid overexercising: It leads to further burnout and insulin resistance.

Step Five

- Take HRT if needed: Work with a medical professional who is well versed in prescribing HRT to patients who are insulin-resistant and have burned-out adrenal glands.

Twenty-One

Frequently Asked Questions

A fter working with patients to heal their metabolisms over the years, I find patients ask some of the same questions over and over again. I have included them here with answers and hope they answer some of the same questions you may have had as you read the book.

FAQs

1. How much protein is needed with each meal and snack?
2. Why do I have to limit caffeine?
3. Is decaffeinated coffee all right?
4. Why are vegetables recommended at every meal?
5. Why can't I eat fruit alone?
6. I've never taken supplements—are they really necessary if I am healthy and eat well?
7. Are sugar substitutes acceptable?
8. Is it okay to eat eggs, including yolks, every day?
9. Don't I have to limit saturated fats?
10. How many calories should I have?

11. What does drinking alcohol do to me?

12. Why can't I eat whole-grain breads, crackers, pancakes and products that are not highly processed and filled with chemicals and/or damaged fats?

13. What happens to the fat I eat along with a high-carbohydrate meal?

14. What is the best way to eat if I am stressed?

15. Why doesn't your food program emphasize the glycemic index of foods?

16. Why do some people want to eat more carbohydrates in times of stress?

17. What is your response to the research that says saturated fats increase insulin resistance?

18. What is your response to the research that says excess calories in any form are converted to fat?

19. What do you think about food combining?

20. What happens if I drink alcohol now and then?

1. **How much protein is needed with each meal and snack?**
   The amount of protein is dependent on your size, weight and activity level. In general, the minimum protein requirement ranges from two to five ounces of protein per meal and one to three ounces per snack.

2. **Why do I have to limit caffeine?**
   Caffeine is limited because it is a stimulant. All stimulants can cause insulin resistance, thereby increasing the metabolic aging process. All stimulants will become depressants because they will end up depleting serotonin. However, if your adrenal glands are burned out, this is not the time to limit your caffeine intake. Try green or black tea.

3. **Is decaffeinated coffee all right?**

If you must drink coffee, water-processed decaffeinated coffee is all right—though there still may be small amounts of caffeine remaining.

4. **Why are vegetables recommended at every meal?**

Vegetables are important for several reasons, including their natural source of antioxidants (which we need in large supplies) and their fiber content, which contributes to helping reduce the glycemic index of a meal and to keeping your intestines healthy.

5. **Why can't I eat fruit alone?**

Fruit is a carbohydrate, and it is important to avoid eating any carbohydrate alone because it raises insulin levels quickly, followed by a rapid rise in adrenaline and cortisol levels. Fruit should ideally be eaten together with a healthy fat, a protein and a nonstarchy vegetable but must *always* be eaten with a healthy fat and a protein.

6. **I've never taken supplements—are they really necessary if I am healthy and eat well?**

If this question had been asked several years ago, I might have agreed that taking supplements was not necessary. Unfortunately, we have damaged our food supply by processing most of our foods and depleting our soil of many essential nutrients. We are surrounded by chemicals and toxins daily, so we require antioxidant protection. Therefore, a pharmaceutical-grade basic regimen of a multivitamin with minerals, calcium with magnesium, stress B-vitamins and omega-3 fats is needed. You may require more than these to help protect you from oxidation as well as heal your metabolism. Check out my Web site at *www.Schwarzbein Principle.com* for more information on vitamins.

7. **Are sugar substitutes acceptable?**

No. Sugar substitutes can cause carbohydrate cravings and they are toxic chemicals. They are made from chemicals or sugars such as mannitol, sorbitol, fructose or xylitol. In the case of Aspartame, this substance actually breaks down into methyl alcohol, which is a chemical poisonous to the human body. It can cause headaches, memory loss, dizziness, depression and confusion. The only sugar substitute that I advocate, besides a small amount of honey, is stevia.

8. **Is it okay to eat eggs, including the yolk, every day?**

Yes. Cholesterol from foods reacts very differently in the body than the cholesterol created in your body does. It is the cholesterol that is created from excessive carbohydrate intake that is damaging to your body and can increase your risk of heart disease. In addition, whole eggs are a good source of essential fatty acids, are a complete source of protein and contain almost every vitamin and mineral.

9. **Don't I have to limit saturated fats?**

Saturated fats can be part of a healthy diet and should be included with monounsaturated and healthy polyunsaturated fats. Remember we are not promoting excessive fat intake but rather a balance of carbohydrates, proteins, nonstarchy vegetables and healthy fats. However, if you do not or cannot decrease your carbohydrate/refined sugar consumption or you do not or cannot exercise consistently you have to eat more monounsaturated and polyunsaturated fats. Refer to the special dietary restrictions in chapter 11 to determine if you need to be on a lower-saturated fat plan.

10. **How many calories should I have?**

Do not count calories. Instead, balance the amount of proteins, healthy fats, real carbohydrates and nonstarchy vegetables in your meals to meet your current metabolism and activity levels.

11. **What does drinking alcohol do to me?**

Alcohol is a toxic chemical that causes an imbalance of all your major hormones. This causes your body to use up its biochemicals more than it rebuilds them. Recent studies have linked alcohol consumption to breast cancer and probably colon and prostate cancer as well.

12. **Why can't I eat whole-grain breads, crackers, pancakes and products that are not highly processed and filled with chemicals and/or damaged fats?**

The answer is you can, but you will probably have to make them from scratch yourself. There are many healthy carbohydrates that you may eat. Stay away from the highly processed ones and eat the right amount for your current metabolism and activity levels.

13. **What happens to the fat I eat along with a high-carbohydrate meal?**

Fat cannot be stored as fat without insulin being present. If you overeat carbohydrates along with fats, the rise in insulin will turn the carbohydrates into fats and store them both in the cells. At this point you can use the fats for energy or store them in your fat cells.

14. **What is the best way to eat if I am stressed?**

Eat smaller amounts of balanced meals more frequently. Stress, including skipping meals, raises adrenaline and cortisol levels, and eating too much at one time raises insulin levels.

15. **Why doesn't your food program emphasize the glycemic index of foods?**

The glycemic index of individual foods will change when they are combined with other foods. It is more important to understand what food category a food belongs to so that you can balance your meals. It is not important to worry about how quickly food is absorbed into your bloodstream and triggers insulin when eaten alone. You are not going to eat foods by themselves on this program.

16. **Why do some people want to eat more carbohydrates in times of stress?**

Stress causes a higher utilization and eventual depletion of serotonin. Low serotonin levels can cause carbohydrate cravings.

17. **What is your response to the research that says saturated fats increase insulin resistance?**

    It is the consumption of damaged fats and the underconsumption of healthy fats that increase the risk of insulin resistance more than the consumption of saturated fats. Refer to the Saturated Fats section on page 244.

18. **What is your response to the research that says excess calories in any form are converted to fat?**

    Excess calories in any form can be converted into fats but only in the presence of excess insulin. My point is that proteins are more likely to become functional and structural proteins (neurotransmitters, enzymes and cell parts), healthy fats are more likely to become functional and structural fats (hormones and cell parts), and excess carbohydrates will always be turned into fats (to be used as energy or stored as fat).

19. **What do you think about food combining?**

    I do not believe in food combining because the proponents of food combining want you to eat carbohydrates and vegetables or proteins, fats and vegetables only. Eating this way causes hormonal imbalances. It is important to eat from the four food groups *together* to regenerate and keep your hormones balanced.

20. **What happens if I drink alcohol now and then?**

    If you are insulin-sensitive and have healthy adrenal glands, a small amount of alcohol will not make or break your program.

If your simple food question was not answered, post a message on the bulletin board on my Web site—*www.SchwarzbeinPrinciple.com.*

Afterword

Now that you have read this book, you know why you need to change your poor nutrition and lifestyle habits, what will happen when you do change them, and how to maintain healthy habits that will ensure your optimum health and successful aging. Have a happy *transition*.

Diana Lynn Schwarzbein, M.D.

References

Genetic and Environmental Components of Aging

Curtsinger, James W., et al., "Genetic variation and aging." *Annual Review of Genetics* 29 (1995): 553–575.

Finch, Caleb E., and Rudolph E. Tanzi. "Genetics of aging." *Science* 278 (October 17, 1997): 407–411.

Fries, James F. "Compression of morbidity in the elderly." *Vaccine* 18 (2000): 1584–1589.

———. "Aging, natural death, and the compression of morbidity." *New England Journal of Medicine* 303 (July 17, 1980): 130–135.

Hayflick, Leonard. "How and why we age." *Experimental Gerontology* 33 (1998): 639–653.

———. "The future of aging." *Nature* 408 (November 9, 2000): 267–269.

Heller, Debra A., et al. "Genetic and environmental influences on serum lipid levels in twins." *New England Journal of Medicine* 328 (April 22, 1993): 1150–1156.

Herskind, Anne Maria, et al. "The heritability of human longevity: a population-based study of 2872 Danish twin pairs born 1870–1900." *Human Genetics* 97 (1996): 319–323.

Jazwinski, S. Michal. "Genetics of longevity." *Experimental Gerontology* 33 (1998): 773–783.

——. "Longevity, genes, and aging." *Science* 271 (July 5, 1996): 54–58.

Kannisto, Väinö. "On the survival of centenarians and the span of life." *Population Studies* 42 (1988): 389–406.

Marenberg, Marjorie E., et al. "Genetic susceptibility to death from coronary heart disease in a study of twins." *New England Journal of Medicine* 330 (April 14, 1994): 1041–1046.

Marmot, M. G., and G. D. Smith. "Why are the Japanese living longer?" *British Medical Journal* 299 (1989): 1547–1551.

Olshanki, S. J. "The aging of the human species." *Scientific American* 268 (1993): 46–52.

Perls, Thomas T., et al. "Siblings of centenarians live longer." *Lancet* 351 (May 23, 1998): 1560.

Stunkard, Albert J., et al. "The body-mass index of twins who have been reared apart." *New England Journal of Medicine* 322 (May 24, 1990): 1483–1487.

Takara, H., et al. "Influence of MHC region genes on human longevity." *Lancet* 2 (1987): 824–826.

Vita, A. J., et al. "Aging, health risks, and cumulative disability." *New England Journal of Medicine* 338 (April 9, 1998): 1035–1041.

Yu, Byung Pal. "Aging and oxidative stress: Modulation by dietary restriction." *Free Radical Biology & Medicine* 21 (1996): 651–668.

Exercise, Strength Training and Aging

Blair, Steven N., et al. "Influences of cardiorespiratory fitness and other precursors on cardiovascular disease and all-cause mortality in men and women." *Journal of the American Medical Association* 276 (July 17, 1996): 205–210.

————. "Changes in physical fitness and all-cause mortality: A prospective study of healthy and unhealthy men." *Journal of the American Medical Association* 273 (April 12, 1995): 1093–1098.

————. "How much physical activity is good for health?" *Annual Review of Public Health* 13 (1992): 99–126.

Evenson, Kelly R., et al. "Physical activity and ischemic stroke risk: The Atherosclerosis Risk in Communities Study." *Stroke* 30 (July 1999): 1333–1339.

Fiatarone, Maria A., et al. "High-intensity strength training in nonagenarians." *JAMA* 263 (June 13, 1990): 3029–3034.

Frontera, Walter R., et al., "Strength conditioning in older men: skeletal muscle hypertrophy and improved function." *Journal of Applied Physiology* 64 (1988): 1038–1044.

Hazzard, William R. "Weight control and exercise: Cardinal features of successful preventive gerontology." (Editorial) *Journal of the American Medical Association* 274 (December 27, 1995): 1964–1965.

Kushi, Lawrence H., et al. "Physical activity and mortality in postmenopausal women." *Journal of the American Medical Association* 277 (April 23, 1997): 1287–1292.

Nelson, Miriam E., et al. "Effects of high-intensity strength training on multiple risk factors for osteoporotic fractures." *Journal of the American Medical Association* 272 (December 28, 1994): 1909–1914.

Paffenbarger, Ralph S., et al. "A history of physical activity, cardiovascular health and longevity: the scientific contributions of Jeremy N Morris, Dsc, DPH, FRCP." *International Journal of Epidemiology* 30 (2001): 1184–1192.

————. "The association of changes in physical-activity level and other lifestyle characteristics with mortality among men." *New England Journal of Medicine* 328 (February 25, 1993): 538–545.

Stress, Mood and Emotions

House, James S., et al. "Social relationships and health." *Science* 241 (July 29, 1988): 540–545.

Kiecolt-Glaser, Janice K., et al. "Emotions, morbidity, and mortality: New perspectives from psychoneuroimmunology." *Annual Review of Psychology* 53 (2002): 83–107.

Krantz, David S., and Melissa K. McCeney. "Effects of psychological and social factors on organic disease: A critical assessment of research on coronary heart disease." *Annual Review of Psychology* 53 (2002): 341–69.

Martin, G. M., et al. "Genetic analysis of aging: Role of oxidative damage and environmental stress." *Nature Genetics* 13 (1996): 25

Sapolsky, Robert M. *Stress, the Aging Brain, and the Mechanisms of Neuron Death,* MIT Press, Cambridge, MA, 1992.

Shanafelt, Tait D., et al. "Burnout and self-reported patient care in an internal medicine residency program." *Annals of Internal Medicine* 136 (2002): 358–367.

Wallace, Robert Keith, et al. "The effects of Transcendental Meditation and TM-Sidhi program on the aging process." *International Journal of Neuroscience* 16 (1982): 53–58.

Williams, Janice E., et al. "The association between trait anger and incident stroke risk: The Atherosclerosis Risk in Communities (ARIC) Study." *Stroke* 33 (January 2002): 13–20.

Effects of Sleep Deprivation

Lusardi, Paola, et al. "Effects of insufficient sleep on blood pressure in hypertensive patients: A 24-h study." *American Journal of Hypertension* 12 (January 1999): 63–68.

Moldofsky, Harvey. "Sleep and the immune system." *International Journal of Immunopharmacology* 17 (1995): 649–654.

Redwine, Laura, et al. "Effects of sleep and sleep deprivation on interleukin-6, growth hormone, cortisol, and melatonin levels in humans." *Journal of Clinical Endocrinology & Metabolism* 85 (2000): 3597–3603.

Diet and Health

Burke, Valerie, et al. "Dietary protein and soluble fiber reduce ambulatory blood pressure in treated hypertensives." *Hypertension* 38 (October 2001): 821–826.

Chen, Y. D. Ida, et al. "Why do low-fat high-carbohydrate diets accentuate postprandial lipemia in patients with NIDDM?" *Diabetes Care* 18 (January 1995): 10.

Cohn, Jeffrey S. "Oxidized fat in the diet, postprandial lipaemia and cardiovascular disease." *Current Opinion in Lipidology* 13 (2002): 19–24.

Gillespie, Sandra J., et al. "Using carbohydrate counting in diabetes clinical practice." *Journal of the American Dietetic Association* 98 (August 1998): 897–899.

King, H., and G. Roglic. "Diabetes and the 'thrifty genotype.'" (Commentary) *Bulletin of the World Health Organization* 77 (August 1999): 692.

Kromhout, Daan, et al. "Prevention of coronary heart disease by diet and lifestyle: Evidence from prospective cross-cultural, cohort, and intervention studies." *Circulation* 105 (February 19, 2002): 893–898.

Liu, Simin, and JoAnn E. Manson. "Dietary carbohydrates, physical inactivity, obesity, and the 'metabolic syndrome' as predictors of coronary heart disease." *Current Opinion in Lipidology* 12 (2001): 395–404.

Nutrition Committee of the American Heart Association. "AHA Dietary Guidelines Revision 2000: A statement for healthcare professionals from the nutrition committee of the American Heart Association." *Stroke* 31 (November 2000): 2751–2766.

O'Dea, Kerin. "Marked improvement in carbohydrate and lipid metabolism in diabetic Australian Aborigines after temporary reversion to traditional lifestyle." *Diabetes* 33 (June 1984): 596–603.

Ravussin, Eric, et al. "Effects of a traditional lifestyle on obesity in Pima Indians." *Diabetes Care* 17 (September 1994): 1067–1074.

Shintani, Terry, et al. "The Waianae Diet Program: A culturally sensitive, community-based obesity and clinical intervention program for the Native Hawaiian population." *Hawaii Medical Journal* 53 (May 1994): 136–147.

Sniderman, Allan D., et al. "Hypertriglyceridemic HyperapoB: the unappreciated atherogenic dyslipoproteinemia in Type 2 diabetes mellitus." *Annals of Internal Medicine* 135 (September 18, 2001): 447–459.

Taubes, Gary. "The soft science of dietary fat." (Editorial) *Science* 291 (March 30, 2001): 2536–2545.

Hormones and Hormone Replacement Therapy

Barrett-Connor, Elizabeth, et al. "A prospective study of dehydroepiandrosterone sulfate, mortality, and cardiovascular disease." *New England Journal of Medicine* 315 (December 11, 1986): 1519–1524.

Col, Nananda F., et al. "Patient-specific decisions about hormonal replacement therapy in postmenopausal women." *Journal of the American Medical Association* 277 (April 9, 1997): 1140–1147.

Colditz, Graham A., et al. "The use of estrogens and progestins and the risk of breast cancer in postmenopausal women." *New England Journal of Medicine* 332 (June 15, 1995): 1589–1593.

Darling, Giselle M., et al. "Estrogen and progestin compared with simvastatin for hypercholesterolemia in postmenopausal women." *New England Journal of Medicine* 337 (August 28, 1997): 595–601.

Grodstein, Francine, et al. "Postmenopausal hormone therapy and mortality." *New England Journal of Medicine* 336 (June 19, 1997): 1769–1775.

———. "Postmenopausal estrogen and progestin use and the risk of cardio-vascular disease." *New England Journal of Medicine* 335 (August 15, 1996): 453–461.

Lamberts, Steven W. J., et al. "The endocrinology of aging." *Science* 278 (October 17, 1997): 419–424.

Morales, Arlene J., et al. "Effects of replacement dose of dehydroepiandros-terone in men and women of advancing age." *Journal of Clinical Endocrinology Metabolism* 78 (1994): 1360–1367.

Nabulsi, Azmi A., et al. "Association of hormone-replacement therapy with cardiovascular risk factors in postmenopausal women." *New England Journal of Medicine* 328 (April 15, 1993): 1069–1075.

Rosmond, Roland, M.D., Ph.D., et al. "Alterations in the hypothalamic pituitary adrenal axis in metabolic syndromes." *The Endocrinologist.* Vol. 11, #6. 12/01, pgs. 491–497.

Stampfer, Meir J., et al. "Postmenopausal estrogen therapy and cardiovascu-lar disease: Ten-year follow-up from the Nurse's Health Study." *New England Journal of Medicine* 325 (September 12, 1991): 756–762.

Women's Health Initiative Investigators. "Risks and benefits of estrogen plus progestin in healthy postmenopausal women." *Journal of the American Medical Association.* 288 (July 17, 2002): 321–333.

Books

Kahn, Robert L., and John W. Rowe. *Successful Aging,* Delacorte Press, New York, March 1999.

Perls, Thomas T., et al. *Living to 100: Lessons in Living to Your Maximum Potential at Any Age,* Basic Books, New York, January 2000.

Snowdon, David. *Aging with Grace,* Bantam Books, New York, May 2001.

Willcox, Bradley J., et al. *The Okinawa Program,* Clarkson Potter Publishers, New York, May 2001.

Glossary

5-HTP/5-hydroxy-tryptophan Derived from the essential amino acid tryptophan, 5-HTP is then converted to serotonin.

Adrenaline One of the major utilization hormones of the body. It is made in the adrenal glands and keeps your heart beating.

ALA/alpha linolenic acid ALA is one of the two essential fatty acids. It heads up the omega-3 family of polyunsaturated fatty acids.

Amino acid An organic compound that links together with other amino acids to form proteins.

Antibodies Proteins produced by the immune system to fight off infections or toxins.

Antidepressant A drug used to treat depression.

Antioxidant A chemical compound that inhibits oxidation.

Armour thyroid A prescription thyroid replacement medication that has both T4 (thyroxine) and T3 (triiodothyronine) in it.

ATP/adenosine triphosphate A form of energy used by cells to provide fuel for biochemical reactions.

Attention deficit disorder (ADD) A syndrome characterized by impulsiveness, hyperactivity and short attention span, which often leads to learning disabilities and various behavioral problems. Also known as attention deficit/hyperactivity disorder (ADHD).

Autoimmune disease A condition brought about by an immune response of the body against one of its own tissues or types of cells.

Biochemical Chemicals that are used for structure, function and energy, which allow you to carry out all your bodily functions—heartbeat, breathing, thinking, eating, etc. Cells, cell membranes, organs, glands, teeth, hair, skin, nails, muscles, bones and connective tissue are examples of structural biochemicals. Hormones, neurotransmitters, enzymes, cell mediators and antibodies are examples of functional biochemicals. Some of the energy biochemicals are sugar, ketones, triglycerides and glycogen.

Bone loss Loss of bone mass caused by inefficient regeneration or disease.

Bone mass The amount of bone an individual has.

Burned-out adrenal glands Occur when your adrenal glands can no longer produce enough of the adrenal gland hormones to keep up with your body's daily demands.

CCK An abbreviation for cholecystokinin, a hormone secreted by the upper intestine in response to incoming fats. CCK signals your brain that food is coming.

Cell The smallest structural unit of an organism that is capable of independent functioning, consisting of a nucleus, cytoplasm and various organelles surrounded by a cell membrane.

Cellular Pertaining to cells.

Central proteins and fats The protein and fat tissues found in the trunk of the body—not on the arms or legs.

Cholesterol A life-giving substance that is found in food and is normally made in the liver. It is vital as a part of cell membranes and cell structure, and to make certain hormones.

Chronic fatigue syndrome (CFS) An illness characterized by debilitating fatigue (experienced as exhaustion and extremely poor stamina), neurological problems and a variety of flulike symptoms. A common cause of CFS is severe adrenal gland burnout.

Cortisol One of the major utilization hormones of the body. It is made in the adrenal glands and keeps your blood pressure from going too low.

Cystic acne Acne with the formation of cysts. One of the most common causes of cystic acne is high insulin levels.

Cytomel A T3 (triiodothyronine) thyroid medication.

Deficiency state The state of not having or not making enough of a biochemical.

Degenerative diseases of aging The metabolic diseases of aging that occur from poor nutrition and lifestyle habits. They include abnormal cholesterol levels, cancer, dementia, depression, early menopause, heart disease, high blood pressure, morbid obesity, osteoarthritis, osteoporosis, stroke and Type II diabetes.

Desyrel A drug that can help your body reset its sleep cycle.

Dexedrine A stimulant drug that has been used to suppress appetite.

DHEA/Dihydroepiandrostenedione A minor growth hormone made mostly in the adrenal glands. Among its many functions, it counters cortisol's effects on the brain.

DNA/deoxyribonucleic acid The carrier of genetic information.

Endocrinology The study of the endocrine system and its role in the physiology of the body.

Enzymes Protein substances that act as organic catalysts in initiating or speeding up specific chemical reactions.

Ephedra A plant stimulant. Another name for ephedra is ma huang.

Ephedrine Derived from ephedra or produced synthetically, ephedrine is used to relieve bronchial spasm and is a central nervous system stimulant.

Essential fatty acids (EFAs) EFAs are polyunsaturated oils that cannot be made by the body and must be obtained from foods or supplements.

Estradiol The female sex hormone made by the ovaries.

Excess state The state of having or making too much of a biochemical.

Fatty acid Any of a number of saturated or unsaturated molecules of fat.

Fibromyalgia A syndrome characterized by widespread pain and tenderness at specified sites, fatigue and unrefreshing sleep. There is abnormally high pain sensitivity. Fibromyalgia is a clinical entity, but should be regarded as a syndrome rather than a disease. The difference between a syndrome and a disease is that a disease is a health condition with a clearly identifiable cause, while a syndrome is a set of symptoms which define the health condition without a single cause on which to place the blame. One of the causes of fibromyalgia is burned-out adrenal glands.

Fight/flight response A sudden release of a large amount of adrenaline in response to a real or perceived stress. The purpose of this response is to get you ready to defend yourself or run away from the stress to increase your chance of survival.

Free radicals Molecules that have an unpaired electron. This makes them very reactive and unstable.

Gland An organ that secretes hormones.

Glandular Pertaining to glands.

Glandular-based endocrine disease/disorder Glandular-based endocrine disorders or diseases are caused by glandular problems and can result in either a hormone deficiency or excess. A deficiency state occurs when a gland produces too little of a hormone; an excess state occurs when a gland produces too much of a hormone.

Glycogen The storage form of sugar in the body made when sugar molecules are joined together by adding a water molecule between them.

High blood sugar The condition of having high sugar levels in the bloodstream.

High-density lipoproteins (HDLs) Protein molecules that carry within their core cholesterol from your cells to your liver.

Homocysteine A biochemical made in the body from the essential amino acid methionine. High levels of homocysteine have been associated with an increased risk for Alzheimer's, strokes and heart attacks.

Hormone A functional biochemical that is produced by a gland and relays messages to your cells, which in turn respond by changing the biochemical reactions that are occurring within those cells.

Hormone replacement therapy (HRT) The treatment and replacement of a missing hormone.

Human growth hormone (HGH) A minor growth hormone produced in the pituitary gland that is important for linear growth during puberty, and increased muscle mass and decreased fat mass during adulthood.

Hyperinsulinemia Excessive levels of insulin in the bloodstream usually caused by poor nutrition and lifestyle habits.

Hyperthyroidism Glandular-based endocrine disease of overproduction of thyroid hormone(s) or the excessive exogenous replacement with too much thyroid hormone(s).

Hypoglycemia Low levels of sugar in the bloodstream.

Hypothyroidism Glandular-based endocrine disease of too little production of thyroid hormone(s) or an under-replacement of thyroid hormone medication.

Immune system The integrated body system of organs, tissues, cells and antibodies that defends the body against pathogens and toxins.

Insulin One of the major hormones of the body. It is made by the pancreas and some of its many functions include regulating blood sugar; rebuilding structural, functional and energy biochemicals; and slowing down the rapid utilization of these same biochemicals.

Insulin resistance The state where your cells are not responding to the normal actions of insulin. It also involves a relative underproduction of insulin compared to the need for insulin, although it is a state of high insulin levels in the bloodstream.

Insulin sensitivity The state where your pancreas produces enough insulin and your cells respond to the insulin in the correct way.

Insulinoma A pancreatic tumor that produces and secretes too much insulin.

Insulin-resistant The description of a person with insulin resistance.

Insulin-sensitive The description of a person with insulin sensitivity.

Irritable bowel syndrome (IBS) A term for any irritation of the bowel that cannot otherwise be categorized as a defined intestinal disease. Symptoms include intestinal bloating, gas pains, constipation and/or loose bowel movements.

Islet cells (beta) The cells of the pancreas that make and secrete insulin.

Ketone A breakdown product of fatty acids.

Ketosis A condition characterized by an abnormally elevated concentration of ketones in the body tissues and fluids. It is a complication of Type I diabetes or starvation and occurs when your insulin effect is too low.

LA/linoleic acid One of the two essential fatty acids. LA heads up the omega-6 family of polyunsaturated fatty acids.

Lifestyle-based endocrine disease/disorder Disease states that occur from the cumulative hormone changes related to chronic over- or under-production and/or secretion of hormones in response to poor nutrition and lifestyle habits.

Low-density lipoproteins (LDLs) The protein carriers of cholesterol from the blood to the cells.

Low-insulin effect The ratio between using up your biochemicals and your ability to rebuild them determines your insulin effect. If you use up more than you rebuild, you have a low-insulin effect.

Lupus/systemic erythematosus A generalized connective tissue disorder found mostly in women characterized by skin rashes, joint swelling and pain, low white-blood-cell count with immunosuppression, organ failure and fever.

Luteinizing hormone (LH) A pituitary hormone that regulates testosterone in men and ovulation in women.

Ma huang The Chinese name for an Asian variety of ephedra.

Metabolism The sum of all the body's regeneration reactions—all the using-up and building-up reactions that occur.

Morbid obesity Weighing 30 percent or more above your ideal body weight.

Neurotransmitters The biochemicals that are needed to perform the functions of the brain such as observing, creating, thinking, multitasking, memorizing, worrying, reading and inventing things.

Nutrient A substance that is provided in your diet to rebuild your biochemicals.

Omega-3 fatty acids A special family of polyunsaturated fatty acids all sharing a similar molecular structure. The omega-3 fatty acids are headed up by the essential amino acid ALA. Other omega-3 fatty acids include DHA and EPO. These fatty acids are used as building material for hormones and other cell mediators that decrease inflammation, reduce your ability to clot your blood and help you dilate your blood vessels. It is the balance between omega-3 and omega-6 fatty acids that is important for good health.

Omega-6 fatty acids A special family of polyunsaturated fatty acids all sharing a similar molecular structure. The omega-6 fatty acids are headed up by the essential amino acid LA. Other omega-6 fatty acids include GLA and arachidonic acid. These fatty acids are mostly used as building material for hormones and other cell mediators that increase inflammation, improve your ability to clot your blood and constrict your blood vessels.

Osteoarthritis One of the degenerative diseases of aging. It involves damage to the tissues that line the joint spaces, causing swelling and pain.

Osteoblasts The cells of the body that rebuild new bone.

Osteoclasts The cells of the body that get rid of old bone.

Osteopenia Loss of bone mass.

Osteoporosis Loss of bone mass resulting in a fracture.

Oxidation The process that forms free radicals in your body. Oxygen or other chemicals can react with other atoms and rob them of an electron, leaving an unpaired electron behind.

Pancreas The organ that produces insulin, glucagon and digestive enzymes.

Peripheral proteins and fats The protein and fat tissues found on the arms and legs—not on the trunk of the body.

pH The way to describe the acid versus alkaline property of a solution.

Phytochemicals A natural bioactive compound found in plant foods that works with nutrients and dietary fiber to protect against disease.

Pilates A full-body conditioning method of exercise that was introduced in the 1930s by Joseph Pilates. It improves strength, flexibility, balance and muscular symmetry. The exercises promote toned muscles and are noted for developing abdomen, lower back and buttocks strength.

Portal vein The part of the circulatory system that links your small intestines to your liver. Insulin is introduced into the bloodstream via the portal vein.

Progesterone The hormone produced by the corpus lutea and adrenal cortex whose function it is to prepare the uterus for implantation of a fertilized egg by stimulating the growth of new blood vessels within the lining of the uterus.

Progestogen A term applied to any substance with progestational activity.

Regeneration The using up and rebuilding of a biochemical. The sum of all the regeneration reactions occurring simultaneously in your body is your metabolism.

REM sleep Rapid eye movement (REM) is the part of the sleep cycle in which your body does most of its rebuilding.

Rosacea A chronic skin disorder affecting the nose, forehead and cheeks, marked by flushing, followed by red coloring of the affected areas and acnelike pustules.

rT3/reverse T3 This inactive thyroid hormone is formed to regulate the action of thyroid hormone.

SAM-e/S-adenosylmethionine A naturally occurring biochemical in the body that helps add methyl groups to tissues. Methylation is one way the body detoxifies chemicals. Methylation is also a way to make new biochemicals. One of the most important functions of SAM-e is in making new neurotransmitters; therefore, it can be taken as a supplement to help depression.

Seasonal affective disorder (SAD) A form of depression with symptoms that occur in the winter months due to a lack of adequate amounts of serotonin in the body.

Secrete/secretion To release a biochemical from a cell or gland.

Serotonin A neurotransmitter made from tryptophan that makes you feel very good and happy.

SSRIs/Selective serotonin reuptake inhibitors A class of antidepressants that help raise serotonin levels.

Stressor Anything that is perceived as stress by the body.

T3 The more biologically active thyroid hormone.

T4 The thyroid hormone secreted in larger quantities than T3 by the thyroid gland. It is converted to T3 to confer activity or deactivated to rT3 to block activity.

Thyroid-stimulating hormone (TSH) A hormone made in the pituitary that regulates thyroid hormone production and secretion.

Trans-fat A damaged fat that is formed when polyunsaturated fats are exposed to high temperatures and the hydrogen atoms around the double bonds are changed from a "cis" (same side) configuration to a "trans" (opposite side) configuration.

Transition (relative to SPII program) A healing process to restore insulin sensitivity and/or heal the adrenal glands.

Triglyceride A compound consisting of three fatty acids attached to a glycerol molecule. It is synthesized from carbohydrates or obtained from eating fatty foods and either used for energy or stored as fat.

Tryptophan An essential amino acid.

Type I diabetes A glandular-based autoimmune disease of insulin deficiency that occurs when the pancreas cells of the body that make insulin are destroyed.

Type II diabetes A lifestyle-based endocrine disorder characterized by high blood sugar due to insulin resistance.

Very low-density lipoproteins (VLDLs) The protein carriers of triglycerides and cholesterol made in the liver. They carry fats to the various cells of the body. They first release all their triglycerides to the cells and become LDLs.

Index

About the Author

Diana Schwarzbein, M.D., graduated from the University of Southern California (USC) Medical School and completed her residency in internal medicine and a fellowship in endocrinology at Los Angeles County USC Medical Center. She founded The Endocrinology Institute of Santa Barbara in 1993. She sub-specializes in metabolism, diabetes, osteoporosis, menopause and thyroid conditions, subjects she lectures on frequently. She lives with her husband in Santa Barbara, California.

Marilyn Brown is a freelance writer.

An Autobiography Filled with Healing, Spirituality and Love

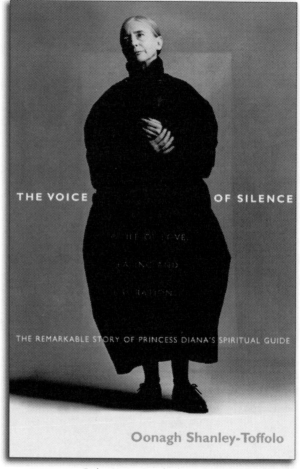

THE VOICE OF SILENCE

THE REMARKABLE STORY OF PRINCESS DIANA'S SPIRITUAL GUIDE

Oonagh Shanley-Toffolo

Code #0340 • Paperback • $10.95
Complete with black and white photographs

England's most sought after healer and confidante to Princess Diana and the Duke and Duchess of Windsor tells her extraordinary story.